Basic Anatomy and Physiology for the Music Therapist

Daniel J. Schneck

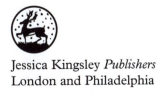

Jessica Kingsley *Publishers*
London and Philadelphia

Figure 5.1 is reprinted with the copyright permission of Geoffrey Rowland, from Figure 8.1 of *The Music Effect: Music Physiology and Clinical Applications*, by Daniel J. Schneck and Dorita S. Berger; Jessica Kingsley Publishers, London and Philadelphia, 2006.

First published in 2015
by Jessica Kingsley Publishers
73 Collier Street
London N1 9BE, UK
and
400 Market Street, Suite 400
Philadelphia, PA 19106, USA

www.jkp.com

Library of Congress Cataloging in Publication Data
Schneck, Daniel J., author.
  Basic anatomy and physiology for the music therapist / Daniel J. Schneck.
      p. ; cm.
  Includes bibliographical references and index.
  ISBN 978-1-84905-756-1 (alk. paper)
  I. Title.
  [DNLM: 1. Anatomy. 2. Auditory Perception--physiology.
3. Human Body. 4. Music Therapy. 5. Music.
6. Physiological Phenomena. QS 4]
  QM23.2
  612.0024'61585154--dc23

                           2014044097

British Library Cataloguing in Publication Data
A CIP catalogue record for this book is available from the British Library

ISBN 978 1 84905 756 1
eISBN 978 0 85700 992 0

Printed and bound in Great Britain

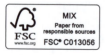

MIX
Paper from
responsible sources
FSC   FSC® C013056
www.fsc.org

This book is dedicated to all of those individuals who have had the wisdom to recognize the value of music in the human experience, and who have thus dedicated and committed themselves to using music to improve the health, comfort, and understanding of humankind.

Contents

PART II HOW DOES "ME" WORK?

List of Tables and Figures

Tables

Figures

Preface

Perhaps William Shakespeare (1564–1616) said it best, speaking through Hamlet in Act II, Scene II of the play by the same name:

> What a piece of work is a man!
>
> How noble in reason! How infinite in faculty!
>
> In form and moving how express and admirable!
>
> In action how like an angel!
>
> In apprehension how like a god!
>
> The beauty of the world! The paragon of animals!
>
> Shakespeare (1603)

Indeed, the human body (male *and* female!) *is* "the paragon of animals"—a model of excellence and perfection in both structure and function; an optimized living organism that can best be described as "express and admirable in form and moving"—when it is working right! Unfortunately, it does *not* always work right! In those instances, medical and allied health-care professionals must intervene to manage the issues that are responsible for such malfunction. Among those health-care professionals are music therapists.

But in order for these professionals to do their job efficiently and effectively, they must have a thorough working knowledge of the structure and function of the biological systems with which they deal. Moreover, it is vital that they are thoroughly familiar with how the human body is likely to respond to clinical intervention therapies within which are embedded mechanisms of action that target specific anatomic/physiologic systems. In the case of music therapy, those mechanisms derive from combinations and permutations of its six fundamental elements: rhythm, melody, harmony, timbre, dynamics, and form. The latter was addressed in a previous publication (Schneck and Berger 2006). This companion volume concerns itself with the former, i.e., a working knowledge of the human body, and it is intended quite specifically for the practicing music therapist.

In the pages that follow, we will take a look at some of the basic principles of anatomy and physiology that make the human body the "piece of work" that it is! In particular, we will concentrate on those attributes of the body that should be of special interest to the music therapist as he or she contemplates the clinical uses of music in the management of diagnosed populations. Thus, the book does not go into the depth and detail that one might expect of a textbook—such as those written by Goss (1966), Jacob, Francone and Lossow (1982), Schneck (1990), and Tortora and Grabowski (1993)—written specifically for an audience of anatomists, physiologists, physicians, physicians' assistants, nurses, and other allied health-care professionals. Rather, it focuses on anatomical and physiological *principles* that are of particular significance to the practicing music therapist. With that in mind, the material explored is divided into two parts. In Part I, "What Is This Thing Called 'Me?,'" we concern ourselves mainly with the body's structure, i.e.:

- how the body is organized (Chapter 1) into essentially six anatomical levels, increasing in size from atoms to molecules, cells, tissues, organs, and systems (*Note:* the latter four levels are often combined into one "continuum" scale of perception)

- how these systems can be made to fit a convenient paradigm for rigorously studying, analyzing, quantifying, and teaching physiologic function. The paradigm is formulated from the facts that the human body can be viewed as being characterized by seven basic features.

These seven basic features are:

1. The fact that the entire organism is an electrochemical, isothermal, *living engine* (Chapter 2), in the sense that it:

    a) takes in fuel

    b) converts part of the fuel into usable energy to drive its metabolic processes

    c) performs its various functions

    d) has a sophisticated subsystem to exhaust the waste products of its various activities.

2. The realization that the living engine has an optimized, mechanical output (Chapter 3), i.e., everything it does, at all levels of organization, involves motion—kinetic energy, and dynamic activity.

3. The observation that all of the body's outputs—everything it does—are monitored through *digitized* (Chapter 4), sensory systems (Chapter 5). These also "check in" and compare *internal* activities (known as *interoception*) with the external environment (known as *exteroception*), in order to confirm and ensure that all is "okay" and the organism is under no immediate threat of extinction.

4. Confirmation and verification of sensory information—and calls for responses (Chapter 6), if necessary—are accomplished through mechanisms of sensory *differentiation/integration*, most of which takes place at a central "command post" (the central nervous system (Chapter 4), consisting of the brain and spinal cord). The living engine is thus fine-tuned by feedback/feedforward control mechanisms that maintain, within prescribed limits, variables critical to life—a process called *homeostasis* (Chapter 6).

5. The control itself (Chapter 7) is accomplished through anatomic systems that respond to homeostatic disturbances by issuing forth "control signals" in the form of, for example, enzymes, neurotransmitters, hormones, and antibodies that attempt to bring system operating variables back in line with prescribed homeostatic reference quantities.

6. Depending on the nature and tenacity of homeostatic disturbances, the human body has the ability to accommodate them (Chapter 12) by:

    a) short-term *reflexive reactions*

    b) medium-term *functional adaptation mechanisms* that result from *entrainment*

    c) long-term *breeding mechanisms* that are embedded in *Feature 7* (i.e., evolutionary processes of natural selection).

7. The human machine has the ability to reproduce—to make other engines just like it—and in so doing, through mechanisms of sexual reproduction, breed, which allows its offspring to improve on the basic design. This last feature of the body is discussed in context throughout the book.

The above seven features become manifest in Part II of the book, "How Does 'Me' work?" through six fundamental *processes* that include:

- metabolism (Chapter 8)
- information processing (Chapter 10)
- consciousness (Chapter 10)
- time perception (Chapter 11)
- physiological optimization schemes (Chapter 12)
- satisfaction of anatomical design criteria (Chapter 13).

The six processes are governed, interpreted or influenced by five fundamental laws of both:

- *physics* (Chapter 8), if viewed from the purely scientific perspective of an academician
- *perception* (Chapter 10), if viewed from the clinical perspective of the music therapist.

Either way, the relevant laws are subject to *four* primary *constraints* (discussed in Chapter 14), imposed at *three* levels of anatomic *organization* (atomic, molecular, continuum, see Chapter 1) on *two sexes* (male and female). They satisfy one *fundamental purpose*— survival! survival of the self (the strongest human drive) and survival of the species (the second strongest human drive, commonly referred to as the drive for sexual fulfillment). Human drives and needs are discussed in Chapters 8 and 9.

This 7–6–5–4–3–2–1 "countdown" paradigm is intended to act as a convenient "guide" for the practicing music therapist, to help him/her understand fundamental principles that govern the anatomical design and physiologic function of the human body. To help in this effort, anatomical considerations endeavor to answer three questions:

1. *What* is it?

2. *Where* (in the body) is it?

3. What does it *do*?"

Answers to the first two are addressed in Part I; question 3 is addressed in Part II. Although every effort is made to define specific terms in context, as they are introduced and used, the reader is encouraged also to have on hand a good medical dictionary (e.g., Cutler and Hensyl 1976; Thomas 1981) to help in this effort. Moreover, the reader interested in more detail regarding "how" and "why" the body does what it does is directed to the plethora of "standard" textbooks in anatomy and physiology—e.g., the previously mentioned *Gray's Anatomy*: Goss (1966); Jacob *et al.* (1982); Tortora and Grabowski (1993)—that are "out there." One can also access the literature references cited at the end of the book—especially Schneck (1990, 1992), and Schneck and Tempkin (1992). Speaking of references, in order to avoid encumbering the reader with a totally inclusive, comprehensive bibliography, I have kept the literature references down to a select few, each of which contains a huge number of citations as well.

For essentially the same reason, I have limited the number of diagrams and figures to a bare minimum, opting instead to summarize important information in tabulated form. I find that tabulated information is easily accessed and convenient to use. Finally, in the Chapter 14 section entitled, "From theory to practice," we tie all of this together to address the fundamental question:

• "As a music therapist, knowing what I now know about the structure and function of the living human body/instrument, how can I intervene clinically to effectively exploit the role of music in affecting physiologic function, in order to treat and manage diagnosed populations?"

Moreover, "How can I exploit the transformative power of music to affect a parallel transformation of my client…from a deprived state to an optimized one?" That's what this book is all about!

But it could never have come to realization without the help and support of many people. Of course, at the very top of the list are family and friends (indeed, writing a book is an obsession that is in desperate need of much unconditional love, limitless help, constant encouragement, counseling, and sacrifice). Next are all of my professional colleagues and many students from whom I have often said I learned more than they ever learned from me! For fear of inadvertently leaving somebody important off the list, I have chosen not to identify any specific individuals, but I am eternally grateful to all of them! Kudos and special thanks to my "editorial assistants"—my dear wife Judi, for her enormous contributions, both in content (keeping me focused, "on track," and relevant), and accuracy (grammar, spelling, typos, etc.) and Nurse Lois Hurd, for reading the manuscript and providing much helpful input from the clinical side. Thanks, of course, to my publisher, Jessica Kingsley—especially Lisa Clark and Jane Evans—for recognizing the need for such a book and graciously agreeing to publish it!

A closing disclaimer: We are all human—to be human, is to be less than perfect, to be less than perfect is to make mistakes. Thus, despite our most valiant efforts, we are all—me included—guilty of both errors of omission and commission. Thus, I would greatly appreciate your bringing to my attention any discrepancies that you come across between what is written in the text and what you know to be factual based on reliable sources. The only thing I would ask is that you be kind in pointing out such discrepancies. Thank you!

Introduction

The Symbiotic Relationship Between
Music and the Human Body

Aristotle recognized it, when he wrote in his *Politics*, "If one listens to the wrong kind of music, he will become the wrong kind of person; but, conversely, if he listens to the right kind of music, he will tend to become the right kind of person" (Taylor 1995). Plato, too, writing in his *Republic* observed, "Music training is a more potent instrument than any other, because rhythm and harmony find their way into the inward places of the soul, on which they mightily fasten, imparting grace, and making the soul of him who is rightly educated, graceful" (Plato 1992). Indeed, the ancient Greeks—including the likes of Pythagoras, Plato, and Aristotle, covering, respectively and collectively, the roughly 235-year period from 582–347 B.C.—saw in mathematics and music the embodiment of all natural phenomena, derived from a cosmic source which they believed to be God (for the Greeks, Zeus; for the Romans, Jupiter). That's why they ascribed divine status to the fine arts and science (in that order!), considering them to be embodied in nine goddesses—sacred daughters of the almighty Zeus. The female deities were called muses, from which the very word "music" is derived.

The ancient Greeks had an incredible respect for music because they recognized its relationship to:

- mathematics—e.g., musical intervals, frequency ratios, patterns of consonance and dissonance, etc. (see Chapter 13)

- nature—e.g., the fundamental principles of order and harmony that prevail throughout the universe (see Chapters 8–13).

Through this relationship, they saw in music the embodiment of sound—acoustic energy—as a mechanism for accessing and influencing a human's physiology (nature) and emotions. Thus, according to the Greeks, music could either corrupt, or enhance "the stillness of one's inner being."

Consider, for example, how they referred to music in their *Doctrine of Ethos*[1], which describes the effects of sound on human behavior, and therefore, its influence on morality. Again, in the words of Plato in *Laws III*, "The Foundations of Music, once established, must not be changed, for lawlessness in art and education inevitably leads to license in manners and anarchy in Society." Thus, with the possible exception of their attributing to a divine source the profound effects of music, the Greeks were not far off in recognizing its symbiotic relationship with the human body, and its immense transformative power! Indeed, there is a very good reason why *music is a universal language!* As we shall see, it is fashioned from the very template that is our own anatomical architecture…and this architecture is universal, essentially the same the world over!

Our bodies are nested hierarchies of vibrational frequencies, mostly in the audible range (20–20,000 cycles per second). These vibrational attributes appear in discrete anatomical structures that function in space and time within larger, more complicated structures, which, themselves, are contained within even larger and more complex vibrational structures (anatomic systems). As we shall see, each structure/ system "prefers" to operate in accordance with specific, optimal frequency patterns. Musicians think of these patterns as defining a state of *physiologic consonance* that is in concordance with the corresponding acoustic energy attribute of *musical consonance*. Indeed, the syntax that is embedded in the six fundamental elements of music— rhythm, melody, harmony, timbre, dynamics, and form—"speaks" this body language and hence enjoys a symbiotic relationship with the very organism that created it in the first place.

Thus, as shall become further apparent in the pages that follow, *all God's creations got rhythm!* Body tissues and organs have a unique shape, size, mass density, state of "tone" (tension), and so on. These unique geometric features and physical properties cause the structures to "resonate" within their own tissue-and-organ-specific range of vibrational energy—sets of "perfect pitches," if you will (see Table 5.2). When anatomical structures drift outside their optimal frequency range of operation, they develop abnormal tensions that result in disturbed physiologic function—states that one can refer to as *physiologic dissonance*. Enter the music therapist!

The role of the music therapist is to *resolve* physiologic dissonance into physiologic consonance, just as a composer does (a good deal of the time, anyway!) in developing the harmonic structure of a piece of music. By externally "driving" the body's organs and tissues—"playing" the *musical instrument*, if you will—using a syntax encoded into musical compositions, this professional health-care provider succeeds in activating processes of *physiologic entrainment* (Schneck and Berger 2006, and Chapter 12). Also

---

1 The *Doctrine Of Ethos* ("ethos" is Greek for "moral character of people") refers to Plato and Aristotle's 4th century B.C.E. writings about the importance and power of music in the human experience. One can learn more about it by referring to: West, M.L. (1992), *Ancient Greek Music*, Oxford: Oxford University Press; or Lippmann, E.A. (1964) *Musical Thought in Ancient Greece*, New York, NY: Columbia University Press; New York, among many others.

called a *frequency-following response*, entrainment refers to the fact that when a weaker anatomic pulsation (which often prevails in states of physiologic dissonance) comes under the influence of—i.e., *entrains*—a stronger one (which "drives" the system from outside), such *forced vibrations* (Schneck and Berger 2006, and Chapter 12). can activate a process called *sympathetic resonance*. This process allows the system to move eventually toward more optimal physiologic operating set points, a state of physiologic consonance arrived at through *physiologic adaptation* (Chapter 12). Thus:

> Under the influence of musical stimulation ("playing" the anatomical instrument that is the human body), misdirected organs and tissues in a state of physiological dissonance (i.e., in need of being "tuned") undergo physiological resolution—through physiological resonance and resulting physiological adaptation. So tuned, they are driven back to the more optimal state of physiological consonance (i.e., they are now in tune"), with a consequent release of the tension which these misdirected organs and tissues had been holding.

And so, exploiting the processes of entrainment and adaptation, the music therapist, thinking of the human body as a sophisticated musical instrument, can effectively *tune* it to a desirable frequency that corresponds to an optimal state of physiologic function, i.e., *health* and *cenesthesia* (defined in Chapter 14). This is not unlike tuning a radio dial to a desired station. The key, of course, is proper *assessment* and *dose-response criteria* (Schneck and Berger 2006), in order to ensure that the right "medicine" is being prescribed for the right "affliction," i.e., that one is tuning in to the right station! It is hoped that this book will help in the development of such criteria.

PART 1

WHAT IS THIS THING CALLED "ME"?

CHAPTER 1

Brief Overview of the Entire Human Body

Six Levels of Organization

Atomic scale: the human body is written in the key of "C" (carbon)

In all, the "typical" adult organism of "average" build is an aqueous ("watery"), organic, complex assemblage of millions upon millions of different atoms. However, note from Table 1.1 that nearly 97 percent of one's body weight consists of just four of them, i.e., oxygen (O), carbon (C), hydrogen (H), and nitrogen (N). The remainder includes at least 40 other elements—more than half of them (the entire right-hand column of Table 1.1) appearing in hardly measurable "trace" amounts (although they play crucial roles in affecting and controlling metabolic processes).

That oxygen and hydrogen should be so plentiful makes sense, considering that at least 60 percent or more of body weight exists as water—and *salt* water, at that. After all, we did originally come from the sea, hence the significant appearance and importance of sodium (Na) and chlorine (Cl) in Table 1.1 (Note: sodium chloride, NaCl, is sea salt). But why carbon and nitrogen? Why is carbon the "key note, C" from which all physiologic processes are "composed?" Why are we *organic* instruments? And what does nitrogen have to do with all of this?

Well, in the case of carbon, the short answer is that, of all the known chemical elements, this one is the most versatile, congenial, "sociable," flexible, and outreaching—easy to deal with, and quite fond of and willing to interact with "others." Thus, when it comes to choosing among all atomic candidates vying for the title of "most likely to succeed in producing complex life forms," carbon is, by far, the clear winner! (For the long answer, see Schneck 2000a.)

As for nitrogen, observe that the air we breath is, by volume, about four-fifths nitrogen. It is not surprising, then, to learn that derived from this colorless, tasteless, odorless gas are some of the most important chemical elements required for the growth of all plants…and that nitrogen is also a necessary ingredient for the manufacture of animal tissue proteins. To address this latter role of nitrogen, we move on to the next level of anatomic organization.

Table 1.1 "Average" elemental composition of the "typical" human adult			
ELEMENT	**% OF BODY WEIGHT**	**ELEMENT**	**% OF BODY WEIGHT**
Oxygen	63.000	Antimony	Trace
Carbon	20.700	Arsenic	Trace
Hydrogen	10.000	Barium	Trace
Nitrogen	2.800	Berylium	Trace
Calcium	1.575	Boron	Trace
Phosphorus	1.050	Cesium	Trace
SUB-TOTAL	**99.125**		
Potassium	0.247	Chromium	Trace
Sulfur	0.207	Cobalt	Trace
Chlorine	0.137	Gold	Trace
Sodium	0.131	Iodine	Trace
Magnesium	0.034	Lithium	Trace
Silicon	0.026	Manganese	Trace
SUB-TOTAL	**99.907**		
Iron	0.0050	Mercury	Trace
Fluorine	0.0037	Molybdenum	Trace
Zinc	0.0033	Nickel	Trace
Rubidium	0.0005	Radium	Trace
Strontium	0.0005	Selenium	Trace
Bromine	0.0003	Silver	Trace
Lead	0.0002	Tin	Trace
Copper	0.0001	Tungsten	Trace
Aluminum	0.0001	Uranium	Trace
Cadmium	0.0001	Vanadium	Trace
SUB-TOTAL	**99.9208**	**TOTAL**	**100.0%**

Combinations of atoms: the molecular level of anatomical organization (musical "notes")

The atoms of the human body are assembled into complex, polymeric, chemical chains that give birth to "the symphony of life." Analogous to musical notes, these molecular chains are classified as follows.

Carbohydrates

Of what kinds of *organic* compounds is the human body "composed?" Well, for one thing, by adding water, H_2O, to carbon, C, i.e., *hydrating* it, one can form compounds called, logically enough, *carbohydrates.* These include all starches and sugars (called *polysaccharides*). In general, one can add "n" molecules of water (where "n" can take on integer number values, i.e., 1, 2, 3…) to "n" atoms of carbon, to form carbohydrates having the general chemical formula, $(CH_2O)_n$. These are *photosynthesized* in green plants from solar-energy-absorbing (hence, "photo-") biochemical reactions, catalyzed by the green-colored enzyme *chlorophyll* (from the Greek *chlōrós*, meaning, "pale green," and *phýllon*, meaning, "leaf"). The reactions combine carbon dioxide $(CO_2)_n$ and water $(H_2O)_n$ to form carbohydrates, $(CH_2O)_n$, releasing oxygen gas $(O_2)n$ in the process. We inhale the oxygen thus released into the atmosphere ("thank you, plants!" Be kind to them!) and return the favor by exhaling for plant use the (CO_2) n that they need for photosynthesis—a truly symbiotic relationship between plants and animals, creating a healthy *ecosystem.*

We animals also *eat* the plants, thereby recovering the energy of the sun. That energy is metabolized into the carbohydrate chemical bonds of the six-carbon (n = 6) sugar (*hexose*) called *glucose*, used both to: (a) charge up our body's "battery," which is *adenosine tri-phosphate* (ATP, described later); and, (b) supply us with energy reserves in the stored, long-chain-coupled form called *glycogen* (literally *"glucose-generating"*).

Carbohydrates also display a generic, organic compound property called *isomerism*—literally, having the property of (-*ism*) being able to exist in any one of a number of different geometric configurations. Thinking in terms of the popular Tinker Toys building set, one can envision each geometric configuration as being built up from the same (*iso-*) parts (*mers*), but having several possible three-dimensional spatial molecular configurations. Thus, the property of isomerism allows certain long-chain, complex polymers (i.e., "having many parts") to share identical chemical formulas, while co-existing in entirely different geometric configurations, i.e., *steric-shapes.* This happens to be particularly true of the four six-carbon sugars: glucose, galactose, mannose, and fructose, all of which have the same chemical formula, but each of which has its own unique spatial-molecular steric-shape.

The ability of human body cells to discriminate among a myriad of different types of organic isomers—because of their unique stereo-chemical and bio-chemical specificity—makes these isomers ideal cell-membrane "markers" that help your body "identify" itself as "you!" The markers themselves are mostly cell-surface antigen-presenting proteins and the process of identifying them is what is sometimes referred to clinically as "typing and cross-matching"—especially in the case of blood transfusions. One's entire set of biological markers is called the body's *major histocompatibility complex* (MHC). The MHC derives from a unique genetic code (the *human leukocyte antigen, HLA system*) embedded on chromosome-6 of the specific individual's genome. Indeed, as we shall see in Chapter 7, both the MHC and HLA systems are at the very heart of how the body's immune system operates.

Moreover, as we shall also see, the fact that carbon atoms can link up with one another, and associate themselves with hydrogen and oxygen, gives carbohydrates the ability to provide a skeletal framework for the manufacture of both: (a) the basic components of protoplasm; and (b) the internal structure of various tissues and organs of the human body; not to mention (c) lubricating its joints; and (d) acting as supporting elements of connective tissue.

Finally, carbohydrates can bond to both lipids (fats) and proteins, and they supply key components of nucleic acids, as well. Indeed, these molecular ingredients of the human body are so versatile, so:

- embedded in the structure of *other* constituents of the body—for instance, as part of the sugar-phosphate backbone of deoxyribonucleic acid (DNA) and ribonucleic acid (RNA)

- necessary as accessory modifiers attached to protein molecules

- transient in both active (i.e., being used up for energy) and inactive (i.e., stored as glycogen) forms

...so fluid, metastable, and labile, that it is difficult, if not impossible, to provide a firm, accurate estimate of the carbohydrate composition of the body at any given moment, or even a reliable "average" for the "typical" adult. Thus, the carbohydrate composition of the body is usually lumped together with that of other anatomic constituents. That having been said, however, given the fact (see Table 1.2) that we can account for more than 98 percent of the entire body, independent of its carbohydrate constituency, we can state with a reasonable degree of confidence that the likelihood that the latter is ever present in quantities exceeding about 1.5 percent of total body weight is essentially zero—hence the value given in Table 1.2.

Table 1.2 "Average" molecular composition of the "typical" human adult	
COMPONENT	% OF BODY WEIGHT
Water	60.0 ± 15
Protein	17.0 ± 8
Fat (lipids)	15.5 ± 3
Minerals (ash)	5.0 ± 2
Carbohydrates	1.5 ± 0.5
Extractives (including RNA)	0.9 ± 0.2
DNA	≈ 0.1

Note: Given the wide ranges shown in the above table, it is obvious that all values are approximate averages convenient only for the purposes of general discussion. Specific values for any given individual, and for the same individual, at any given time, might vary significantly from those shown in the table, but the values are at least representative of what one is likely to encounter.

Fatty acids

In the general carbohydrate formula, $(CH_2O)_n$, if we isolate oxygen, O_n, and limit it to just n = 2, to create a compound having the general chemical formula $(CH_2)_nO_2$, we have created *fatty acids*—the building blocks of *fats*, or *lipids* (from the Greek *lipos*, meaning "fat"). Among the many functions of fats in the body (other than providing an incentive for dieting!) are:

- Thermal insulation: more than two-thirds of the body's fat content is stored just below the skin surface (i.e., *sub-cutaneously*), and in other self-contained *adipose tissue.*

- Energy storage: fats act as an alternative fuel when needed. A quarter of the body's fat content is stored mainly as a type of fat known as *triglycerides*—a major component of very low density lipoproteins (VLDL), found mostly in *musculoskeletal tissue.*

- Cell structure: types of fat called *phospholipids*, along with some *cholesterol*, serve as the primary structural component of cell membranes.

- Hormones: many fats are precursors of *hormones* (from the Greek, *ormanein*, meaning "to excite")—chemical substances conveyed by blood to specific "target organs," which are thus stimulated to increased functional activity. Among these are:

  ○ anti-inflammatory *steroids* derived from cholesterol

  ○ various *stress hormones*, also derived from cholesterol, including *catecholamines* (such as epinephrine, or adrenalin, and norepinephrine, or noradrenalin). For reasons we shall discuss in Chapter 7 and Part II of this book, the music therapist should endeavor to become particularly familiar with and conscious of the role of stress hormones in the clinical management of a client (see also Schneck and Berger 2006).

- Emulsifying agents (*bile acids*): as we shall see, these assist in the digestion/ absorption of lipids. Indeed, the very word, *cholesterol*, derives from the Greek *cholē*, meaning "bile," and *sterós*, meaning "solid, stiff," undoubtedly referring to the consistency of this fatty substance manufactured in and secreted by the liver.

- Surfactant activity: *surfactants* are chemical substances that help to maintain the *surface tension* that acts to prevent collapse of the tiny air sacs in the lungs.

So you see, contrary to the bad rap that fats get as risk factors for cardiovascular disease and all sorts of other terrible afflictions, they are, in fact, a very important component of human body structure and function and we should not minimize their role in keeping us healthy and well! We need them, especially those *essential fatty acids* that are not synthesized in the human body, but are required for normal, healthy metabolism. Hence, we must ingest them from a diet containing, in particular:

- cold water fish such as salmon, herring, and mackerel

- nuts, such as almonds and walnuts

- dark green leafy vegetables, such as broccoli and spinach

- eggs, whole-grain foods, and olive oil—to name a few.

Included among the essential fatty acids are: linoleic and linolenic acid, and arachidonic acid.

Nucleic acids and the human genome

As promised, let's now add nitrogen, N, into the mix of carbon, hydrogen, and oxygen. We will include it either: (a) attached to a carbon atom as a side chain consisting of the *amino group*, NH_2, or (b) attached all alone directly to the carbon atom. Thus, if we let n = 1 in our general carbohydrate formula, i.e., start with CH_2O and add to it $(CHN)_3$ to construct a compound having the general chemical formula $C_4H_5N_3O$, we have given birth to the *pyrimidine* base called *cytosine*, which shall be designated by the symbol C_y to distinguish it from pure carbon, C.

On the other hand, if we add instead to CH_2O the combination, $O(CH)_4N_2$, to construct a compound having the general chemical formula $C_5H_6N_2O_2$, we have synthesized the *pyrimidine* base called *thymine*, T. (*Note:* if we replace the *methyl group*, CH_3, in thymine by just a single hydrogen atom, H, thymine becomes the pyrimidine base called, *uracil*, U = $(CH)_4(NO)_2$. Going one step further, let's now add to our basic carbohydrate CH_2O, the combination $N(CN)_4H_3$ to create compounds having the general chemical formula $C_5H_5N_5O$, with their molecules linked together in contiguous fashion. We have thus created the *purine* base, *guanine*, G. Finally, shedding the oxygen from guanine and rearranging the molecular configuration somewhat yields the *purine* base, *adenine*, A, which has the chemical formula: $C_5H_5N_5$.

Remember in discussing carbohydrates, our previously mentioning *adenosine triphosphate*, our body's "battery?" Well, here we are, i.e., if we now attach the five-carbon, pentose sugar, *ribose*, $(CH_2O)_5$, to adenine, discarding a water molecule, H_2O, in the process, we get a product called *adenosine*, $C_{10}H1_3N5O4$. Adenosine becomes *adenosine triphosphate* (ATP) when it combines in the *mitochondria* of human cells with three phosphoric acid groups, $(H_2PO_4)_3$. The latter chemical reaction takes place via an aerobic process—which is why we need oxygen!—called *oxidative phosphorylation*. During this process, three *hydroxyl groups*, i.e., 3(-OH), are given up, to yield the chemical compound ATP = $C_{10}H_{16}N_5O_{13}P_3$. It is the subsequent splitting off (*hydrolysis*) of the phosphate groups from ATP that releases the large amounts of chemical energy that drive all metabolic reactions.

Now, if we combine our ribose sugar instead with *any* of the four bases, A,G,C_y,U, we produce four types of *nucleoside;* and…if we add phosphoric acid to these nucleosides, we generate what are called *nucleotides*. Nucleotides can be bonded to one another to create long, *single*, linear strands. These non-branching strands are called *nucleic acids*, as in: *ribonucleic acid* (RNA). If we replace U in RNA by T, and exchange ribose for *deoxy*-ribose, then the bases on a nucleic acid strand will pair up with an equal number of partners (bases) on a neighboring strand, due essentially to electrostatic attractions, forming what are called *polar bonds*. We have thus produced the *double* strands of *deoxyribonucleic acid* (DNA).

DNA is a long-chain, branched, double-stranded (as opposed to RNA, which consists of just single strands) polymer. Moreover, the base pairing that creates the double strand is not random: it always involves a purine base, A or G, hooking up with a pyrimidine base, T or C_y, in that order, respectively—i.e., A with T and G with C_y; and the base pairs, in turn, follow one another along the chain in specific sequences, each sequence "coding" for the composition of a corresponding chemical species. The two paired strands of DNA form a coiled (twisted) double-helix configuration— like a spiral staircase. The sugar-phosphate complex forms the backbone, or "sides" of the staircase, and the base pairs form its "steps."

Base-pair sequences of DNA are organized into functional units called *genes*, from the Greek "to be born." There is a specific gene that "codes" for every anatomic feature/physiologic attribute of the organism. Variable numbers of genes are further assembled and distributed among rod-shaped bodies called *chromosomes*. There are long-size chromosomes and short-size ones. They are all contained in the *nucleus* of a cell. However, although variable in *size*, chromosomes are of a definite *number* for each species, and they usually occur in pairs. There are 23 pairs in human cells that contain a nucleus (red blood cells do not)—46 chromosomes all together: one set of the pair from your biological mother, another set from your biological father. The only exception is the gametes—sperm cells in men, egg cells in women—which contain only 23 to be passed along to the offspring of a biological mother and father. In total, the chromosomes of the human body contain some 20,000–25,000 genes. Collectively, these comprise the human *genome*—the blueprint for one complete, unique human being.

Among many inherited genetic disorders, one of particular interest to music therapists is *Down syndrome*—named after the English physician, John L. Down (1828–1896), who first described it. This congenital condition results from an extra number-21 chromosome in the child's cells. It is characterized by severe mental deficiency and specific physical features. Music is particularly effective in caring for individuals affected by Down syndrome.

Table 1.3 RNA codes for the 20 amino acids					
AMINO ACID	**CODON**				
Alanine	GC_yU	GC_yC_y	GC_yA	GC_yG		
Arginine	C_yGU	C_yGC_y	C_yGA	C_yGG	AGA	AGG
Asparagine	AAU	AAC_y				
Aspartic acid	GAU	GAC_y				

Cysteine	UGU	UGC_y				
Glutamic acid	GAA	GAG				
Glutamine	C_yAA	C_yAG				
Glycine	GGU	GGC_y	GGA	GGG		
Histidine	C_yAU	C_yAC_y				
Isoleucine	AUU	AUC_y	AUA			
Leucine	C_yUU	C_yUC_y	C_yUA	C_yUG	UUA	UUG
Lysine	AAA	AAG				
Methionine	AUG					
Phenylalanine	UUU	UUC_y				
Proline	C_yC_yU	$C_yC_yC_y$	C_yC_yA	C_yC_yG		
Serine	UC_yU	UC_yC_y	UC_yA	UC_yG	AGU	AGC_y
Threonine	AC_yU	AC_yC_y	AC_yA	AC_yG		
Tryptophan	UGG					
Tyrosine	UAU	UAC_y				
Valine	GUU	GUC_y	GUA	GUG		
A = Adenine	C_y = Cytosine		G = Guanine			U = Uracil

Amino acids

Amino acids are the building blocks of *proteins*—the "stuff" of which we are made. There are 20 of these (Table 1.3) manufactured on the basis of an RNA code derived from the DNA recipe. That is to say, looking closer at the DNA chain, we note that a sequence of three consecutive bases on it—called a *codon*—"codes" for the manufacture of a specific one of the 20 amino acids. A *gene*, then, is defined more formally to be "that DNA segment of a nucleic acid chain that contains a sufficient number of codons to synthesize all, or a significant portion of a protein." Now, four bases, taken three at a time, can produce 64 triplets (i.e., $4^3 = 64$), more than three times as many possibilities as there are amino acids (20). Thus, as indicated in Table 1.3, there is considerable redundancy in the DNA coding for amino acids. Sixty-one possible triplets are accounted for in the table; the remaining three, UGA, UAA, and UAG, are used as "stop" codes that signal the end of a protein synthesis chain. In summary, then, a specific set of codons—called an *exon*—"book-ended" by stop codes, is strung together in different lengths, but in a specific sequence along a nucleic acid chain. This establishes a corresponding sequence of amino acids that, together, are the components of a specific protein molecule. The "stringing together" takes place on cellular bodies called *ribosomes*.

Several exons (often just one), separated by "spacers" called *introns*—included within the "stop codes" on the nucleic acid chain—form the functional unit called a *gene*. As mentioned earlier, there are an estimated 20,000–25,000 (perhaps as many as 30,000) *functional* genes in the human genome. Hypothetically, any nucleated cell in the human body is coded to produce one entire human being! That is the theoretical basis for the very exciting possibilities afforded by the relatively new field of stem cell research.

An amino acid has a central carbon atom to which are attached four side chains: a hydrogen atom, -H, an amino group, $-NH_2$, a *carboxyl group*, -COOH, and an "-R" group. The constituents and chemical properties of the R-group determine which of 20 possibilities the amino acid is, as shown in Table 1.3, where, again, the redundancy in many cases should be noted. Any linkage between two (or more) amino acids is called a *peptide*. Sequential repetition of this process yields *polypeptide linkages*—long-chain polymers called *proteins*, from the Greek *prôtos* (since polypeptide chains were once thought to be the essential "first" constituents of all animals and plants). The genetically coded 40,000 or so different types of protein make them the most abundant class of organic compounds in the healthy, lean human body, accounting for more than half of its cellular dry weight and up to a quarter of its total body weight. Their multi-faceted functions include:

- *catalysis:* metabolic enhancement through *enzymes*
- *communication: information* transport and processing through *neurotransmitters* and *membrane receptor sites*
- *active mass transport:* in the form of *carrier molecules*
- *muscular contraction:* via *actomyosin-filament* complexes
- *protection:* in the form of the immune system's *immunoglobulins* and *antigens* and the integumentary system's *skin*
- *structure:* in the form of an interlacing fabric composed of combinations of proteins and carbohydrates called *glycoproteins*
- *joint lubrication:* via "slippery" *synovial fluid*
- *metabolic regulation* in the form of the activity of *hormones*

...to name but a few!

Again, the linear sequence of amino acids that uniquely identifies any given protein is encoded into a specific gene. When that protein's presence is called for, the corresponding gene is *activated*, i.e., the portion of the DNA chain (between introns) that contains that protein's exon ("recipe") "opens up," like a piece of zipper. The exon's genetic codon information is then *transcribed* ("copied")—in the nucleus of the cell—from the exposed DNA-site onto a *messenger RNA (mRNA)* complex. mRNA's codon sequence mirrors the precise placement of amino acids in the protein molecule. In other words, mRNA is the mirror pattern from which the corresponding protein will ultimately be assembled, in a process called *gene expression*.

Since DNA never leaves the nucleus, it is left up to messenger RNA to *transport* the protein recipe from the transcription site into the cytoplasm of the cell. But before the right protein can be expressed from this recipe, the mirror image on mRNA must be reversed if it is to correspond exactly with what the DNA code is calling for. Thus, *transfer RNA (tRNA)* molecules—generally manufactured in the *nucleolus* located inside the nucleus of the cell—taking their cue from the mRNA pattern, now scamper about in the cytoplasm, collecting the specific amino acids that will be required to express the corresponding protein. They *transfer* these amino acids to, and place them at—*in the exact, unique sequence called for by the DNA code*— at the sites of protein synthesis, which are cellular *ribosomes.* Here, the sequence is formally coupled together (*translated*)—which is to say, the amino acids are "zipped up" by the ribosome, sliding along the contiguous elements to finally express the desired protein and release it to do its job. Protein synthesis, or *gene expression*, is thus essentially a three-step process: (a) *transcription* (DNA-to-mRNA); (b) *transportation* (mRNA cuing tRNA); and (c) *translation* (ribosome coupling of amino acids). The *uniqueness* of every living organism is the result of its having been endowed with the ability to manufacture a *specific* set of proteins—unlike any other that has ever existed and, more than likely, *will* ever exist. Indeed, *each of us is a minority of one*, as is proven mathematically in Schneck (2001a).

In summary

The *atoms* of which the human body is composed are organized into *molecules.* Most of them are in the form of water. About one-third are divided between body fats and proteins. The remainder consist mostly of inorganic minerals, with lesser amounts of various inorganic and organic (carbon-containing) compounds—more than half of which are in the form of carbohydrates and DNA. What's left after all of the above are sorted out includes such "extractives" as RNA, urea, carbon dioxide, coloring pigments, and anything else that does not fit into one of the other categories.

Before we move on, it is worth emphasizing that numerical values quoted in the tables and text throughout this book should be considered to be approximations based on averages measured and accumulated for a wide variety of "typical" individuals (e.g., see Duck 1990; Jacob *et al.* 1982; Lentner 1981, 1982, 1984, 1986, 1990; Schneck 1990). Thus, *specific* values for any *given* individual will vary, but statistically speaking, they should lie within a reasonable range of the means quoted. Furthermore, anatomic data varies between adult men and women, between adults and children, and among adults of different ages, anthropometric build, hereditary lineage, diet, lifestyle, state of health, and so on. Moreover, even for a *given* individual, body composition goes through cyclical changes as often as daily, but certainly during the course of a lifetime. Keeping all of this in mind, let's now explore the next level of anatomic organization of the human body, which is the *cell*, its basic functional unit, illustrated in Figure 1.1 (on the following page).

Cellular level of organization:
the functional unit of life

We have already mentioned some parts of a living human cell (derived from the Latin, *cella*, meaning "a small room")—namely, its *cytoplasm* (internal granular matrix), *mitochondria* (the site of ATP synthesis), *nucleus* (the "safety deposit box" that houses DNA), *nucleolus* (the "home" of RNA), and *ribosomes* (the site of protein synthesis). Indeed, looking at Figure 1.1, we note that a cell may be thought of as being a tiny, self-contained village, surrounded by a "picket fence"—the bi-lipid layer, semi-permeable, porous *plasma membrane*—inside which are contained all of the services that are necessary for the village to function. It has its own:

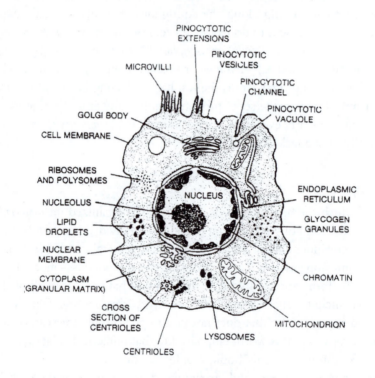

Figure 1.1 Schematic representation of the essential features of a "typical" nucleated human cell containing various cytoplasmic organelles

- government and government services—housed in the *nucleus* of the cell, which is surrounded by its own protective membrane, and within which is contained its:
  - *executive branch*, which derives its authority from a "constitution and by-laws"—the DNA genome
  - *legislative branch*—i.e., "functioning agencies" operating through the *nucleolus* and its messenger RNAs

- utility services to:
    - provide power (ATP) to the village, by as few as two, to as many as 2500 *mitochondria* ("power plants") per cell—tiny generating stations that charge up its "battery"
    - dispose of sewage and waste products of metabolism through 300 or so *lysosomes* ("sewage plants") and 200 or so *peroxisomes* ("metabolite disposal units") per cell. These take care of detoxification activities, destruction/ digestion of unwanted material—such as foreign substances and cellular debris (the main function of lysosomes)—recycling, and the potential harmful effects of "stray" oxygen molecules (the main function of peroxisomes). It is these many, tiny *organelles* ("little organs") that give the cytoplasm its characteristic "granular" appearance when examined under a microscope.
- internal highway networks: the *endoplasmic reticulum* and *cytoskeletal microtubules*
- external ports and loading docks—*pinocytotic extensions, vesicles,* and *channels*; *microvilli,* and *cell membrane receptor sites* for specific hormones, neurotransmitters, and enzymes
- industries that make all of the unique products—*proteins*—for which the village is world famous, manufactured by some 15,000 (to millions of) *ribosome* plants per cell
- packaging and distribution centers—the cellular *Golgi complex*
- storage facilities embedded in visible *glycogen granules, lipid droplets, vacuoles* and *secretory vesicles*
- necessary architecture by which to reproduce itself—including *chromosomes,* the *chromatin DNA protein complex, centriole pairs,* and *mitotic spindles*
- additional *organelles* that individual cells might need to perform their assigned function—which also determines *how many of each organelle* any given cell will contain.

The latter is determined early on in gestation through the process of *cellular differentiation.* This is the biological process by which the single fertilized cell that is destined to become "you"—the *zygote* that is inherently coded to produce one entire human being—goes through a series of divisions that produce varieties of cells programmed to perform very different, specific functions. We mentioned this briefly when we introduced the idea of stem cell research in our earlier discussion of amino acids.

Thus, when all is said and done, the "typical" adult human body consists of some one hundred trillion, give or take a trillion, cells that are of approximately 210 different types, a few of which are shown in Table 1.4. On average, about *50 million* of these cells are replenished *per second*! However, individual cell lives vary—from mere seconds (e.g., some white blood cells (WBC) only live that long) to 120 days (a red blood cell generally lives that long), to 25 years (the average lifespan of a typical bone cell), to an entire life span (as is true for some nerve cells). About 98 percent of most of your cells are replaced annually; and every five years or so they may have undergone a complete turnover. Again, cells are self-contained *units of life*—tiny masses of animated, functional *protoplasm* (from the Greek *prôtos*, meaning "first," and *plasma*, meaning something "molded," see Figure 1.1, page 34). Their classification into some 210 different types is based on:

- their *morphology*, i.e., external structure and form, such as:
  - what they look like—their size, shape, color, geometrical configuration, "granular" or "agranular" appearance, etc.
  - where and/or in what organ of the body they are located, including—as is the case for *lymphocytes*, for example—the anatomical location where they matured
  - what stage of development they are in
- their *physiology*, i.e., what these cells do, as in:
  - their *function*—which depends on how many organelles they contain, the nature and quantity of their constituency, and the various biochemical reactions in which these constituents participate
  - the *rate* at which they do what they do
  - whether or not they are doing what they are designed for and *supposed* to be doing, i.e., their state of health
- their *heritage*, i.e., the name of the person who first identified or described them, as in, for example, *Kupffer's* cells of the liver. Such terminology goes by the name *eponyms*, from the Greek for "named after")
- the way in which they are *identified* in the laboratory, usually connoting a staining mode, as in:
  - are the cells "acid loving," i.e., *acidophilic?* And, if so, to what specific acidic stain(s) (as in, for example, *eosinophils*, in the case of a certain type of white blood cell)?
  - are they "alkaline loving," i.e., *basophilic?* And, if so, to what specific alkaline stain(s)?
  - are they *neutral*—indifferent to the type of stain (as is the case for *neutrophils*)?

In many cases, the above considerations are embedded in the *prefix* that identifies the cell, to which is attached—for mature cells—the suffix -*cyte* (from the Greek *kytos*, meaning "hollow vessel"). Some of these are illustrated in Table 1.4. For example, a *fibrocyte* (or a "desmocyte") is a type of cell found in most connective tissue (from the

Latin *fibra*, meaning "fiber," or the Greek *desmós*, meaning "chain, bond"). In fact, note from the numbers in parentheses in Table 1.4, that almost half (46%) of all the cells in the human body are fibrocytes (or precursors of fibrocytes, called *fibroblasts*) that have to do with the basic *structure* of the organism. Of the other 54%:

- more than half of them (27.5%) are various types of blood cells
- just under half (24.5%) are *epithelial* cells (to be described later).

The remaining 2 percent is divided in a ratio of about 3:1 among muscle cells (1.5%) and nerve cells (0.5%). As we shall see in the next section, all the other types of cell can be shown to fall into one or more of the above classifications. "But," you may ask, "where do body *fluids*—i.e., liquids and gases—fit in to the various levels of organization of the human body? Some fluids are inside the cells...some are outside...what gives?" I'm glad you asked!

Table 1.4 A few of the 210 types of human cells		
TYPE (% OF TOTAL)	PREFIX-*CYTE*	MEANING
Ingesting Cells	PHAGO-	Greek, "To eat"
Connecting Cells (46)	FIBRO-	Latin, "Fiber, band"
Blood Cells (27.5)	HEMATO-	Greek, "Blood"
• Oxygen-carrying	ERYTHRO-	Greek, "Red"
• Immature red cell	RETICULO-	Latin, "Net"
• Elongated red cell	STOMATO-	Greek, "Mouth"
• Immune function	LEUKO-	Greek, "White"
◦ Phagocytic	GRANULO-	Latin, "Little grain"
◦ Scavenger	AGRANULO-	Non-granulated
	MONO-	Contains one nucleus
	LYMPHO-	Latin, "Clear water"
• Clotting	THROMBO-	Greek, "Lump"
• Spleen	SPLENO-	Greek, "Spleen"
Epithelial (24.5)		
• Alveolar lining	PNEUMO-	Greek, "To blow"
Skin	DERMATO-	Greek, "Skin"
• Structural protein	KERATINO-	Greek, "Horn"
• Pigment	MELANO-	Greek, "Black"
• Fat	ADIPO-	Latin, "Fat"
• Phagocytic	HISTIO-	Greek, "Web"

cont.

TYPE (% OF TOTAL)	PREFIX-*CYTE*	MEANING
Skeletal		
• Bone	OSTEO-	Latin, "Bone"
• Cartilage	CHONDRO-	Latin, "Gristle"
• Ligament	DESMO-	Greek, "A bond"
• Marrow/Spinal cord	MYELO-	Greek, "Marrow"
Muscular (1.5)	MYO-	Greek, "Muscle"
• Heart	CARDIO-	Greek, "Heart"
Nervous (0.5)	NEURO-	Greek, "Sinew"
• Supporting cells	GLIA-	Greek, "Glue"
• Neuro-glia fibers	ASTRO-	Greek, "Star-shaped"
• Type of neuroglia	PITUI-	Latin, "Phlegm"
Reproductive Gametes		
• Male	SPERMATO-	Greek, "Seed"
• Female	OÖ-	Greek, "Egg"
Liver	HEPATO-	Greek, "Liver"
Germ Cells	BLASTO-	Greek, "Germ"

Human body fluids and fluid distribution

About 60 percent or so by weight of the "typical," lean, relatively fat-free human body is water. As you aptly observed, some of this liquid—in fact *most of it* (two-thirds to three quarters)—is confined, cumulatively, to the interior spaces of all of the cells of the body, i.e., the regions collectively bounded by cell membranes. This confined volume is called the *intracellular fluid compartment* (ICF), of the body. The cumulative amount of fluid that lies outside the ICF is then called, logically enough, the body's *extracellular fluid compartment* (ECF), amounting to one-quarter to one-third of total body water.

The ECF includes mainly two sub-compartments: (a) a *vascular* (blood plasma volume)/*lymphatic* region, accounting for about 25 percent of the ECF; and (b) a "bathing," *interstitial fluid* space, literally "standing between" the *extra vascular* (outside the vascular region) cells of the body. Interstitial fluid accounts for about 75 percent of the ECF.

To be "safe," the ICF/ECF ratio should be maintained fairly close to the range 2:1–3:1. Suffice it to say for now that to be "safe" means an ICF/ECF ratio that balances body fluid distribution in a way that is both optimal and critical for the proper life-sustaining transport of materials into (mostly oxygen and nutrients) and out of (mostly carbon dioxide and other waste products of metabolism) the cell (Schneck 1990).

Continuing with our discussion of body levels of organization, note that if we combine *blood* cells—thinking of them in an abstract sense as a type of structural anatomical "connection" among body parts—with *actual* structural "connective" cells (see Table 1.4), then the 210 cell types bathed in a supporting interstitial liquid may actually be grouped into four broad categories, i.e.:

1. *connective* (structural, including "skin and bones," and blood)

2. *epithelial* (cells that externally "cover" and/or internally "line")

and two categories of "excitable," meaning that the cells have electrical properties, namely:

3. muscle cells

4. nerve cells.

Collectively, each category is called a type of *tissue*, from the Latin *texere*, meaning "to weave," as in cells "woven" together as explained below.

Tissue level of organization: building an entire body

If one envisions atoms and molecules to be the *chemical ingredients* of which the human body is composed, and cells to be its basic *functional components*, then tissues assume the role of primary *structural building blocks*—i.e., combinations of cells that are "woven together" to be the "bricks and mortar" from which the body's organs and systems are constructed. Tissues are assembled and designed to have a very specific, desired effect—for example, to *cover* or *line* various body structures; to *support* and *connect* anatomical components; to produce *movement*; or to receive, transmit, and process *information*. Thus, we have, respectively: *epithelial*, *connective*, *muscular*, and *nervous* tissue.

Epithelial tissue

The word *epithelial* has a rather interesting etymology, being derived from the Greek *epi-*, meaning "on," and *thēlē*, meaning "nipple," as in a small projection or appendage. Thus, literally, *epithelial* means "on the nipple," suggesting "a covering" (use your imagination!). The tissue consists of epithelial cells arranged in continuous sheets, either to wrap around (encase or cover) surfaces—thereby providing a *sheathing* to protect body structures—or to line cavities and canals (in which case they are called *endothelial cells*, from the Greek *endon*, which means "inner"). Much of this tissue is *squamous*—flat, "scale-like" (from the Latin, *squama*), and smooth (as in the *skin*)—but a good deal of epithelial cells have:

- finger-like projections called *microvilli* that increase the tissue's surface area to maximize absorption (as in the lining of the small intestines)

- contractile properties, as in the hair-like projections called *cilia* that adorn *myoepithelium*, from the Greek, *mys*, for "muscle." The movement of cilia helps to propel things along (for example, air in the respiratory tract and eggs in the female Fallopian tubes).

- the ability to manufacture and secrete chemical compounds, as in the *glandular parenchymal* (functional, as opposed to structural) *epithelium* of the endocrine and exocrine glands

- the ability to be otherwise *excitable*, i.e., capable of being stimulated—as in the *neuroepithelium* of the functional layers of the sense organs

- *phagocytic* capabilities, i.e., they are "eating" cells (from the Greek, *phagein*, meaning "eat"). These cells can engulf things, either to: (a) transport them, like taxis (in a process called *active transport*), to places they would not go otherwise (or not get there fast enough); or (b) to digest and destroy them (as in, the *reticulo-endothelial system* of the spleen) when their presence is undesireable or no longer desirable, as is the case for outdated red blood cells (which have no nucleus and hence cannot reproduce).

Table 1.5 Classification of epithelial tissue	
CLASS: SIMPLE (one cell layer)	**SOME TYPICAL LOCATIONS**
Squamous (flat)	
Endothelium	Lining of the heart and blood vessels
Mesothelium	Lining of pleural (lung), peritoneal (abdominal), and pericardial (heart) cavities
Mesenchymal	Lining of subarachnoid and subdural cavities, chambers of the eye, and perilymphatic spaces of the ear
Cuboidal (tube-shaped)	Lining of renal tubules Germinal coverings for the ovaries Pigmented layer of the retina Parenchymal (functional, as opposed to supportive): secretory glands
Cuboidal (tube-shaped)	Lining of renal tubules Germinal coverings for the ovaries Pigmented layer of the retina Parenchymal (functional, as opposed to supportive): secretory glands
Columnar (cylindrical pillars)	

Nonciliated	Lining of the urethra, mucosa of the stomach, bile ducts, uterine tubes and upper respiratory tract
Ciliated	Microvilli of the intestines and respiratory tract
Myoepithelium has contractile properties	
Neuroepithelium has electrical properties, forming the terminal nerve endings of the special senses	
Glandular parenchymal	Exocrine and endocrine glands
Phagocytic	Reticuloendothelium of spleen
CLASS: STRATIFIED (multiple cell layers)	**SOME TYPICAL LOCATIONS**
Squamous	Digestive, respiratory, urinary, and reproductive tracts; conjuctiva of the eye; and middle ear
Cuboidal	Ducts of parotid gland near the ear
Columnar	Ocular conjuctiva of the eye
Pseudostratified (simple, with stratified *appearance*) Columnar	
Ciliated	Respiratory tract
CLASS: TRANSITIONAL (alternating distention/relaxation cell patterns)	**SOME TYPICAL LOCATIONS**
	Lining of the kidney pelvis, urethra, urinary bladder, and the upper part of the urethra

Because of the wide variety of functions that epithelial cells can perform, epithelial tissue is technically broken down into two basic divisions: a covering and lining *membrane* division and a *secretory glandular* division. In Table 1.5 is illustrated four basic sub-divisions of the former, i.e., *simple* (one cell layer), *stratified* (multiple cell layers), *transitional* (*seemingly* alternating among several geometric configurations, depending on *when* one looks at the cell), and *pseudostratified* (*appearing* to be stratified, depending on *how* one looks at the cell). The two *glandular* sub-divisions include the epithelial tissue of the *endocrine* and *exocrine* glands (to be described in Chapter 7).

In turn, based on their geometry, epithelial cells are further classified as being: *squamous* (flat), *cuboidal*, (tube-shaped), or *columnar* (cylindrical pillars having or not having cilia). For further details on all of these types of epithelial tissue, see Jacob *et al.* (1982) and Tortora and Grabowski (1993). In general, by *mass*, epithelial tissue accounts for some 12.5 percent of the total body—the vast majority of it being housed in the skin.

Connective tissue

Connective tissue (which includes body fluids and fat (*adipose*) tissue), as the name implies, consists of conglomerations of cells arranged in configurations that *support* and *connect* (or bind) body parts, either directly—through contiguous contact—or indirectly—through fluid transport. Thus, as is illustrated in Table 1.6, in addition to body fluids and fat, connective tissue includes the:

- *cartilage* (gristle) and trans-cellular *synovial* (joint, ECF) fluid that allow bones to glide smoothly over one another

- 206 bones of the skeletal system that form a "scaffolding" to support body structures, and "levers" to provide them with both mobility, and a "mechanical advantage" in performing work

- bone *marrow* that has *hemopoietic* (or *hematopoietic:* "blood-cell forming") properties, occupying the *medullary* (inner) *cavity* of bones

- *tendons* that connect muscles to bones

- *ligaments* that secure bones to one another where they articulate, helping to maintain their proper alignment

- interlacing networks of fibers that provide a structural framework for muscles, bone marrow, the spleen, liver, lungs, kidney, and other body organs (*viscera*)

- band-like coverings (*fascia*) that envelope the body beneath the skin (like plastic-wrap), and also separate layers of muscles nested within one another.

Table 1.6 Classification of connective tissue	
CLASS	**SOME TYPICAL LOCATIONS**
General Supporting/Binding	
Loose (areolar)	Interstitial substance of most organs; adventitial layer of major blood vessels
Dense (fibrous, collagenous)	
Yellow fibrous	Intimal and medial wall layers of arteries
Irregularly arranged	Dermis (skin) Fibrous membranes Capsular enclosures
Regularly arranged, white fibrous	Muscle tendons Cartilage; aponeuroses; ligaments Lamellated structures
Special Supporting/Binding	
Fibrous elastic Lymphatic tissue	Muscle fibers Lymph nodes Spleen; thymus gland

Adipose	Fat tissue
Mucous	Mucous membranes of the gastrointestinal tract
Reticular (fibrous, adipose, mucous combined)	Liver; lungs; larynx; trachea; kidney
Pigmented	Skin and choroid coat of eye
Cartilage	
Articular	End surface layers of bones
Hyaline, white	Trachea; nose septum; larynx
Elastic, yellow	Epiglottis; external ear; auditory tube
White fibrous	Joins bones together
Bone	
Osseous tissue	
Compact, lamellar cortical	Outside surface of bone
Spongy cancellous	Inner regions of bone
Trabecular	Ends of bones
Myeloid Tissue: Bone Marrow	Active Red Bone Marrow
	Inactive, Yellow Bone Marrow
Body Fluids	Blood; lymph; ICF/ECF

Because of this impressive variety of functions, one finds an equally impressive variety of connective tissue classifications. In the broadest sense, the tissue is classified as being either *ordinary* (general) or *special* (see Table 1.6). The "ordinary" classification includes:

- fibrous, loose, *areolar* tissue, which makes up the interstitial substance of most organs, and the outer layer (*adventitia*) of major blood vessels
- *dense*, regularly and irregularly arranged tissue.

The "special" connective tissue classification includes (a) *generic*, (b) *supporting*, and (c) *fluid* categories. The *generic* one includes:

- *mucous* ("jelly-like"), *reticular* ("net-like"), and *fibro-elastic* matter
- *adipose* (fat), and *hemopoietic* ("blood-cell-forming") substance
- *pigmented* ("colored-matter")
- some *supporting* tissue fibers.

The hemopoietic sub-category is broken down further into *lymphatic* and *myeloid* divisions. The former includes non-encapsulated and encapsulated—e.g., lymph nodes, spleen, thymus gland—sub-divisions; while the latter (shown separately in

Table 1.6) includes active "red" and inactive "yellow" connective tissue cells present in bone marrow.

Supporting "special" connective tissue includes:

- *cartilage*—articular, hyaline, fibrous, and elastic types

- *bone*—immature, and mature compact, spongy, and trabecular types.

Body *fluids*, as discussed earlier (and will be covered again in Chapter 2) include, broadly, extracellular and intracellular fluid compartments.

Together, epithelial and connective tissue make up about half of one's total body mass, in roughly a 3:1 (connective/epithelial) ratio which breaks down, approximately, as follows: blood and lymph, 8.25 percent + other connective tissue, 29.25 percent = 37.5 percent = 3 x epithelial tissue @ 12.5 percent. The other half of one's total body mass consists basically of muscle and nerve tissue, in a ratio of about 4 or 5 to 1 (muscle/nerve).

Muscle tissue

Along with myoepithelium and neuroepithelium, muscle and nerve tissue have the property of being *excitable*. This means that they are capable of generating an electrochemical signal—called an *action potential*—when provoked by an *adequate stimulus* of sufficient strength. "Sufficient strength" means that there is a *threshold level (electrical "potential")* below which the tissue will be unresponsive (Junge 1981; Schneck and Berger 2006). "Adequate stimulus" means that the tissue will respond only to a *specific* type of energy—sound, heat, light, electricity, magnetism, mechanical force, etc.

In the case of muscles, the action potential incites to a working state excitable cells that are concerned with generating *movement*, both internal and external. Internal movement is accomplished by:

- involuntary *smooth muscle tissue*. It comes in two types:

  ○ *vascular*, in blood vessel walls

  ○ *visceral*, in various body organs

- involuntary *cardiac* (heart) *muscle tissue*

- involuntary/voluntary *striated skeletal muscle tissue*, such as the diaphragm and gluteus (of the buttocks).

External movement is accomplished entirely by the 639–656 (depending on how one counts them, Schneck 1992) voluntary *striated skeletal muscles*. All three types of muscle—smooth, cardiac, and striated skeletal—transform chemical energy (mainly derived from the aforementioned ATP), into mechanical work (Schneck 1992). The work appears as the effort required to:

- maintain postural balance and/or locomote parts or all of the animal body
- maintain the "tone," "undulating motion," and internal milieu of visceral organs and tissues
- keep the heart beating and the individual breathing!

In Chapter 3 we will elaborate a bit more on why we need these three different types of muscle tissue which, for a "typical" adult, may represent up to 41 percent of the total body mass.

Nerve tissue

Rounding out our brief discussion of body tissues, we come to the fourth basic type, nerve tissue. This tissue provides the structural architecture for the human body's communications network. Nerves transmit information, encoded into *action potentials*, in three ways:

- *to* (*afferent*) the brain and spinal cord, from sensory receptors
- *from* (*efferent*) these *central nervous system* centers, as motor signals to "target" organs and tissues
- *among* (*internuncial*) themselves, via interneuron networks.

Indeed, any given nerve can interact at various *synaptic junctions* with as many as 10,000 other nerves en route to (afferent) or from (efferent) the central nervous system (CNS). Thus are formed complex *neural networks* that "wire" the body like an elaborate telephone system. Armed with nearly 50 miles of such "cable," the body's nervous tissue (amounting to some 9 percent of total body mass) can serve all of its "customers" (the cells of the body). Such service can be provided either *directly* to the customer (i.e., a single nerve is attached uninterrupted to a "target" cell) or *indirectly*, via a "middle-person" that may include an intervening nerve network or glandular secretion. Either way, not one of the cells of the body is without service; and the lines are constantly "buzzing" with information about the "state of the organism," and the need to intervene when that state is being disturbed or threatened. We shall have much more to say about all of this in Chapters 3–7, for we must now move on to the organ level of anatomical organization.

Organ level of anatomical organization

Some—but not all—tissues are *organized* into *organs*—a word that is actually derived from the Greek *érgon*, which means "work."[1]

Among those tissues that are *not* organized into "organs" are striated skeletal muscles, certain nerve networks, and those comprising blood vessels. Having said that, we note that an organ is formed by the combination of any two or more tissues that are *organized*—integrated and coordinated to do (as the name implies) *work*— more to the point: to perform a specific, well-defined *task*. That task (function) is determined by which ones of the organ's constituent tissues dominate its structure, both in quantity and activity. For example:

- some organs—like the lungs, kidneys, and spleen—might have the primary task of *processing* the materials they deal with, e.g., the:

  - lungs oxygenate the blood that courses through them, while removing carbon dioxide and water vapor

  - kidneys cleanse the blood of toxic waste products of metabolism, especially those containing nitrogen

  - spleen rids the blood of worn out red blood cells (at the incredible rate of two to ten million per second!)

...and so on. Such organs, then (see Table 1.5), are heavily inundated with types of *epithelial* and *endothelial* tissue that: (a) offer relatively large *surface areas* for mass transport and the exchange of materials across cell membranes; and (b) line the many channels that course through the respective organ to optimize its performance.

- Other organs—like the liver and certain glands—might have the primary task of *manufacturing* things, such as:

  - *bile* (liver), which is used in the small intestine to neutralize acids and emulsify fats for subsequent absorption. The liver is both the largest *gland* and the largest single organ inside the body.

  - *hormones*—e.g., the endocrine glands—to affect or control the activity of other cells, tissues and/or organs.

These, then, are heavily endowed with *glandular parenchymal epithelial* tissue that has chemical manufacturing capabilities.

---

1 The etymology is the same for the "organ" that is a musical instrument. Apparently, the earliest musical "organs" required a great deal of "work" to play them—what with having to pump away vigorously on foot bellows, and all that "effort" stuff! Moreover, the organ itself also *does* work in producing sound energy. In fact, originally, the word "organ" referred to any *musical* instrument. Since then, however, in usage it has come to refer to *any* instrument, musical or otherwise, that is capable of performing a specific task.

- Still other organs, like the body's senses, have the primary responsibility of *transducing* energy, i.e., converting it from one form—the *adequate stimulus* to which they respond (such as heat, light, or sound)—into another—the body's electrochemical syntax: *action potentials.* Thus, such organs contain a great deal of *nervous* tissue of various kinds.

- Organs like the skin—the largest single organ of the entire body (inside or out)—and those included in the body's immune system, have the primary task of *protecting* the body from invasion, from "losing its insides," or from yielding to *foreign organisms.* It is not surprising, then, to note that these organs have an ample supply of *reticuloendothelium, phagocytic,* and *lymphatic* tissue.

- Organs like the heart are primarily responsible for *pumping* things—moving them from one part of the organism to another; and so, also not surprisingly, are endowed with a good deal of *muscle* tissue.

- The organs of reproduction (breasts, ovaries, prostate gland, testes, uterus, etc.) have the primary task of giving the human body the ability to *procreate*—to make other "yous" [but not exactly *like* you! (Schneck 2001a).

All organ tasks are concerned ultimately with:

- the maintenance of the life of the particular individual involved—survival of the self, the single strongest of all human drives

- perpetuation, as a whole, of the breed of animal to which that particular individual belongs—survival of the species, the second strongest of all human drives.

Note the conspicuous use of the word "primary" in the discussion of organ tasks. Virtually all of the organs of the body can (and do) perform more than one task—i.e., they are quite adept at *multitasking*—so that classifying them as being purely regulatory, manipulative, secretory, productive, propulsive, reproductive, etc., is somewhat simplistic, even misleading. Furthermore, many organs are able to assume each other's task(s) if any of them should "go down" or have to be removed for whatever reason—i.e., they are quite *multitalented,* as well, in their capable, diverse abilities. In that sense, there are many "back-up" arrangements and a great deal of redundancy built in to the structure and function of the human body (see *Anatomical design principle number 2* in Chapter 2).

Table 1.7 Some organs and tissues included in the body of a "typical" human adult			
PHYSIOLOGIC STRUCTURE	**% OF BODY WEIGHT**	**PHYSIOLOGIC STRUCTURE**	**% OF BODY WEIGHT**
Two adrenal glands	0.023	Pancreas	0.143
Arterial system	0.291	• Women	0.102–0.146
Urinary bladder	0.066	• Men	0.108–0.154
Blood	8.050	Four parathyroid glands	Negligible
	Blood cells (3.773)	Paraganglia	0.005
	Blood plasma (4.277)	Pineal gland	Negligible
Brain	2.070	Pituitary gland	0.001
	• Women 1.95	Spinal cord	0.044
	• Men 2.15	Spleen	0.254
	Gray matter (0.828)	Stomach	0.214
	White matter (1.242)	Thyroid gland	0.029
RUNNING SUB-TOTAL	10.500	**RUNNING SUB-TOTAL**	18.540
Cerebrospinal fluid	0.175	Skeleton	14.611
Esophagus (food pipe)	0.058	• Bone	(7.963)
Two eyes	0.025	• Compact	(6.371)
Gall bladder	0.015	• Spongy	(1.592)
Gall bladder bile	0.090	Cartilage	(1.751)
Hair	0.029	Bone marrow	(4.796)
Heart	0.473	• Red	(2.183)
• Women	0.335–0.408	• Yellow	(2.613)
• Men	0.408–0.495	32 teeth	(0.067)
Intestines	1.428	• Enamel	(0.015)
Two kidneys	0.440	• Dentin	(0.051)
• Women	0.335–0.451	• Pulp	(0.001)
• Men	0.364–0.495	Synovial fluid	(0.001)
Larynx (voice box)	0.041	Ligaments	(0.033)
Liver	2.571	Trachea	0.015
• Women	1.747–2.183	Thymus gland	0.029
• Men	2.183–2.620	Female breasts	0.527

Lungs	1.66	Two ovaries	0.018
• Right lung	(0.870)	Empty uterus	0.060
• Left lung	(0.790)	Range:	0.04–0.12
Lymphatic system	0.341	Male prostate gland	0.023
Nails	0.004	Two testes	0.051
RUNNING SUB-TOTAL	**17.850**	**AVERAGE TOTAL:**	**33.8 ± 0.2 %**

There are some 40 or more organs in the human body, some of which are itemized in Table 1.7. Note, in particular, that only about 8 percent of total body mass is comprised of the *viscera*—the soft, internal organs of the *torso* of the body, which usually include the:

Adrenal glands	Urinary bladder	Gall bladder
Heart	Liver	Lungs
Kidneys	Spleen	Stomach
Pancreas	Small and large intestines	Reproductive organs (including gonads)

Indeed, note further, that *all* of the entries in Table 1.7 add up to just over a third (~34%) of total body mass. Contributing roughly another quarter, in somewhat equal amounts, are skin (~12%) and adipose (fat) tissue (~14%); and rounding out the remaining 40% or so of total body mass distribution are, as previously mentioned, mostly muscle (~33%), with significantly lesser amounts of nerve tissue (~7%)—in both of the latter cases, quantities over and above those that are already embedded in the tabulated values. But…*caution:* yet again, we emphasize that these numbers are not to be taken as literal and firm, even though it would appear so from the fact that they are carried to three decimal places! The values listed in Table 1.7 are just "typical" of what one is likely to measure—on average—across a wide population spectrum. Specific numbers for any given individual could vary widely from those tabulated. Always keep that in mind and be careful not to generalize.

So…thinking of *organelles* as being cellular structures that allow it to function as a little village, then on a larger scale, organs take on the role of an *organic* fabric that manifests itself as an *entire country*—one functioning human being! The components of the fabric are called *systems*—the next level of anatomic organization.

System level of organization: "orchestrating" an entire living human being

A collection of organs assembled—like the instrumental sections of an orchestra—to work together towards the accomplishment of a common goal that could not be achieved by any one of the organs (orchestral sections) acting alone is referred to as a *system* of the body, its final level of organization. One can easily develop an analogy between the anatomical systems of the living human body, and the instrumental sections of a major symphony orchestra. As we shall see, each anatomical system has specific tasks to perform. Likewise, each instrumental section, too, has specific tasks, i.e:

- to produce sounds of different frequencies (*pitches*)
- having different sound qualities (*timbre*)
- assembled in specific patterns (*melodic contours*)
- using differing ways of creating vibrations (*acoustic energy*):
    - string "systems," consisting of "organs" that include violins, violas, cellos, basses, and harps, generate vibrations by the *quivering* action of cords (*strings*) pulled taut between two fixed supports and displaced from an equilibrium position
    - wind "systems," consisting of: (a) woodwind "organs" that include flutes, piccolos, oboes, English horns, bassoons, clarinets, saxophones, etc.; and (b) brass "organs," consisting of trumpets, trombones, tubas, flugel horns, bugles, French horns, etc.—all of which generate vibrations by imposing an oscillating motion to columns of air of different lengths
    - percussion "systems" that generate vibrations by having one strike *membranes* (as opposed to strings) pulled taut across a fixed boundary *(drums)* or a variety of other objects, such as triangles, cymbals, tambourines, castanets, chimes, keyboards, and so on, that create characteristic acoustic energies when struck with appropriate utensils (like mallets or drum sticks) (Schneck and Berger 2006).

In a traditional symphony orchestra, then, we have varieties of instruments ("organs") and instrumental sections ("systems") that all work together to generate, it is hoped, a pleasing ("healthy") experience for an audience. Carrying this reasoning over to its anatomical analog, the human organism ("symphony orchestra"), too, has "sections"—*systems*—made up of specific organs ("instruments") that, it is hoped, function in a *healthy* way to produce a "pleasing resonance." Thus, one specific goal of music therapists, akin to the *conductor* of a symphony orchestra, is to work with clients to produce such an anatomical/physiological pleasing resonance—by understanding and exploiting systemic responses to musical stimulation.

Collectively, over two dozen anatomical *systems* are assembled to create an entire functioning human being. In the chapters that follow we shall examine most of these, including, for example, in Chapter 2, the:

- Respiratory system: a collection of organs and passages through which oxygen is taken into the body in exchange for carbon dioxide, water vapor, and heat being expelled.

- Digestive system: a collection of organs and passages through which food, beverages, and nutrients are taken into the body and desirable ingredients from them are made absorbable.

- Circulatory system: a collection of organs and passages through which various biochemical substrates, nutrients, oxygen, and hormones are delivered to the cells and tissues, in exchange for various undesirable substrates, waste products of metabolism, carbon dioxide, and heat being carried off for subsequent disposal through the excretory system.

- Lymphatic system: a collection of organs and channels through which lymph flows throughout the body, carrying absorbed nutrients to the cells, picking up fats (*chylomicrons*) from the small intestine, and transporting body wastes back into the blood.

- Excretory system: a collection of organs and tissues responsible for ridding the body of the waste products of metabolism and other substances (including heat and foreign matter) that need to be disposed of.

In Chapters 3 and 4, we cover the neuro-musculoskeletal systems: collections of organs and tissues responsible for moving parts or all of the animal body. Chapters 4, 5, 6, and 7 explore the:

- Nervous/Sensory system: a collection of organs and tissues responsible for keeping the human body in contact with the world outside (*exteroception*), and in touch with the environment inside (*interoception*). This is the *information-procuring system* of the human body, including its sensory organs of sight, smell, taste, touch, hearing, and others.

- Central information-processing systems—the brain (*cranial* portion) and spinal cord (*rachis* portion).

- Peripheral information-processing systems—12 pairs of cranial nerves; 31 pairs of spinal nerves.

- Autonomic ("automatic") protecting neural systems—consisting of *sympathetic* and *parasympathetic* divisions.

- Endocrine system: a system of *ductless glands* producing secretions (*hormones*) that pass directly into the bloodstream or lymph, to be carried to *target organs and tissues* in order to produce a desirable effect.

- These target organs and tissues also include those of the following three systems:

- Reproductive system: a collection of organs and tissues by which the body can propagate the species by giving birth to offspring.

- Exocrine system: a system of glands whose secretions leave the body as a result of being transported directly, or through a duct, to an epithelial surface.

- Immune system: a collection of biochemical factors, cells, tissues, and organs responsible for the body's resistance to, or recovery from, invasion by microbes and foreign matter.

We shall also revisit these systems in Part II of the book.

All of the various parts of the body are considered to be contained within specific *regions* and/or *cavities* of the body. These are itemized in Table 1.8, where *dorsal* refers to the rear (*posterior*) or back-side of an organ or body part, and *ventral* refers to the front (*anterior*) or stomach side of an organ or body part. Toward the "top" or head end, and "bottom" or tail end are designated, respectively, as *superior* (above, upper), and *inferior* (below, lower), while *medial* and *lateral* refer, respectively, to locations *toward*, or *away from* the midline of the body or any particular organ. Additional terminology will be defined in context when necessary.

Table 1.8 Regions and cavities of the body	
REGION/CAVITY	**MAJOR STRUCTURES CONTAINED**
Head: *Cranial* part of *dorsal (back)* cavity	Most major sense organs
	Some food gathering and respiratory structures
	brain
Neck: *Vertebral canal* of *dorsal* cavity	Larynx, trachea, esophagus, parathyroid and thyroid glands
	spinal cord (extends down to pelvic cavity)
Trunk: Ventral (stomach side):	Thorax plus abdomen
Thoracic cavity:	Large blood vessels; esophagus (food pipe); trachea (wind pipe); bronchi; thoracic duct; breasts
Pleural cavity	Lungs
Pericardial cavity	Heart; thymus gland
Abdominal cavity:	Stomach, small intestine, most of large intestine; liver; pancreas; spleen; gall bladder; kidneys; adrenal glands; urinary tract
Pelvic cavity:	Urinary bladder; sigmoid colon; rectum; reproductive organs: Male: seminal vesicles; part of the vas deferens; prostate gland. Female: ovaries; uterus; vagina; uterine tubes

Extremities:	Fingers; hands; wrists; forearms; elbows; upper arms; shoulders (Pectoral Girdle); toes; feet; ankles; lower legs; knees; thighs; hips

A final thought

Again, using the symphony orchestra analog, one can appreciate the fact that the entire human organism—as an integrated, functioning unit—relies on the *collective* mission of all organ systems acting in concert. Imagine what it would sound like, and the chaos that would result if every section of an orchestra simply went off on its own to "do its thing" without regard for whatever else the rest of the orchestra was doing. Talk about a cacophony and musical dissonance! Indeed, just like each section of the orchestra, no one organ system is self-contained and independent of any other; no one of them could exist without the help of the others. One string section does not an orchestra make! It's a team effort among strings, winds, and percussion— cooperative, controlled, integrated, coordinated, optimized, fine-tuned, holistic! The human body is, indeed, a "symphony orchestra" attempting to harmonize at its finest—to create a *physiologic consonance!* Therefore, as a music therapist, you must view the entire organism *holistically*—not concentrating your clinical intervention or management of a client on any one system of the body to the exclusion of any other. With that in mind, and considering the hierarchy of anatomic levels of organization, let us take a closer look at some of the elegant and unique design principles that are exploited in this marvelous "piece of work that is a human being."

CHAPTER 2

The Living Engine/Instrument

In the Preface, we pointed out that *Feature 1* of the seven attributes—on the basis of which, a convenient paradigm to study the anatomy and physiology of the human body can be formulated—is that we recognize it to be a *living engine* (or, to the music therapist, a sophisticated musical instrument). Indeed, our body:

- takes in and creates an air (oxygen)/fuel (food) mixture

- derives useful energy from this mixture by "burning" (oxidizing, metabolizing) some of it

- uses that energy to do work, i.e., to drive all of the body's processes and activities

- exhausts the waste products of metabolism to the environment.

In fact, no less than five major organ systems, occupying:

- virtually all of the trunk—i.e., the thoracic, or chest cavity, plus the abdominal, or "belly" cavity, separated from one another by the muscular *diaphragm*

- much of the extremities (arms and legs)

- significant portions of both the head (face, skull, brain) and neck

are concerned with this one single attribute shared by all living organisms (Schneck 2005a). This attribute, in the context of the useful mechanical work output of the human organism (Chapter 3), "officially" classifies it as an *electrochemical* engine.

Notice, I did *not* say a "heat" engine—which is what your automobile is—I said an *electrochemical* engine. The distinction has to do with the *temperature* at which the engine operates. Our "engine" operates at a relatively constant temperature—37° Celsius, or 98.6° Fahrenheit—i.e., it is an *isothermal* engine. Automobile engines are not—in fact, they *cannot* operate at a constant temperature (Schneck 2005b). So basic is this isothermal requirement to how our body works, that it deserves some special consideration.

An isothermal living engine

When we say that an organism is "living," we mean several things, among them that it is *able to convert energy into usable forms that drive controlled, purposeful activities in support of both its, and its species' survival*. Indeed, "living" is all about energy conversions, called *transduction*, and the "activities" driven by energy transduction concern, first and foremost, those that are directly concerned with survival of the self! Moreover, such activities can be attributed to the function of the human body as a sophisticated *electrochemical* engine that produces a mechanical output (Chapter 3). But…why an *isothermal* (constant temperature) engine? Why are we warm-blooded *homeotherms*, creatures that maintain a (nearly) *constant* internal temperature at all times? Why does the adult "me" that we are talking about here operate at a relatively *constant* core temperature of 37°C, plus or minus about 1°C? Indeed:

- "plus 2°C" (i.e., 39°C or 102.2°F) in the adult organism already defines a condition of *hyper-* (too much) *-thermia* (heat)
- plus 3°C is a severe *fever* (Latin, *fervere*, "to grow warm")
- 41°C is critical, including the potential for severe brain lesions
- 43°C results in *heat stroke*
- 44°C is usually fatal
- a sustained body core temperature of 45.6°C (114°F) is the highest recorded limit at which an individual could actually survive, but for only a brief period of time.

Going the other way:

- "minus 2°C" (i.e., 35°C or 95°F) in the adult organism defines a condition of *hypo-* (too little) *-thermia* (heat)
- minus 5°C results in unconsciousness
- 26°C (78.8°F) is usually fatal
- a sustained body core temperature of 23.3°C (74°F) is the lowest ever recorded in an individual who actually survived, but could do so for only a brief period of time in the absence of carefully controlled and monitored cryogenic conditions.

Again, "Why must the human engine be isothermal?" you ask. The answer begins by first noting that if left unto their own, critical biochemical reactions involved in human body metabolism would not proceed at a rate compatible with the sustenance of life, for two basic reasons:

1. there is no guarantee that the right biochemical reactions will occur, at the right time, in the right place, involving the right substrates, to successfully meet the instantaneous metabolic needs of the organism

2. even if (1) were not an issue, there is no guarantee that appropriate metabolic reactions—if allowed to occur at a spontaneous, random rate—would be taking place fast enough to ensure that the metabolic needs of the organism were being adequately met for survival. In fact, the likelihood is exactly the opposite, i.e., that these reactions would probably be taking place much too slowly for that to be the case.

Thus, enter the physiologic equivalent of the Yiddish, "Yenta, the matchmaker"— the *enzyme!*

Enzymes are proteins produced in living cells that catalyze (without being themselves affected) biochemical reactions, such that these reactions proceed at rates as high as a *trillion times* (or more!) the uncatalyzed rate! (Schneck 1990). These biochemical "matchmakers" are manufactured from "recipes" encoded into the cell's "cook book," i.e., the human genome. The *right* (substrate-specific) recipes in the genetic code are activated to expression by the appearance in the cell of the corresponding substrates to be metabolized. In other words, the substrates themselves trigger their own demise! Thus, enzymes not only speed up biochemical reactions, but, by being species-specific, also ensure that the right reactions will be occurring, at the right time, in the right place. *However*, in order for the appropriate enzyme to "do its thing," it must not only be manufactured—as an *inactive apoenzyme*—but must also be properly "activated."

Being "active" means that the physical geometric configuration of an enzyme (i.e., the geometry of its "binding sites") is exactly congruent with the geometry of the substrate molecules that it serves, so that these molecules can properly "dock" to the biochemical catalyst. Several factors contribute to activating biochemical enzymes, among them:

- *co-enzymes*, including *vitamins* of the B-complex. The combination of an activating coenzyme with an inactive apoenzyme forms an active complex known as a "complete," or *holoenzyme*

- *co-factors*, including inorganic *mineral ions*, such as magnesium, iron, zinc, chromium, and some others of the "trace" elements listed in Table 1.1

- substances that mediate electron transfer—such as *quinones* that are chemically similar to vitamins E and K

- you guessed it—*temperature!*

The stereochemical (geometric) architecture (configuration) of enzymes is strongly temperature sensitive. Temperatures not too far on either side of 37°C can quickly *denature* (make "unnatural") biochemical enzymes, by rendering their structural characteristics totally impotent for catalytic purposes. In other words, heat or cold can "warp" enzyme structure in a manner that destroys their proper physical integrity. Such destruction deactivates enzymes, effectively bringing body metabolism to a grinding halt, with obvious consequences. So…bottom line: *maintaining body temperature at or near 37°C is critical for keeping biochemical enzymes from becoming denatured*, and thus helping to ensure that they will function properly in catalyzing those reactions that guarantee efficient and effective metabolic function.

"But," you continue, "how does the body avoid generating heat as it goes about the process of living?" The answer is, "it doesn't!" What it *does* do (as elaborated on further in Chapter 3) is operate according to optimization principles of *cascading reactions* and *reaction coupling* (Schneck 1990, 1992, 2005b) to develop a paradigm that (a) encourages the *storage*, as opposed to dissipation, of useful energy; (b) minimizes the *rate* at which heat is generated (or lost); and (c) optimizes the rapid *removal* of what heat *is* generated—especially when the environmental temperature is high (as in panting, sweating, etc.)—so that heat doesn't "hang around" long enough to raise body core temperature by a significant amount (see Chapter 3). Conversely, when environmental temperature is low, i.e., under "cold stress," the body endeavors to conserve body core temperature by (a) "pouring more coal on the fire" (this is a thyroid-gland-mediated *calorigenic effect*); and (b) minimizing the loss of heat to the environment (mostly via cardiovascular-mediated *peripheral vasoconstriction*). For the interested reader, details can be found in Schneck (1990, 1992, 2005b) and we shall have a bit more to say about this in later chapters. For now, we return to our examination of the five organ systems that have to do with *Feature 1: The living, isothermal, electrochemical engine:*

1. Alimentary (digestive) system: *ingestion, digestion*

2. Respiratory system: *respiration*

3. Circulatory systems (cardiovascular and lymphatic): *circulation*

4. Renal (urological) system: *urination/excretion*

5. Excretory: *egestion*

The alimentary (digestive) system

As illustrated in Table 2.1, the alimentary canal (from the Latin *alimentum*, meaning "nourishment"), otherwise known as the digestive system (from the Latin *digestio*, meaning "taking apart"), is a collection of organs and passages by which food is taken into the body and desirable ingredients contained in it are made absorbable by mechanically and enzymatically "taking them apart." What we are dealing with in Feature 1 of our anatomy/physiology paradigm is essentially a five-step "-tion," process, i.e., ingestion/digestion, respiration, circulation, urination/excretion, and egestion. The alimentary canal handles at least two of them, and a part of the third, to wit: ingestion/digestion, egestion, and excretion.

Table 2.1 Major anatomical features of the alimentary system

ANATOMICAL STRUCTURE

- System inlet: lips; tongue; mouth; Epiglottis (leafy valve)
  - ° 32 permanent teeth:
    - › 8 incisors
    - › 4 canines
    - › 8 premolars
    - › 12 molars
  - ° 6 salivary glands; 2 each:
    - › Parotid (near the ear)
    - › Submaxillary (beneath the lower jaw)
    - › Sublingual (under tongue)
  - ° Auxiliary buccal glands
  - ° Pharynx (throat)
  - ° Uvula and soft palate
  - ° Fauces
- Esophagus (food pipe):
  - ° Cardiac orifice
- Stomach ("mixer"):
  - ° Cardiac portion
  - ° Fundus
  - ° Main body
  - ° Pylorus portion
  - ° Pylorus sphincter
- Small intestine:
  - ° Duodenum
  - ° Ligament of trietz
  - ° Jejunum
  - ° Ileum
  - ° Mesentery (attaching "middle of intestine" to rear of abdomen)
  - ° Ileocecal valve
  - ° Cecum
- Peritoneum (abdominal cavity lining)
- Vermiform appendix
- Large intestine

  - › Ascending colon
  - › Transverse colon
  - › Descending colon
  - › "S"-shaped sigmoid colon
  - ° System outlet:
    - › Rectum
    - › Anal canal
    - › Anus
- Auxiliary organs:
  - ° 4 lobes of liver
  - ° Gall bladder (stores bile)
  - ° Common bile duct
  - ° Pancreas
  - ° Duct of Wirsung
  - ° Pancreatic Islets of Langerhans
- Major secretions:
  - ° Ptyalin (salivary amylase for starch)
  - ° Stomach hydrochloric acid
  - ° Stomach pepsin for protein
  - ° Liver bile for lipids
  - ° Amylopsin (pancreatic amylase for starch)
  - ° Pancreatic maltase
  - ° Pancreatic sucrase
  - ° Pancreatic lactase
  - ° Trypsin (pancreatic enzyme for proteins)
  - ° Pancreatic chymotrypsin
  - ° Pancreatic peptidases
  - ° Steapsin (pancreatic enzyme for fats)
- Serviced by splanchnic (visceral), mesenteric (intestinal), hepatic (liver), renal (kidney) and Celiac ("belly," abdominal) Circulatory pathways

The alimentary canal

INGESTION

Food (nutrients) enters the body—is *ingested*—through the mouth, and is partially prepared to be absorbed by being mechanically and chemically broken down into very small sizes.

- The *mechanical* breakdown is accomplished by chewing—utilizing the jaw (*mandible,* from the the Latin, *mandibulum*) muscles and 32 permanent teeth to bite, crush, and grind the food to a pulp, in a process called *mastication* (from the Greek *mastichân,* meaning "gnash the teeth").

- The chemical breakdown is accomplished by the action of various enzymes contained in the *saliva* secreted by the body's three pairs of salivary glands. Most of it (70%) is derived from the *submaxillary glands,* with lesser amounts being secreted by the *parotid* (25%), and *sublingual glands* (5%). Also contributing to the manufacture and secretion of saliva are small, auxiliary *buccal* (Latin, "cheek") *glands* situated in the mucous membranes of the mouth. Saliva contains the enzyme *ptyalin* (salivary amylase), that begins the breakdown of carbohydrates—specifically, starch—into the sugar, *maltose.*

The chewed, partially digested food is now swallowed—i.e., passed through an aperture called the *fauces* (from the Latin for "throat")—into a cavity called the *pharynx* (from the Greek for "windpipe," or "throat"). From there, it continues over the *epiglottis*—the thin, leaf-shaped "valve" located immediately behind the root of the tongue that guards the entrance to the larynx (voice box)—and into the *esophagus,* the food pipe. Travelling down this 23–25.5 cm (9–10 inch) long pipe, the soft food mass exits through a *cardiac orifice* into a 50 ml—but able to expand to a capacity of as much as a liter (in some cases, even more!)—chamber called the *stomach.* It is located in the abdominal cavity, just under the diaphragm.

The stomach serves primarily as a storage ("gas") tank. The partially digested food will spend several hours here, being further churned and mixed as it passes through three regions—the *cardiac, fundus,* and *main body* chambers—while being subjected to still more digestive enzymes. This organ secretes two to three liters per day of hydrochloric acid and gastric juices that mostly change proteins into peptones—via the enzyme *pepsin*—and curdle milk. Some ptyalin is also secreted to convert starch (Greek, *amylum*) into maltose, but otherwise not much digestion of fats and carbohydrates takes place in the stomach. Rather, the vast majority of the digestive process continues as the churned food, now called *chyme,* passes from the stomach through the *pylorus sphincter* (the circular muscle constricting an opening) into the long (as much as 9m, or 29.5 foot), 1–4 cm-wide coiled tubing called the *small intestine.*

DIGESTION

Before we take a closer look at the small intestine, where virtually all of digestion proper takes place, we note that it is assisted in its digestive function by three major *auxiliary organs*:

- Four-lobed *liver*, weighing some 3.5 lbs, located in the upper right part of the abdomen, under the dome of the diaphragm, almost straddling the stomach. As mentioned in Chapter 1, the digestive function of the liver is to manufacture *bile*, a *lipolytic* enzyme that emulsifies (breaks down large globules of) fat so that it can be easily absorbed. This organ manufactures some 500–1000 mls of bile daily, which is sent to, concentrated by, and stored in the *gall bladder*.

- *Gall bladder*—the bile manufactured by the liver is sent to a pear-shaped storage sac located on the undersurface of the right lobe of the liver. The capacity of the *gall bladder* is some 50–75 ml of concentrated bile, which is equivalent to 1.5 pints (just under 750 ml) of liver bile. As needed during the digestive process, the gall bladder dispatches bile to the duodenum of the small intestine via the *common bile duct*, which joins the *pancreatic duct* as they enter this first portion of the small intestine.

- *Pancreas*—this second largest gland in the body is located behind the stomach, lying in a horizontal position just in front of the first and second lumbar vertebrae. It secretes about two liters per day of pancreatic juices that enter the small intestine through the above-mentioned *pancreatic duct* (*Duct of Wirsung*). These juices help in the digestion of proteins (via the *proteolytic* enzymes *trypsin*, and *chymotrypsin*), carbohydrates (via the enzymes *amylopsin, lactase, maltase,* and *sucrase*), and fats (via the *lipolytic* enzymes *lipases*—specifically one known as *steapsin*). The pancreatic *Islets Of Langerhans* also have important endocrine functions that shall be addressed more specifically in Chapter 6.

So…continuing down the alimentary canal, the milky chyme—now called a *bolus*—tootles along the elongated small intestine which itself manufactures and secretes into its interior (*lumen*) various *intestinal juices* (mainly *succus entericus*). *Succus entericus* helps to digest proteins—via the enzyme *erepsin*—and carbohydrates—via the enzyme *invertase*. The "tootling along" is helped by progressive undulations of the intestinal wall. These are of two types:

- Local *rhythmic segmenting muscular contractions* provide "sectional" impetus to the contents of the intestine.

- Regional *peristalsis*, generated by periodic, regularly alternating contractions of longitudinal and circular smooth muscle tissue embedded in the intestinal wall, sends waves propagating down the entire length of the intestine every few seconds. Each wave only lasts a few seconds and typically travels along the tube at speeds of only a few centimeters per second, but collectively, the waves help mix the intestinal contents as they move it along.

Speaking of which, from *duodenum* (entrance) to *ileum* (exit):

- proteins in the bolus are broken down into amino acids

- carbohydrates are broken down into simple sugars

- fats are broken down into small droplets (*chylomicrons*) containing short-chain fatty acids

- glycerol, vitamins, minerals, and certain other products of digestion are all made small enough to be absorbed.

The absorption takes place across the thin walls of arteriolar/capillary/lymphatic networks of vessels that permeate the *villi* of the intestinal lining. Recall from our discussion in Chapter 1 of *cell membranes* and *epithelial tissue*, that *villi* and *microvilli* are tiny, finger-like microscopic projections, each coated with a single layer of epithelial cells that, themselves, have on their surface, as many as 3000–6000 *microvilli*. All together, the microvilli, villi, and circular folds (called *Folds of Kerckring*) of the wall of the small intestine increase its ability to absorb nutrients by a factor of about 600, compared with what the internal surface area for absorption would be for the same size vessel if it was simply a cylindrical tube having smooth internal walls. Keep that in mind—it's a basic design principle that is exploited throughout the body, i.e.:

> *Anatomical design principle number 1: A very effective way to "squeeze" huge geometric regions into very confined spaces is to make the boundary of the regions very irregular, i.e., fold it, make it very tortuous or "crumple" it up (as you would do with a large sheet of paper when you wish to compress it into a small ball).*

While we're at it, keep something else in mind, too: although the alimentary canal is a continuous tube that is "typically" around 26 feet long or more from lips to anus, *only the duodenum and a very small initial segment of the jejunum are absolutely essential to the body.*

The former is the first 20–30 cms (just under a foot) of the small intestine, measuring roughly three times the width across four extended fingers of the hand—hence its name *duodenum*—derived from the Latin, *duodo-* (a prefix meaning, "twelve") and *numerare* (meaning "to count"). The *jejunum* (Latin, "empty," because of its presumed state after death) is the next 8 feet (~2.4 m) of intestinal tubing—but we only "need" about the same initial length of it as are the "twelve fingers" of duodenum, i.e., just under a foot. The jejunum is demarcated from the duodenum by the *Ligament of Trietz*. At its other end, it is connected to the final three-fifths of the small intestine—the 2–4 m *ileum*. It, along with most of the jejunum, *may be removed with no significant impairment of digestive function!* This illustrates another anatomical design principle:

> *Anatomical design principle number 2: The human body is endowed with redundancy and back-up systems.*

Thus, we have the ability to remove entire (or significant portions of) anatomical organs—such as the *tonsils*, and small *vermiform appendix* opening into the *cecum*—without seriously impairing overall physiologic function. Also, when necessary, another organ or tissue can take over the function of the organ that has been lost. This is typically the case, for example, when the liver takes over for the gall bladder, or the spleen, should either or both of these have to be removed for whatever reason.

Finally, re-emphasizing our need to be an *isothermal* engine, take special note of the fact that all digestive processes are *enzymatically controlled*—which is to say, for proper digestion:

> *The right enzyme must be manufactured, at the right time, in the right amount; and it must appear in the right place, in an activated form, ready to go to work.*

If any of these criteria should fail, then the nutrient that depends on that enzyme for proper disposition will either:

- not be absorbed at all

- be absorbed in only a partially digested form that the body's immune system might/will interpret as a "foreign body," thus triggering an immune response to that nutrient (Frazier 1974; Graedon and Graedon 2007; Schneck 2004). In turn, the recipe for an enzyme is coded into the genome, so if the code is missing, or otherwise corrupted, or adversely mutated, the individual so afflicted will suffer from food allergies or various levels of intolerance (Graedon and Graedon 2007).

Thus:

> *As a music therapist, in your clinical assessment of a client you should always be on the look-out for such adverse reactions to food. It's a diagnostic parameter that is all too often overlooked or completely ignored…and certainly not fully appreciated when evaluating a patient.*

That having been said, it is also important to note that ingested food usually contains some *indigestible*, non-usable, or otherwise undesirable material that has no useful purpose in metabolism and so must be discarded (egested). This is also true for things inadvertently swallowed, like paper clips, benign poisons, chewing gum, tobacco products, and other strange objects that seem to find their way into the esophagus. Thus, enter the large intestine.

EGESTION

Leaving the small intestine, whatever has not been absorbed continues through the *ileocecal valve* into the *cecum*, a pouch-like outpocketing at the junction of the *ileum* with the *ascending colon*, lying slightly below the ileocecal valve. Attached to the lower part of the cecum is the *vermiform* ("worm-shaped") *appendix*, that is endowed with a large amount of lymphoid tissue.

The cecum is the very first portion of the *large intestine*—a 150 cm (about 5 foot) long channel that extends from the ileum to the anus, and also includes the colon and rectum. The colon has a sort of upside down U-shape, with a vertical *ascending* portion, a horizontal *transverse* portion (the longest part), a *descending* portion, and a terminal *sigmoid* ("s-shaped") portion which acts as a storage tank. The sigmoid colon can hold material for as long as 9.5 hours before releasing it into the *rectum*—the terminal inch or so of which is called the *anal canal*. Finally, we reach the alimentary canal exit, the *anus*, which exhausts the contents—*feces*, or "stool"—of the large intestine to the exterior. Total travel time through the entire alimentary canal, from lips to anus, can vary from as little as 12 hours, to as many as 24 hours, depending on the nature and consistency of the food being digested. Moreover, this passageway is the only part of the body that is open to the environment at both ends, so technically it is not really an "internal" system/cavity of the body.

Okay, so through our digestive system—also referred to as the *gastrointestinal*, or "GI" tract—we have now secured our engine's "fuel." We have "gassed-up," harnessed the energy derived from food sources (which in turn got theirs originally by *transduction* of solar energy or some other means of *ingestion*). But in order to use this fuel—which you will recall from Chapter 1 is eventually *stored* in the high-energy bonds of adenosine triphosphate (ATP, our body's "battery")—we must add air to it to produce an "air/fuel" mixture that can be metabolized. Indeed, metabolism requires that an *oxygen-dependent*, enzyme-catalyzed splitting of high-energy ATP bonds takes place in order to *release* the stored energy that drives all physiologic processes. Our source of oxygen is the *respiratory system.*

The respiratory system

This system, itemized in Table 2.2, is a collection of organs, tissues, and passages by which air is taken into the body (*inspired*) and oxygen is extracted from it, in exchange for carbon dioxide, water vapor, and heat, all being expelled (*expired*).

Table 2.2 Major anatomical features of the respiratory system

ANATOMICAL STRUCTURE

- Upper respiratory tract:
  - Nasal cavity, mouth, nose
    - Sinuses: paranasal groups
    - 2 frontal; 2 maxillary; Paired sphenoidal; Paired ethmoidal
  - Epiglottis; Uvula; Pharynx:
    - nasopharynx
    - oropharynx
    - laryngopharynx
  - Tonsils:
    - palatine
    - pharyngeal (adenoids)
  - Cartilage:
    - arytenoid; cricoid
    - cuneiform; epiglottic
    - Thyroid ("Adam's Apple")
  - Larynx ("voice box")
    - Ventricular/vestibular folds ("false" vocal cords)
    - Vocal folds/glottis ("true" vocal cords)
    - Vocal ligaments
  - Glottis ("back of the tongue")
  - Trachea ("wind pipe"); carina
- Lower respiratory tract:
  - Left and right primary bronchi
  - 16 generations of lobar bronchi
  - 66,000 bronchioles
  - 3 transitional generations of bronchi
  - 525,000 respiratory bronchioles
  - 3 respiratory generations of bronchi
  - 14 million alveolar ducts
  - 300 million air sacs (alveoli)
  - Three-lobed right lung
  - Two-lobed left lung
  - Mediastinum (middle wall)
  - Diaphragm/chest muscles
  - Pleural lining of the chest
- Lung volumes:
  - TLC = total lung capacity; Maximal *inspiration* = VC + RV
    - (Male/female = 6/4 liters) VC = vital capacity:
  - VC = vital capacity: TV + IRV + ERV Maximal *expiration* = (5/6)TLC
  - RV = residual volume = (1/6)TLC
  - ERV = expiratory reserve
    - Volume ≈ (1/3) x TLC FRC = functional residual
    - Capacity= RV + ERV = 0.5 x TLC
  - IRV = inspiratory reserve
    - Volume ≈ 0.4167 x TLC
  - TV = tidal volume ≈0.0833 x TLC
    - approximately 500 mℓ Air
  - IC = inspiratory capacity =
    - TV + IRV ≈ 0.5 x TLC
- Respiratory zones/volume percent:
  - Non-respiratory = 10 percent (trachea down to 17th generation)
  - Respiratory alveoli = 52 percent
  - Respiratory bronchioles = 32 percent
  - Remaining 6 percent = tissue and blood Vessel respiratory capacity
  - TLC = Non-respiratory + alveoli + bronchioles + tissue and blood vessel zones = VC + RV
- Serviced by: main, left, and right bronchial arteries branching into tissue-*feeding* networks; Pulmonary artery dividing into 6 main branches down to 3.25 billion capillary networks involved in blood *processing*

Upper respiratory tract

INSPIRATION

Air enters and leaves the body through the mouth (*oral cavity*) and/or nose (*nasal cavity*). At rest, each "entering"—*inspiration* or *inhalation*—takes in about 500 ml of air. This is called the *tidal volume* (TV). During inspiration, air is literally *sucked* into the body as a result of the activity of the musculature of the rib cage (*costal inspiration*) and the *diaphragm* (*abdominal inspiration*). The latter results in deeper breathing.

Indeed, 500 ml of air is a mere twelfth of the six-liter *total lung capacity* (TLC) for men. TLC is about four liters for women. Thus, if one tries really, really hard, one can *forcibly* inhale much more air, over five times as much as is inspired during quiet breathing. This *additional* amount of air inspired, over and above the TV during deepest breathing, is called the *inspiratory reserve volume* (IRV), which can be as high as 2500 ml for men and 1667 ml for women. Note, however, that the sum of TV plus IRV, called one's *inspiratory capacity* (IC), is still only about 50 percent (up to 60%) of TLC. We shall address the remaining 40–50 percent—which has to do with air that is already occupying lung space and therefore preventing further inspiration—in the next section.

EXPIRATION

The diaphragm and rib-cage muscles can also *force* air out of the body in a process called *expiration* or *exhalation*. At rest, this cyclic inhalation-exhalation breathing in the adult generally ranges between 16 and 18 breaths per minute, the so-called *breathing rate;* it is an important "vital sign." Again, though, if one tries really, really hard, one can *forcibly* expel much more air than is normal during quiet breathing. That *additional* amount of air exhaled over and above TV is called one's *expiratory reserve volume* (ERV), which is typically around a third of TLC—i.e., 2 liters for men; 1.33 liters for women.

Thus, one's *vital capacity* (VC), which is the sum of IRV, TV, and ERV, is the maximum amount of air that one can *expel*, forcibly, from the TLC during a single breath. Note that it amounts to only five-sixths of TLC because it is virtually impossible to completely empty the lungs of air. To do so would cause them to collapse. Thus, to keep the lungs at least a sixth inflated at all times, a certain amount of *residual volume* (RV) is always left trapped behind in the lungs during maximal, forced expiration. The sum of RV and ERV then accounts for the remaining 50 percent of TLC that we were missing above. This sum is called the *functional residual capacity* (FRC) of the lungs, it being the amount of air typically left behind in them during quiet breathing.

ANATOMICAL FEATURES OF THE UPPER RESPIRATORY TRACT

As the TV passes through the nasal cavities and epithelium-lined paranasal group of *sinuses* (see Table 2.2), it is filtered, moistened, and warmed en route to a musculo-membranous, elliptical, resonating chamber in the back of the throat, called the *pharynx*. Along its major, front-to-back/top-to-bottom axis, it is divided into three sections:

- a *naso-pharynx* originating at the back of the nose near the base of the skull, which leads into

- an *oro-pharynx*, which carries the TV past the *hyoid* (Greek, "U-shaped") bone at the root of the tongue, en route to

- the *laryngo-pharynx* that includes the *larynx* ("voice box")—located in the neck at about the level of the sixth vertebra—and below which the pharynx becomes continuous with the food pipe, i.e., the *esophagus*, located behind the cartilaginous wind pipe, or *trachea*.

Along the way, one encounters:

- a 3–4 cm-long auditory, or *eustachian* tube connecting the naso-pharynx to the middle ear in order to equalize the pressure on both sides of the ear drum

- an *epiglottis* valve located just above the laryngo-pharynx, guarding the entrance to the larynx (and wind pipe), so that food will be directed into the food pipe when one swallows

- *pharyngeal* ("adenoid") and *palatine tonsils* that help to both filter invading bacteria from the tidal volume, and aid in the formation of white blood cells.

THE LARYNX

Of particular interest to musicians, the larynx is a perfect example of a biological, "double-reed" wind instrument—a sound-generating organ that gives voice to the body! Anatomically the "voice box" is a musculo-cartilageneous enlargement of the upper end of the trachea, just below the pharynx. It is constructed of nine cartilages—three single ones and three paired ones—all connected by an elastic membrane (see Table 2.2). Mechanically, the larynx is moved by a sophisticated set of both extrinsic ("from without") and intrinsic ("from within") muscles.

The sound-generating portion of the wind instrument is the two pairs of folds (hence, "double-reed") located in the cavity of the larynx—the *ventricular folds* or "false vocal cords," and the *vocal folds* or "true vocal cords." Separating the true vocal cords is a very narrow slit between them, the *rima glottidis* or simply, *glottis* (from the Greek for "back of the tongue"), which is the actual sound-producing apparatus of the larynx. If you have ever held two blades of grass tightly between your thumbs, and blown forcibly through a narrow slit between them to produce a sound, then you know how the vocal cords work.

In the larynx, exhaled air is blown forcibly through the rima glottidis between the vocal cords ("blades of grass"), causing them to vibrate at a frequency determined by their state of tension at the time, and the velocity and intensity of the air passing through them. The variable tension is controlled by the musculature of the larynx, helped along by *vocal ligaments* interspersed among the cartilage. The higher the tension, the higher the pitch of sound produced, and vice versa.

Similarly, the shorter and thinner the vocal cords are, the higher the pitch of sound produced, and vice versa. That's why women—with vocal cord lengths varying from 9 to 13 mm—have higher-pitched voices than do men, whose vocal cord lengths vary from 15 to 20 mm, and within each gender, there are basses, baritones, tenors, altos, various types of sopranos, and so on.

The typical lips-to-vocal cords distance is about 17 cm (some 6.7 inches). The voice box itself is divided into *vestibular, ventricular*, and *inferior* regions, the latter being the actual *entrance to the glottis*. After leaving the larynx, the tidal volume continues into the 11 cm long (about 4.33 inches) *trachea*, or "wind pipe," that terminates at the *carina*, leading into the *lower respiratory tract*. Before examining the latter, let's pause briefly here to mention that, in addition to the music therapist being sensitive to and looking for food allergies that derive from a dysfunctional *alimentary canal*, he or she must also recognize that some clients—especially those that are totally non-verbal, or otherwise suffering from various speech impediments—might very well have subtle anatomical/physiological issues that derive from a dysfunctional *respiratory system*. Thus, be on the lookout for troubled or asthmatic breathing, and/ or impaired air flow through the larynx due to a compromised musculoskeletal system airway obstructions, and/or congenital birth defects that may have led to a malformed laryngeal architecture.

ANATOMICAL FEATURES OF THE LOWER RESPIRATORY TRACT

As was the case for the alimentary canal, the respiratory tract, too, is concerned with maximizing the trans-cellular area available for absorbing or discharging material into or out of the body respectively—but also doing so in a very restricted space (basically the thoracic or chest cavity). The lower *digestive* tract—confined to the abdominal cavity—uses *Anatomical design principle number 1* to accomplish this goal effectively—i.e., making the walls of the canal tortuous and endowing it with a plethora of "fin-like projections" (villi and microvilli). The lower *respiratory* tract employs yet another effective design principle to accomplish this same goal:

> *Anatomical design principle number 3: Hollow out the interior of the confined region using a complex branching pattern that generates a network of increasingly larger numbers of smaller and smaller vessels.*

This is a design principle that, as we shall see, is also exploited in the branching networks of the kidney, cardiovascular and lymphatic systems, and the nervous system.

Thus, starting at the trachea, the "bronchial tree," as it is called, progresses through 16 generations of bifurcating "forks" as it descends systematically into the various lobes of the two (right and left) lungs. These include the *right and left superior* ("towards the head") *lobes, right middle lobe,* and *right and left inferior* ("towards the feet") *lobes.* Note that the right lung has three lobes, accounting for 55 percent of the TLC, whereas the left lung has only two, accounting for 45 percent of the TLC. It is smaller and more confined because it needs to leave room for the heart on the left side of the thoracic cavity.

The first branching fork has the trachea dividing into *right and left primary bronchi* that conduct the tidal volume into the right and left lungs, respectively. This is followed by 15 downstream bifurcations that ultimately generate over 65.5 thousand *lobar bronchi.* These are strictly *conducting* pathways—no gas exchange occurs anywhere along this network, which is why it is designated as the *conducting zone* of the respiratory system. In fact, from the trachea, down to the 17th generation, we have a *non-respiratory zone* accounting for only about 10 percent of the volume of the respiratory system.

Generations 17–18–19 are called the *transitional zone,* which now includes both bi- and tri-furcating networks that create 525,000 *respiratory bronchioles* that account for another 32 percent of the respiratory system volume. Continuing, generations 20–21–22 are called, collectively, the *respiratory zone.* This is an irregularly branching region that terminates in some 14 million *alveolar ducts.* Added to the volume occupied by respiratory tissue and blood vessels, we have now accounted for nearly half (48%) of the volume of the lungs.

The other half (52%) is attributed to what takes place by the last, 23rd generation, where we find that the alveolar ducts have finally distributed themselves into grape-like clusters containing a total of approximately 300 million *alveoli,* from the Latin, *alveolus,* meaning "a small hollow or cavity." Indeed, alveoli are tiny, 100–350-micron-diameter "air sacs" (*note:* a micron is one millionth of a meter). These are inundated with about ten times that many tiny blood vessels—*capillaries*—averaging 7–9 microns in diameter, by about 0.5–1.00 mm in length. Thus a network is formed that facilitates the absorption of oxygen from the TV, and the release into it of carbon dioxide and water. Oxygen is not very water soluble, and so is "carried" by red blood cells as an *oxyhemoglobin complex.* Water is exhaled as water vapor, which takes with it, 20 percent or more of the heat generated by physiologic metabolic processes.

Some three quarters of the tidal respiration is attributable to the activity of the muscular diaphragm that separates the thoracic and abdominal cavities. The diaphragm flattens out with each inspiration, allowing the bases of the lungs to descend in the thoracic cavity as they "suck" air in; it assumes a convex-upward configuration with each expiration, forcing up the bases of the lungs. About 25 percent of the TV results from the expansion and contraction of the chest wall.

Two last points on respiration:

- Recall that the alimentary canal has a built-in redundancy (*Anatomical design principle number 2*) that allows us to live a full life with huge portions of it removed. The same is true for the lungs. For example, we have *two* relatively *large* ones (see Table 1.7). The fact is, that if necessary, one entire lung can usually be removed with only a minimal impairment of physiologic function; and in extreme cases, even significant portions of the remaining lung can be excised before the situation actually becomes life threatening.

- *Unlike* the alimentary canal, however, the respiratory tract only opens to the environment at one end—operating very much like a bellows. It expands to take in air and contracts to expel it, both events taking place through the same *tracheal* tube. During the swallowing process, the larynx is mechanically raised to push it up, so that it seats firmly against the *epiglottis.* Thus is sealed-off the entrance to the larynx, preventing food or liquids from entering the trachea. You can feel this if you hold your forefinger in front of your throat, at the top of the "Adam's Apple" (the laryngeal prominence), and swallow. As you do so, you will feel the trachea rise and then fall.

Okay, so thanks to the alimentary canal and respiratory tract, we now have our air/ fuel mixture. But how do we get it to all of the cells and tissues of the body? Answer: through a sophisticated transportation system—the *circulation.*

The circulatory system

The *circulatory system* is actually three systems in one (see Table 2.3): a *cardiovascular division* that includes: (1) a *pulmonary circulation* connected in series to a (2) *systemic circulation;* and (3) a parallel *lymphatic division* that eventually drains back into the venous side of the systemic circulation. There are also *auxiliary organs and tissues,* such as the *spleen, liver,* and *bone marrow.*

Table 2.3 Major anatomical features of the circulatory system

ANATOMICAL STRUCTURE

- Heart (~7 percent of total blood volume)
- Systemic circulation: ~84 percent of total blood volume
  - Aorta—32 main branches
  - Arterial system
    - 5,000 Blood vessels divide into ~500,000 terminal branches
  - Microcirculation—down to >16 billion capillaries
  - Venous system—nearly 500,000 collecting branches Converge to form ~21,000 various sized veins
  - Vena cava—collect blood from about 500 branches
- Pulmonary circulation (lungs): ~ 9 percent of total blood volume
  - Pulmonary artery—6 main branches eventually lead to ~140,000 terminal branches
  - Microcirculation—down to ~3.25 billion capillaries
  - Venous system—about 35,000 collecting branches
  - Pulmonary veins—4 of them Collect blood from about 64 branches and veins
- Blood (5.2 Liters)
  - Erythrocytes (~5.2 x 10^6/mm^3) Leukocytes (~7500/mm^3); WBC
    - Granulocytes (5175/mm^3)
      - Neutrophils (65 percent WBC)
      - Basophils (1 percent WBC)
      - Acidophils (3 percent WBC)
    - Agranulocytes (2325/mm^3)
      - Lymphocytes (25 percent WBC)
      - Monocytes (6 percent WBC)
  - Thrombocytes (~2.675 x 10^5/mm^3)
- Blood plasma (~ 2860 mℓ)

- Lymphatic system:
  - Lymphatic capillaries originate as microscopic, open-ended, funnel-like "blind" entrances in the tissue spaces of body
  - Capillary collecting plexuses
  - Lymphatic channels
  - Terminal collecting lymphatics
  - Large collecting vessels equal in number to (2x) blood vessels
    - Deep set
    - Superficial set
  - Five major trunks:
    - Bronchomediastinal
    - Jugular
    - Subclavian
    - Intestinal
    - Lumbar
  - Lymphatic ducts
    - Thoracic
    - Right lymphatic
  - 600–700 lymph nodes in:
    - Cervical region (neck)
    - Axillary region (under arm)
    - Inguinal region
  - Tonsils
  - Thymus gland (near heart)
  - Spleen (near stomach)
  - Kupffer cells of liver
  - Microglia of nervous system
  - Connective tissue macrophages
  - Lymph (~10 liters)
- Blood flow distribution (percent)
  - Head (13)/neck-arms-thorax (25)
  - Abdominal circulation (50.1):
    - Splanchnic circulation (20.6)
    - Hepatic circulation (6.0)
    - Renal circulation (21.5)
  - Legs and lower body (11.9)

The cardiovascular division

The cardiovascular division includes several sub-systems that comprise a collection of organs and passages by which oxygen, nutrients, hormones and other biochemical substrates are delivered to the cells and tissues of the body, in exchange for various waste products, heat, and undesirable substances being removed for subsequent disposal. The major organ of this division is a pump—the *heart*, or *cardiac portion*, which is illustrated in Figure 2.1.

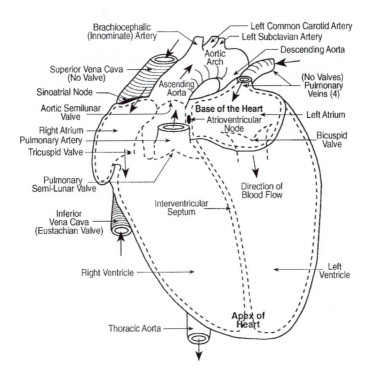

Figure 2.1 Anterior view of the human heart, showing the four chambers, the inlet and outlet valves, the inlet and outlet major blood vessels, the wall separating the right side (pump 2) from the left side (pump 1), and the two cardiac pacing centers—the sinoatrial (SA) node and the atrioventricular (AV) node. Bold-face arrows show the direction of flow through the heart chambers, the valves, and the major blood vessels

THE PUMP: HEART

Barely the size of the clenched fist of the individual in whom it resides, the heart is a four-chamber, hollow muscular organ having an inverted-cone configuration—with its base at the top (toward the head) and its apex at the bottom (toward the feet). Weighing about three-quarters of a pound, it measures 12–13 cm from base to apex and 7–8 cm at its widest point, making it about the size of a 3 x 5-inch index card. The organ occupies a small region between the third and sixth ribs, in the center of the thoracic cavity. Situated in between the lower parts of the two lungs, it rests just above the diaphragm, its base-to-apex axis leaning mostly toward the left side of the body and slightly forward.

The heart is actually two, self-contained pumps sitting side by side, but, as we shall see, connected in series, i.e., it is divided by a tough muscular wall (the *interatrial/interventricular septum*) into a somewhat crescent-shaped, low-pressure right side (right atrium plus right ventricle) that drives blood through the *pulmonary circulation*, and a cylindrically-shaped, high-pressure left side (left atrium plus left ventricle) that drives the fluid through the *systemic circulation*. Thus, consider how the *cardiac cycle* is generated:

- It begins when the *ventricle* of the *left heart* (output chamber of pump 1) contracts, forcefully driving oxygen-rich blood through the *aortic semilunar valve* into the *aorta*—the main blood vessel of the *systemic circulation*. This forceful contraction is called *ventricular systole*, and is reflected in the top number of a blood-pressure reading, expressed, for example, as "120 mm of mercury." It also makes a characteristic "dup" sound under clinical *auscultation* (i.e., stethoscopic listening to cardiac acoustics).

- The systemic circulation transports blood to within a differential neighborhood of every cell in the body—from which it returns via the *superior* and *inferior vena cava* to the *atrium* (Latin, meaning "corridor"), or "dog-ear-shaped" *auricle* (*input chamber*) of the right side of the heart (pump 2), now low in oxygen but rich in carbon dioxide.

- The right atrium now contracts, called *atrial systole*, accompanied by a "lub" sound, forcing blood through the *tricuspid valve* into the *right ventricle*.

- Next, the *right ventricle* (output chamber of pump 2) contracts ("dup" again, actually in unison with the left ventricle), forcing blood through the *pulmonary semi-lunar valve* into the *pulmonary artery*—the main blood vessel of the *pulmonary circulation*.

- The latter transports blood to the lungs, where its oxygen supply is replenished and its carbon dioxide content is purged before four *pulmonary veins* return the blood to the somewhat spherical, dome-shaped *atrium (input) chamber* of the left side of the heart.

- The left atrium now contracts ("lub" again, actually in unison with the right atrium), forcing blood through the *bicuspid* (or *"mitral"*) *valve* into the left ventricle, and the cycle begins all over again—60–80 times per minute at rest, making the characteristic "lub-dup"—*long-short*—rhythmical sounds that define, respectively, a relatively longer atrial systole ("lub"), followed by a much shorter ventricular systole ("dup").

The complete journey—out of the left ventricle (pump 1)…through the systemic circulation…back into the right atrium (pump 2)…and then out of the right ventricle…through the pulmonary circulation…back into the left atrium—takes from as little as 18–24 seconds, to as long as a minute. This is called the *circulation time*.

Some important observations:

- Contraction of the heart's four cardiac chambers (two atria, two ventricles) is accomplished by special *cardiac muscle tissue* that is activated electrically by signals originating in the *sinoatrial (SA) node*, located at the junction of the superior vena cava with the right atrium (see Figure 2.1, page 71). The propagation of these electrochemical impulses throughout the walls of the heart is measured clinically by an *electrocardiogram*.

- Although *both atria* contract at the same time ("lub"), as do *both ventricles* ("dup"), contraction of the *atria and ventricles* is *not* simultaneous—given their roles in the cardiac cycle, that would be counter-productive. Thus, in order to allow the atria to "do their thing" in filling the ventricles, ahead-of and unimpeded by simultaneous contraction of the latter to empty the heart, the impulses travelling through the atria all finally converge on an *atrioventricular (AV) node*—a small mass of *slowly* conducting tissue located in the right atrial wall near its junction with the interventricular septum (see Figure 2.1). Being slow to transmit a signal, the AV-node creates an electrochemical "bottle-neck" that acts to *delay* the electrical impulses propagating through the cardiac musculature, so that the ventricles will contract *after* the atria do.

- In summary, there are four phases to the cardiac cycle:

  1) A *filling phase*, called *diastole* (usually associated with the lower (bottom) number in a blood-pressure reading), wherein both ventricular "inlet valves" (tricuspid and mitral) are open and both "outlet valves" (pulmonary and aortic semi-lunar) are closed. This phase continues until the end of atrial systole and the beginning of ventricular systole, which snaps the inlet valves shut.

  2) An *isovolumetric contraction phase*, during which all valves are closed as pressure is building up in the contracting ventricles. This phase continues until the pressure is high enough to force open the ventricular outlet valves.

  3) An *emptying (ejection) phase*, called *systole* (usually associated with the higher (top) number in a blood pressure reading). In this phase, the tricuspid and mitral inlet valves are closed; the pulmonary and aortic semi-lunar outlet valves have been forced open; and a bolus of fluid, called the *stroke volume*, is ejected into the pulmonary artery and aorta, respectively. This phase continues to the end of ventricular systole, when all valves close again as blood pressure drops off.

4) An *isovolumetric relaxation phase*, wherein all valves remain closed again as the pressure continues to fall off during ventricular diastole. This phase continues until the inlet tricuspid and mitral valves open and filling starts all over again.

- The *cardiac output* (CO) is defined to be the mathematical product of *stroke volume* (around 70 ml at rest) and *heart rate* (on average, 75 beats/minute at rest), yielding a CO of around 5.25 liters of blood per minute. However, in extreme cases of vigorous exertion, under the influence of both the autonomic nervous and endocrine systems, heart rate can more than triple, to as high as 240 beats per minute. This is called a *chronotropic* effect. Furthermore, stroke volume can more than double, to as high as 175 ml—an *inotropic* effect. Under these circumstances, CO can increase to as much as 42 liters/minute, which is eight times "normal!" Keep in mind, though, that this can *only occur for very brief periods of time—it is not sustainable!*

- Also keep in mind that the filling ("lub") and emptying ("dup") times of the cardiac cycle, as mentioned, are not equal. In general, nearly two-thirds (64%) of a "typical" cardiac cycle is attributable to ventricular diastole, during which time the heart is mostly "resting." Thus, contrary to popular belief, your ventricles are actually *not* working most of the time! That's why they can go seemingly "non-stop," 24/7, for an entire lifetime—they are only active just over a third (36%) of the time.

THE FLUID: BLOOD

Averaging 5200ml in total volume, blood—the *hematic portion* of the cardiovascular division of the circulatory system—is the fluid pumped throughout the body by the *cardiac portion*, i.e., the heart. Blood is a complex, heterogeneous liquid composed of *formed elements*—the blood cells (*hematocytes*)—suspended in a continuous, straw-colored *plasma*.

Hematocytes

There are 32 different types of blood cell—20 in various stages of development at their source, which is *bone marrow*, and 12 in the circulating fluid, per se. Of these 12, seven are of particular interest (see Table 2.3). The seven are divided into three main types of *hematocyte*:

1. *Red blood cells (erythrocytes)*, numbering some 5.2 million/mm^3 of blood, account for nearly 95 percent of the formed elements, and about a quarter of the total number of cells in the entire human body. The term *hematocrit* refers to the percentage by volume of erythrocytes in blood; it ranges from 30–54 percent for "healthy" adults—higher in men, lower in women, averaging 45 percent. The primary function of erythrocytes is to aid in the transport of blood gases—oxygen—by the formation of an iron-dependent *oxy-hemoglobin*

complex in the cell; and carbon dioxide, by the *carbonic-anhydrase*-catalyzed formation of carbonic acid, which dissociates into water-soluble bicarbonate and hydrogen ions.

2. *Platelets* (*thrombocytes*) account for considerably less, coming in at about 268,000/mm³ of blood, which amounts to about 5 percent of all blood cells. The primary function of platelets is to participate in the blood-clotting process. For example, among other things, they form "knots" to which the filamentous protein *fibrin* adheres.

3. *White blood cells* (*leukocytes*) account for even less, averaging 7500/mm³ of blood, or something on the order of 0.15 percent or less of all hematocytes. The primary function of leukocytes is to endow the human body with the ability to identify and dispose of foreign substances (such as infectious organisms) that do not belong there. One type of leukocyte—*agranulocytes* (mostly *lymphocytes*, with lesser amounts of *monocytes*)—essentially does the "identifying;" and a second type—*granulocytes* (mainly *neutrophils*, with sparingly little amounts of "acid-loving" *acidophils* and even less "alkaline-loving" *basophils*)—is primarily concerned with the "disposing."

Hematopoietic system

This is a blood-cell-forming system that includes mainly red ("active") bone marrow, but also certain lymphatic tissue (hence the designation *lymphocytes*), and organs (e.g., the *spleen*). In a typical lifetime, *myelocytes* ("bone marrow cells," from the Greek *mŷelós*, meaning "marrow") will manufacture over three-quarters of a ton of anuclear red blood cells (*note:* erythrocytes lose their nucleus just as they reach maturity). Each takes six to seven days to complete and survives about 100–120 days in the circulation.

When they become "worn out," senescent erythrocytes are removed from the circulation by the spleen—the largest lymphatic organ—an ovoid body located in the upper left quadrant of the abdomen, behind and below the stomach. In addition to *purging* the blood of senescent erythrocytes—after recycling their innards—the spleen can also *store* and *discharge* red blood cells *into* the vascular system as necessary. The daily turnover rate of these cells is about one percent, but that amounts to over three million cells per second, the remains of which show up in the stool as "ghost cells" and the pigment *bilirubin*, which contribute to its characteristic brown color.

Blood plasma

Removal of all hematocytes from blood leaves behind the aqueous (91% water by weight), saline (salt) suspending medium called *plasma* (from the Greek for "a thing formed or molded"). Some 6.5–8 percent by weight of plasma consists of the *plasma proteins* (TP), of which there are four major types:

- *Albumin* (56% of TP) is a large protein that does not readily pass through capillary walls. Thus, it serves mainly:

    o to help maintain the transmural (*osmotic*) pressure differential that ensures proper mass exchange between blood and interstitial fluid, at the microcirculation level

    o as a transport carrier molecule ("taxi cab") for several water-insoluble hormones and other small biochemical constituents, such as some metal ions.

- The *globulins* (38% of TP) are a *class* of proteins that serve mainly to:

    o act as transport carrier molecules for large, water-insoluble biochemical substances, such as: (i) fats—in the form of high-, low-, and very-low density *lipoproteins:* HDL, LDL, and VLDL respectively (these account for 6% of total protein); (ii) certain carbohydrates—in the form of *muco-and-glyco-proteins;* and (iii) heavy metals—in the form of *mineralo-proteins.* The latter two account for 18 percent of total protein.

    o work, as *immuno-globulins*—antibodies—14 percent of total protein, together with leukocytes, in the body's immune system.

- *Fibrinogen (*4% of TP) works together with thrombocytes, the fourth major plasma protein—*prothrombin* (0.25% of TP)—and several "clotting factors," to form blood clots. Removal of fibrinogen from plasma leaves behind a clear, slightly yellowish fluid called *serum.*

Of the remaining 2 percent or so by weight of plasma:

- just under half (0.95%) consists of: (i) minerals (inorganic "ash"); (ii) trace elements (silicon, iron, sulfur, protein-bound iodine, etc.); and (iii) electrolytes—mainly the *cations* sodium, potassium, calcium, and magnesium; and the *anions* chlorine, bicarbonate, phosphate, and sulfate, the latter three *buffering* the fluid to maintain its slight 7.4 pH alkalinity

- just over a third (0.76 percent) includes three major types of *emulsified fats: cholesterol* (a major component of HDL and LDL, in free and esterified forms); *phospholipid* (a major component of cell membranes); and *triglycerides* (alternate forms of energy, and a major component of VLDL), with lesser amounts of the fat soluble vitamins A, D, E, and K; and free fatty acids, chylomicrons, and other lipids

- the remaining 0.29 percent that completes the 2 percent consists of: (i) mainly (0.25%) "extractives," of which two-thirds are glucose and other carbohydrates (the balance is made up of the water-soluble B-complex and C vitamins); and (ii) traces of certain enzymes; non-nitrogenous and nitrogenous waste products of metabolism (including urea, creatine, and creatinine); nearly a dozen additional *clotting factors*; organic acids; hormones; and many even smaller amounts of other biochemical constituents.

In other words, the list of plasma ingredients seems virtually endless…and indeed, it is! In fact, the very brief description of blood given in this section should give the reader an immediate appreciation for why this circulating fluid is often referred to as "the river of life!" But where does this river flow? Let's take a look at a very sophisticated piping network.

THE PIPING NETWORK: VASCULAR SYSTEM

Impelled by the heart, blood flows through the *vascular portion* of the cardio*vascular* division of the circulatory system. It includes major passages called *arteries*, which carry blood away from the heart, and *veins*, which bring it back—the two comprising a *macro-vascular network* of blood vessels and a much smaller group of channels that comprise the *micro-vascular network* of blood vessels, i.e., *arterioles, capillaries,* and *venules.*

Major anatomical features of the macrocirculation

Referring to Table 2.3 and our previous discussion of the heart, we note that two major circulatory pathways have already been introduced—namely, the *pulmonary* and *systemic circulations.* The former illustrates an important feature of vascular networks, i.e., some are intended to be primarily blood *processing*—"operant" pathways; others, organ and tissue *servicing (nourishing* and *sanitizing)*—"nutritive" networks. Thus, for example, the *pulmonary circulation processes* blood, oxygenating it and removing carbon dioxide and heat (absorbed into water vapor), but a totally separate *bronchial circulation* actually *services* lung tissue itself. Similarly, blood is *processed* by the *portal circulation* coursing through the liver. Here, certain blood constituents are removed, such as:

- glucose derived from digestion (to be converted into glycogen)
- waste products from the metabolism of amino acids (to be "deaminized" and converted into urea)
- "toxic" substances that might inadvertently have been absorbed into the blood from the intestine
- the previously mentioned senescent erythrocytes extracted by the spleen (to be disposed of in the stool).

The liver itself, however, is *serviced* by a totally separate *hepatic circulation.*

Another important point to be made about vascular networks is that there is a hierarchy of priority as to *which* networks receive blood: *when, how much,* and *composed of what.* Thus, under normal circumstances (see Table 2.3), blood flow distribution in the *systemic circulation* "typically" breaks down as follows:

- 13 percent is sent to the brain via the *cerebral circulation*

- 15 percent is directed to the head, neck, and arms via the three main blood vessels that originate in the *aortic arch* (see Figure 2.1, page 71)

- 10 percent is distributed as follows: 5 percent to the *coronary circulation* that *services* the heart; 3 percent to the *bronchial circulation* that *services* the lungs, and 2 percent to the *thoracic circulation* that *services* the remainder of the thoracic cavity

- 20.6 percent flows through the *splanchnic circulation* that divides as follows: spleen (*splenic*), 5.6 percent; and *mesenteric* (pancreas, stomach, small and large intestines), 15 percent—all branches of these two networks eventually merging to form the *portal vein* that feeds into the *portal circulation*, which is a blood-processing network

- 21.5 percent flows through the *renal circulation* that both *services* the kidney while having its blood supply *processed (dialyzed)*

- 8 percent is directed to the *hepatic circulation* (6%) that *services* the liver, and *abdominal circulation* (2%) that services the remainder of the abdominal cavity (*Note:* the hepatic and portal circulations both empty into the hepatic vein)

- 11.9 percent is directed to the legs and lower extremities via the *femoral arteries* that derive from the left and right *common iliac arteries.* The latter two originate from the abdominal aorta at its bifurcation near the *inguinal* ("groin") *region* of the body.

All well and good…*but*…when you are being chased by a lion, the last thing your body is concerned with is digesting a meal! When you are freezing cold, the last thing you want is for blood to flow to the periphery, where so much heat is lost through the large surface area of the arms and legs. In other words, when extenuating circumstances require the body to *redistribute* blood flow, it has the ability to do so, and makes decisions based essentially on three criteria:

1. The first one has to do with *Anatomical design principle number 2*, i.e., we can survive without arms, legs, a stomach, a large portion of the small intestine, the spleen, the gall bladder, tonsils, adenoids, a large chunk of the liver, eyes, ears, one kidney, and even one lung. But we cannot survive minus a brain, a heart, and at least one functioning kidney and lung. Thus, when necessary, the body exploits its redundancy by cutting off the flow of blood to these regions, figuring if the worst comes to the worst, we can live without them, so let them fend for themselves.

2. Related to criterion 1, the body also knows that certain tissues—such as striated skeletal and smooth muscle—can survive for long periods of time under *anaerobic conditions*; others—such as several types of connective tissue—can function quite effectively at a significantly *decreased metabolic rate*; and still

others—such as a vast majority of endothelial, connective, nerve and muscle tissue—are much more *massive* than they really need to be, and so blood flow to them, too, can be significantly compromised with no really serious consequences.

3. Finally, blood flow to any given region of the body is ultimately determined by how essential the perfused region is:

    a) to the *maintenance of life* under the given circumstances

    b) in allowing the organism to *respond effectively to a perceived* (that's the operative word here) *life-threatening situation*.

Such distribution, or re-distribution of blood flow is accomplished at the arteriolar level of the circulation, by the activity of smooth muscle tissue in "closing down" the entrances to downstream capillary beds. Before getting to this level, blood flows through bi- and tri-furcating networks of vessels that again illustrate *Anatomical design principle number 3*, i.e., the vessels progressively increase in number as they decrease in geometric size. Thus:

*   Derived from the 32 main branches of the 1–3 cm-diameter *aorta* are nearly 300 "large" (4–5 mm-internal diameter, D, by 1.4–2.8 cm long, L), and over 1100-"medium-size" (2.5–4.0 mm-D by 1.0–2.2 cm-L) arteries.

*   These spawn about 3500 "small" (1.0–2.5 mm-D by 0.6–1.7 cm-L) arteries that distribute themselves into nearly 21,000 tributaries, having mean internal diameters of 0.5–1.0 mm and average lenths of 0.3–1.3 cm.

*   Tributaries divide into about 83,000 *small rami* (0.25–0.5 mm-D by 2–8 mm-L), which, in turn, yield about 500,000 *terminal branches* (0.1–0.25 mm-D by 1–6 mm-L) en route to the microcirculation.

On the other side of the microcirculation:

*   Some 500,000 *terminal branches* of collecting veins (0.2–0.6 mm-D by 1–6 mm-L) merge into 20,000 "small" (0.6–1.1 mm-D by 2–9 mm-L) and 500 "medium-size" (1–5 mm-D by 1–2 cm-L) veins.

*   The latter continue to combine into about 250 "large" (5–9 mm-D by 1.4–3.7 cm-L) veins and an equal number of *venous main branches*, averaging 0.9–2.0 cm-D, and 2–10 cm-L.

*   Main venous branches eventually merge into the two 2.0–3.5 cm-D by 20–50 cm-L *vena cava* that drain into the right atrium en route to the pulmonary circulation. The *superior vena cava* returns blood from regions above the heart; the *inferior vena cava* does the same from regions below the level of the heart.

Because they operate at significantly lower blood pressures than do their arterial counterparts, veins are, in general, larger than arteries and have much thinner, less muscular walls. Blood, then, tends to "pool" on the venous side of the circulation. Indeed, of the average 3.25 liters of blood that is typically in the *systemic macro-circulation* at any given time, over 75 percent of it resides on the venous side, less than 25 percent on the arterial side. This 3:1 ratio is not quite that dramatic in the 343 ml or so of blood that typically comprise the *pulmonary macro-circulation*, where about 57 percent is found in veins and 43 percent in arteries—a ratio of only 4:3. Together with the 338 ml of blood that typically resides in the chambers of the heart, we have thus far accounted for about 75 percent of the 5.2 liters of blood that is a "typical" value for *total* blood volume; most of the remaining 25 percent can be found in the *microcirculation*.

Major anatomical features of the microcirculation

Arteries and veins are connected by a vascular network that begins with tiny blood vessels called *arterioles* on the artery side. These empty into *capillaries*, which merge into collecting *venules* on the venous side. Collectively, arterioles, capillaries, and venules comprise the *micro-circulation*, across the vascular walls of which the transport of mass and energy to and from the interstitial fluid that bathes the cells of the body takes place. For the purposes of this discussion, the *microcirculation* is defined to include blood vessels on the arterial side having internal diameters of 0.1 mm or less, and those on the venous side being smaller than 0.2 mm-D. The former includes:

- ~ 18.6 million *arterioles* (0.025–0.1 mm-D by 0.2–3.8 mm-L)
- ~ 239 million *metarterioles* (0.01–0.025 mm-D x 0.1–1.8 mm-L)
- > 16 *billion capillaries* (3.5–10 *micro*-m, μmD, by 0.5–1.1 mm-L).

The latter includes:

- ~ 4.5 *billion post-capillary venules* (8–30 μm-D by 0.1–0.6 mm-L)
- ~ 160.5 million *collecting venules* (30–50 μm-D x 0.1–0.8 mm-L)
- ~ 32 million *muscular venules* (0.05–0.10 mm-D x 0.2–1.0 mm-L)
- ~ 10.25 x 10^6 *small collecting veins* (0.1–0.2 mm-D x 0.5–3.2 mm-L).

The significance of the microcirculatory anatomy is two-fold: first, the sheer *number* of blood vessels involved ensures that any given cell will be no further away from the nearest capillary than a distance equal to a typical cell size. Second, the fact that the *wall thickness* of these tiny blood vessels decreases—to something to the order of 0.5–1.0 *millionths* (micro-) of a meter—ensures that mass and energy can be transported easily out of or in to the circulation at the cellular level. The only exception is *arterioles*—which have relatively thick, 20–30 μm walls—comparable with their 25–100 μm internal diameter. This is because the walls of arterioles are heavily inundated with smooth muscle tissue, endowing them with the ability alluded to in our earlier discussion of blood distribution, i.e., to "shut down" when necessary, flow to the downstream vascular beds that they service. Thus, arterioles serve as *control points* for blood distribution. But that's not all.

A further note about the anatomy of the circulatory system

A closer look at the geometric configuration (*morphometry*) of the circulatory branching networks reveals yet again an anatomical design principle that we already encountered in our discussion of the respiratory system—and that, indeed, prevails throughout the body. Recall that in order to optimize the effective use of a very confined thoracic space, the respiratory system exploits the idea of hollowing out the interior of the region into a complex, branching pattern of exactly 23 generations that produce increasingly larger numbers of smaller and smaller air-conducting vessels...and the branching patterns are *not random*, they are highly predictable. Sound familiar? Well...as it turns out...the anatomical branching patterns of the circulatory system, too, are not random. Like the lung, they follow a pattern that we shall elaborate on further in Part II, and that also has significant relevance to musical patterns, in general, and to the role of the music therapist, in particular. Suffice it to say for now, that in the arterial network of blood vessels, one finds that the total number of generations from parent-trunk to terminal capillaries is remarkably consistent, being, for example, 12 for the *bronchial circulation*, 13 for the *renal* (kidney), *coronary* (heart), and *cerebral* (brain) *circulations*, and 17 for the *pulmonary circulation*.

Moreover, it is also observed that vascular branching configurations typically start out *binary*, i.e., a parent vessel bifurcating into two daughter branches, for the first two or three generations. The pattern then becomes *tertiary*—the daughters each "sprouting" three branches—for several generations beyond that; after which they become increasingly complex as the progeny approach the microvasculature. On the venous side, the patterns simplify again as the vascular networks reconverge en route back to the heart. Details are beyond the scope of this book, but the reader interested in learning more about this is directed to Singhal, Henderson and Horsfield (1973), Tortora and Grabowski (1993), Schneck (1990, 2009a and b), Schneck and Voigt (2006), and Jacob *et al.* (1982).

Moving on, then, we note further that the cardiovascular division of the circulatory system handles mainly small, microscopic particles. Larger ones—such as absorbed fat particles *(chylomicrons)* from the small intestines, macroscopic plasma proteins that have "leaked" out of broken capillaries, large body wastes, and "foreign invaders"—are handled by the lymphatic division of this system.

The lymphatic division of the circulatory system

During the processes of microcirculatory transport, it turns out that the outflow from this vasculature exceeds the inflow by about 10 percent—the resulting excess tissue fluid being eventually returned to the blood by a special auxiliary *lymphatic* transport system (see Table 2.3). Although somewhat simplistic, one might think of the lymphatic system as the body's *sewage disposal unit*—a collection of organs and channels akin to blood vessels, but carrying instead of blood, a transparent, slightly yellow, somewhat opalescent, viscous, mucous-like fluid called *lymph*, similar to blood plasma. The "sewer-line" analogy derives from the fact that the lymphatic division of the circulatory system is responsible for removing body wastes and toxic materials from extracellular tissue spaces. Among the ways it does this are: (i) *phagocytosis*, i.e., the ingestion and digestion of bacteria and particles by "eating" cells ("garbage trucks") called *phagocytes*; and (ii) the similar activity of *lymphocytes*. Most of the waste products are transported through the lymphatic "sewer lines," eventually dumping back into the bloodstream for subsequent disposal by the body's exhaust systems. However, don't minimize the important role that this system plays as well in helping to carry certain food products from the blood to the cells, themselves.

As indicated in Table 2.3, *lymphatic capillaries* originate as microscopic, open-ended, "funnel-like," blind (i.e., with no identifiable origination site) entrances scattered throughout the extracellular tissue spaces of the body. These entrances allow ECF—of which most lymph is composed—access to the lymphatic network of pipes, channels, and glands.

Lymphatic capillaries thus created eventually converge to form larger *lymphatic vessels*—more than twice as many as there are comparably sized arteries. The vessels continue to merge into five major *trunks:*

1.   *bronchomediastinal* (around and between the lungs and chest)

2.   *jugular* (in the neck)

3.   *subclavian* (beneath the collar bone)

4.   *intestinal* (in and around the abdomen)

5.   *lumbar* (at the lower part of the back and sides).

Lymphatic trunks eventually coalesce into two main *lymphatic ducts:*

- the *thoracic duct* that empties into the left subclavian vein
- the *right lymphatic duct* that empties into the right subclavian vein.

Thus, the lymphatic system is a *unidirectional* (not re-circulating) flow system that begins in the interstitial fluid spaces and ends on the venous side of the systemic circulation. Along the way, one encounters some 600–700 bean-shaped *lymph nodes* ("sewage plants"), mostly in the neck (*cervical nodes*), groin (*inguinal nodes*), and armpits (*axillary nodes*). Lymph nodes are active as a source of lymphocytes, and thus contribute to filtering out from the lymph, bacteria and other harmful micro-organisms. Tonsils and adenoids are among the lymph glands.

Finally, a system closely related to the lymphatic system is one known as the *reticuloendothelial system*. The latter is a generic term for the collection of all anatomic cells—e.g., *phagocytes*—that have the ability to ingest (Greek, *phagein* means "to eat") and ultimately digest or otherwise dispose of particulate matter such as bacteria and colloidal particles. Included are:

- *macrophages* (*histiocytes, clasmatocytes,* and resting "wandering cells") of loose connective tissue

- *reticular* ("net-like") cells of lymphatic organs such as the spleen (cells lining its blood sinuses); liver (*Kupffer cells*); and thymus gland

- some *myeloid tissue cells* found in bone marrow

- certain cells lining the blood sinuses of the adrenal cortex and hypophysis cerebri (pituitary gland)

- the *microglia* of the central nervous system

- the *adventitial cells* surrounding major blood vessels

- the so-called "dust cells" of the lungs.

While we are on the subject of waste disposal, it seems appropriate to move on to talk about the last set of organ systems that have to do with the *engine feature* of the human body, i.e., its various *exhaust systems.*

Anatomical exhaust systems

When I think of physiologic waste disposal, several "-tions" come to mind. The first and most encompassing, of course, is elimina*tion*—which refers to exhausting refuse, debris, and the undesirable products of metabolism through the:

- intestines (*digestive system*)

- lungs (*respiratory system*)

- skin (*integumentary system*)

- lymph nodes (*lymphatic system*)

- kidneys (*renal-urological system*).

Each of these handles its own, unique exhaust function; and with the exception of skin and kidneys, we have already addressed the other three. The respective "-tions" involved are:

- **Eges***tion:* the elimination by the digestive system of indigestible residue, excess liquid water, worn-out red blood cells, bacteria, heat, and other wastes through *defecation*—from the large intestine, through the rectum. anal canal, and anus.

- **Expira***tion:* the elimination by the respiratory system of carbon dioxide, gaseous water vapor, and heat.

- **Convec***tion:* the elimination (by transport of lymph through the lymphatic system) of excess plasma proteins, fats extracted from interstitial fluid, overflow capillary seepage, "ghost" erythrocytes filtered from blood by the spleen, dead disease-producing microorganisms that have been phagocytized in lymph nodes or deactivated by antibodies, and other sewage.

- **Evapora***tion:* the elimination through the integumentary system (skin) of excess heat, through *perspiration.* Also eliminated through the skin are certain salts (mostly dissolved in sweat), and a small amount of urea. Contributing to heat dissipation from the skin surface are three more "-tions:" *radiation, conduction,* and *convection.* You might be interested to know that even in the dead of winter we perspire, generating as much as several pints of imperceptible *sweat* a day. Indeed, were it not for our vascular system's *thermoregulatory function*— i.e., blood acting like the coolant flowing through the coils of an automobile radiator—and the six "-tions": defeca-, expira-, perspira-, radia-, conduc-, and convec-, the metabolic heat generated by routine *activities of daily living* would cause body core temperature to rise 1.0–1.25°C per hour! In less than three hours, this rate of heat production would raise the core temperature to critical levels (see Table 5.5 of chapter 5); and, in just six hours, would probably kill you. That's why we must have elaborate heat-dissipating systems—remember, as we said right at the beginning of this chapter, *we are an isothermal living engine!* No heat! Thus, under conditions of extreme physical exercise or exertion, to help eliminate heat more effectively, we:

  - breathe more heavily (pant, hyperventilate)

  - increase blood flow to the periphery (via increased blood pressure—an *inotropic* effect; accelerated heart rate—a *chronotropic* effect; widening of the peripheral blood vessels—by *relaxing peripheral arteriolar smooth muscle;* and, *contracting* arteriolar smooth muscle more centrally, to divert flow toward the periphery)

  - sweat profusely

  - experience enhanced urination—which brings us to the last organ system that we will address in this chapter.

- **Urina***tion:* the elimination by the *renal-urological system* of excess liquid water, nitrogenous substances—urea, uric acid, creatine, creatinine, and other products that result from the metabolism of proteins and nitrogenous compounds—and mineral salts, through *micturition,* i.e., voiding the urinary bladder. A summary of the anatomical features of the renal-urological system is given below and in Table 2.4. Details may be found in Goss (1966), Jacob *et al.* (1982), Kinne (1989), McGovern and Waldbaum (1985), Schneck (1990, 2006a), Seldin and Giebisch (1985), and Tortora and Grabowski (1993).

Table 2.4 Major anatomical features of the renal-urological system

ANATOMICAL STRUCTURE

- Renal system:
  - Two kidneys (gms each):
    - Women: 115–160
    - Men: 125–180
    - › 11.5 cm L x 2.5 cm thick x 5–7.5 cm wide; left longer and narrower than right
  - Nephrons: 1.25×10^6 per kidney x 30–38 mm total length each
    - › Bowman's capsule; 0.2 mm-D
    - › 20–50 glomerular capillary loops per nephron, each
    - › capillary measuring 300– 500μm L x $(32/\pi)$μm D
    - › Proximal convoluted tubule 14 mm L x 59μm D
    - › Thin, short Loop of Henle
    - › Distal convoluted tubule 5mm L x 35μm D
    - › Collecting tubule, 20–22 mm L x 40μm D
  - Renal corpuscle (malpighian body)
  - The hilum opening
  - Inner portion of kidney:
    - › Renal medulla
    - › Renal pyramids and papillae
    - › Major and minor calyces
    - › Renal pelvis
  - Outer portion of kidney:
    - › Renal cortex
    - › Renal columns
    - › Medullary rays
    - › Fibrous capsule
  - Renal sinuses
  - Glomerular filtration rate:
    - › 125ml/min protein-free Plasma; 180 liters/day 99.5% reabsorbed daily

- Renal circulation:
  - Right and left renal arteries
    - › 5.5 mm-ID x 6.8 cm-L nominal
  - 4 posterior and anterior branches
    - › ~ 3.4 mm-ID x 4.66 cm-L
  - 8 segmental arteries
    - › 2.1 mm-ID x 3.2 cm-L nominal
  - 16 polar branches
  - 32 interlobar arteries
  - 160 arcuate arteries
  - 800 interlobular arteries
  - 4000 perforating capsular vessels
    - › 20,000 terminal branches
  - 100,000 71μm-ID x 2.27mm-L sprigs
    - › 500,000 pre-arterioles
    - › 2,500,000 afferent arterioles
    - › 12,500,000 glomerular tufts metarterioles
  - 125,000,000 glomerular capillaries
    - › 2,500,000 efferent arterioles
    - › 19,687,500 cortical nephron peritubular capillaries
  - 500,000 vasa recta
    - › Venae rectae; collecting venules; venules; venous branches and veins

- The urinary system:
  - Two ureters
  - (28–34 cm-L; one from each kidney leads to urinary bladder)
  - Urinary bladder: (urine storage; up to 500 ml when moderately full; 12 cm D)
  - One urethra (17.5–20 cm-L male; 4 cm-L female; excretes urine from bladder to environment)

- The penis (male)
- Micturition (urinary excretion)
  - up to 1–1.5 liters per day

Major anatomical features of the renal-urological system

Interestingly, were it not for nitrogenous wastes that are the products of protein metabolism, we probably wouldn't need a kidney! The respiratory system is quite adept at exhausting carbon dioxide, water vapor and heat—the by-products of carbohydrate and fat metabolism. Whatever the lungs can't handle, the large intestines, lymphatic system, and skin can. But when it comes to nitrogenous wastes…well… nitrogen cannot be converted to its gaseous forms—nitrogen dioxide and ammonia gas—for expulsion by the lungs, because both are highly toxic, so that won't work. For the same reason, the liquid form of nitrogen—ammonium hydroxide—won't work either, because the skin cannot simply "sweat it out." Indeed, most gaseous and liquid forms of nitrogen, unlike the pure gas found in our atmosphere, are simply not able to be handled and disposed of easily by the human body. So…what to do?

Answer: convert nitrogenous wastes into relatively benign forms that the body *can* handle—at least long enough to get rid of them—and then invent an organ that can do just that. The "benign" forms are *urea* and *creatinine*, and the pair of glandular organs that function as an elaborate creatinine/urea filtering system are the bean-shaped *kidneys* (from the Anglo-Saxon, *cwith*, meaning "womb, belly" and *nyra*, later Middle English *ey*, meaning "egg" …hence "belly-eggs" because of their shape and location). The size of each kidney is given in Table 2.4. One is located on each side of the spinal column, at the back of the abdominal cavity, between the twelfth thoracic and third lumbar vertebrae. The right kidney is slightly shorter, thicker, and lies a bit lower than the left.

The functional unit of the kidney is the *nephron*, from the Greek, *nephros*, for "kidney." Between them, the pair of organs contain some 2.5 million "U-shaped" nephrons. At the top of one side of the U is a funnel-like entrance region called *Bowman's capsule*. It empties into a twisted mass of coiled, convoluted tubing called, logically enough, the *proximal* (nearest to the entrance) *convoluted tubule*. The collection of Bowman's capsules and proximal convoluted tubules lies mainly in the outer part—the *cortex*—of the kidney.

Proximal convoluted tubules eventually straighten out to become the thin, 9 mm long *descending limb* of the U-shaped nephron, and the limb promptly makes a sharp, 180° hairpin turn at the bottom of the "U." This turn is called the *Loop of Henle*, which continues up the other side of the "U" as a somewhat wider, 5–10 mm-long *ascending limb*. Both descending and ascending limbs of all nephrons, along with the Loops of Henle, extend into the inner, *medulla* portion of the kidney. The ascending limbs soon become again coiled masses of tubing that continue back into the cortex, this time, being called *distal* (furthest from the entrance) *convoluted tubules*. Each one of the latter drains into a 2 cm-long (just under an inch) by 0.04 mm-diameter *collecting tubule*.

Collecting tubules join to form *collecting ducts* that pass back down into the renal medulla. Here, several ducts fuse to form a *papillary duct*, through which the duct contents—now called *urine*—drains into the *renal pelvis*. In the renal pelvis, papillary ducts converge to form first *minor calices* (singular "calyx," from the Greek for "cup"), then *major calices*, and eventually the *ureter*, through which urine leaves the kidney en route to the *urinary bladder*. The urinary bladder will store urine until enough of it forms to warrant voiding (*micturition*) through the *urethra*. So…how is urine formed to begin with?

It is basically formed from *serum*—a blood-cell-free, protein-free, essentially fat-free fluid that is filtered out of blood as it courses through the *glomerular capillary network* that derives from the *renal circulation* servicing the kidneys (see Table 2.4). This capillary network engulfs Bowman's capsule (20–50 capillary loops per capsule), forming a structure loosely called the *juxtaglomerular apparatus*. Thus, entering the descending limb of the nephron tubule is a plasma ultrafiltrate called *tubular urine*, which amounts to about 19 percent—the so-called *filtration fraction*—of the total plasma volume that actually entered the glomerular capillary network. The *total* tubular urine formed in *all* of both kidneys' Bowman's capsules is called the *glomerular filtration rate* (GFR), which is "typically" around 105 ml/min for women, and 140 ml/min for men. However, most of it, as we shall see, is *reabsorbed*, leaving behind to be excreted daily only about 1–1.5 (to as much as 2.0) total liters of urine.

Tubular urine contains most of the crystalloid solids formerly present in blood (i.e., urea, hippuric acid, uric acid, and creatinine), along with other substances that were inadvertently carried along in the filtration process because of their small size. These include sodium, chlorine, potassium and bicarbonate ions, glucose, amino acids, and some albumin. We must endeavor to put these back! So, as the tubular urine continues down the descending limb of the nephron, around the Loop of Henle, and on into the ascending limb en route to the collecting duct, the renal *tubular capillary network* that winds its way around the various portions of the nephron tubules *reabsorbs* virtually 100 percent (including 98–99.75% H_2O) of everything *but* urea and creatinine, leaving at least half of the former and all of the latter to be expelled, along with miniscule amounts (if any) of the other substances "caught" in the ultrafiltrate.

The entire cardiac output is filtered through the kidneys 300–400 times per day, thus purifying blood in a process called *dialysis*. Finally, as a group, the collection of organs and tissues responsible for ridding the human body of things (including heat) that need to be disposed of are sometimes referred to as the *excretory system*.

Some closing remarks

To the music therapist, this "engine" of ours can be viewed as a sophisticated musical instrument. For example, in the section dealing with respiration, we talked about the analogy between the larynx and a double-reed wind instrument. Taking this one step further, our body is an instrument that is animated by the physiologic process of breathing (Sanskrit *prana*). In that sense, again, we are not unlike a wind instrument that "comes to life" when one breathes into it. Moreover, this "human instrument" is driven by bodily energy (Chinese *ch'i*) that combines with the "breath of life" (*prana*) to resonate along anatomical lines of energy ("strings"), called meridians, and tonification points, called access nodes (Prophet and Spadaro 2000; Shiffrin and Bailey 1976; Tsuei 1996). And as we shall also see in Chapter 5, the basic architecture of the human ear is such that hearing, itself, derives from the internal *harp* that is the basilar membrane of the inner ear.

Thus, in both structure and function, the body combines the essential features of the major three families of musical instruments—string, wind, and percussion. Indeed, fundamental to all physiologic function are *biorhythms*—the rhythms of life which, like the percussion instruments of any musical ensemble, maintain a certain periodicity to the output of this finely-tuned, complex "human instrument." We shall have more to say about this in Part II of the book. But now, let's take a closer look at the "output" of our engine.

CHAPTER 3

The Mobile Engine/Instrument

In the preface to this book, we listed a second feature of our "living engine," namely, that its *output* is *mechanical*. Indeed, everything it does, be it voluntary locomotion of parts or all of the animal body, or involuntary activities related to metabolic processes, involves movement at various scales of perception. In fact, if movement ceases...life ceases!

Thus, four major organ systems (three discussed in this chapter) are the ones most responsible for our perception of how the kinematic feature of life becomes manifest. They include the:

- three nervous systems: central, peripheral, and autonomic (discussed separately in Chapter 4)
- three muscular systems: striated, smooth, and cardiac
- skeletal system of bones and levers
- articular system of joints.

Before examining these systems, let's say a few more words about *metabolism* and how it relates to the idea of our being an *isothermal* engine—specifically, how the heat invariably generated by "movement" is handled by the body without jeopardizing its *isothermal* property.

Our optimized living engine

In physiology, when one speaks of *metabolism*—from the Greek *metabolē*, meaning "change" and *ismos*, meaning "state of"—the "change of state" referred to is either a building up of complex molecules from simpler ones—*anabolism*—or, conversely, a breaking down of complex molecules into simpler ones—*catabolism*. The latter, like the breakdown of ATP, often results in a release of chemical energy and so, is called *exergonic*—"energy releasing." The former, like muscular contraction, usually *requires* energy to drive it, and so is called *endergonic*—"energy absorbing." In a process called *reaction coupling*, the body minimizes the metabolic conversion of chemical energy into thermal energy (heat, which, you will recall, it cannot use) by arranging for exergonic biochemical reactions to drive endergonic ones and thus *pairing* these reactions to conserve *chemical* energy as much as possible.

> *Reaction coupling* is *physiological optimization principle number 1*, one of several *optimization* schemes that the body employs to allow it to operate most effectively (not necessarily efficiently!). We encountered a few others in Chapter 2, when we introduced anatomical design principles 1–3.

Another scheme, intended to minimize the biochemical production of heat is:

> *Physiological optimization principle number 2:* principle of cascading reactions, wherein the process of going from initial substrates to final products is not accomplished in one single step.

Instead, the desired products are manufactured via an extended sequence of many intermediate steps—like "pumping" your car brakes to stop the vehicle, rather than "slamming" them on.[1]

Of course, a significant price you pay for *pumping* your car brakes rather than *slamming* them on abruptly is that it takes longer and a greater distance to stop the vehicle…so…again, enter activated enzyme kinetics in isothermal physiologic systems, to alleviate the time-and-distance problem by expediting otherwise slow, complex biochemical reactions. However, there is one notable exception to the optimization schemes of reaction coupling and cascading reactions intended to conserve energy. That is, what happens when the body *needs heat*, i.e., when it is cold!

Enter the thyroid gland to the rescue! This is a bi-lobed, "butterfly-shaped" (the wings look like "shields," hence the Greek *thyreoeidēs*), endocrine organ located in the front of the neck, straddling the middle to lower part of the larynx and the upper part of the trachea. The thyroid gland is the body's thermostat. Thus, under conditions of "cold stress," this organ secretes its major hormone, *thyroxin* (T^4). The most striking effect of thyroxin in intact homeothermic animals is both the stimulation of increased oxygen consumption and the interference with reaction coupling. In what is called the *calorigenic effect*, thyroxin uncouples the symbiotic connections between paired exergonic-endergonic reactions. It thus causes:

- the *exergonic* ones—intensified by increased oxygen consumption—to *convert into heat* all of the chemical energy released in the reaction

---

1 The principle of cascading reactions also presents more opportunities for the body to intervene at any intermediate step, thus giving it more *control* over the outcome of biochemical processes, i.e., the processes can "switch tracks" at any of a number of key junctions in the metabolic pathways. The more intermediate steps employed in the cascading reaction scheme, the more control the body has to determine the outcome of those reactions. That's among the reasons that biochemical pathways are so numerous, elaborate, and seemingly cumbersome.

- the *endergonic* ones to be simultaneously *blocked from absorbing this energy* to manufacture, for example, ATP. The result of impaired ATP synthesis is a drained "dead battery." Among other things, muscular contraction is thus impaired, leading to malaise, fatigue, and total musculoskeletal shutdown.

In this respect, I have often wondered how history might have been changed if Napoleon was more aware of the temperature-dependent limitations of musculoskeletal function. You see, at the height of his power in 1812 he unadvisedly declared war against Russia and invaded Russian territory—with disastrous results! The winter setting, and the failure of his soldiers to be acclimated to the bitter Russian cold, brought his army to its knees. Musculoskeletal function was reduced to zero, and severe dehydration set in; the men were so fatigued and weakened by famine, disease, and cold that they had not even the strength to carry their fallen comrades off the battlefields. By the time Napoleon reached Moscow he was forced to retreat—barely 50,000 of his original 550,000-man army making it back alive. The rest of the story, as they say, is history.

Moreover, how might the course of history also have been changed if, over 125 years later, Hitler had learned from Napoleon's fatal mistake? You see, Hitler, too, at the pinnacle of his power, chose to violate his 1939 "treaty of friendship" with Russia, invading it instead. But his failure to capture Moscow before winter set in caused him to make the same fatal mistake that defeated Napoleon—with the same result! Hitler's army was miserably wiped out, mostly by the cold weather; and from then on, his fortunes declined: the end was in sight!

The moral(s) of these two anecdotes:

- Military leaders—indeed, all of us, but especially music therapists—should have a better understanding of basic physiologic function.

- We should have a greater appreciation for the lessons to be learned from the mistakes of history!

More to the point, the music therapist, often having to deal with musculoskeletal issues (Berger 2015) in clients, should be conscious of the environmental climate within which the therapy is being administered, and the possible role of the thyroid gland in affecting such function. For instance:

- Hypothyroidism—a deficiency of thyroid secretions—can result, among other things, in a lowered metabolic rate, a feeble pulse, constantly feeling cold, and, as we shall see in Part II, a serious distortion of one's sense of time (especially important when dealing with music!). A serious form of this condition is congenital hypothyroidism, a congenital condition characterized by a lack of physical and mental development due to thyroid insufficiency.

- Conversely, hyperthyroidism—excessive thyroid secretions—too, can distort one's time perception, while causing autonomic imbalance, exaggeration of all functions, psychic disturbances, increased metabolic rate (and hence, hunger), rapid pulse, restlessness, a constant feeling of being "flushed" and hot—and, in extreme cases, exophthalmic goiter and/or Graves' disease, named after the Irish physician Robert J. Graves (1796–1853) who first described it.

Keeping all of the above in mind, let's return to *metabolism* by recalling from Chapter 2 our description of how the enzymatically catalyzed degradation of complex nutrients allows them to be absorbed and delivered to the cells of the body. In turn, the cells *catabolize* these nutrients—break them down—to release the *chemical* energy stored in the bonds of the respective molecular entity. But, this energy is not used directly or immediately. Instead, you will also recall from Chapter 1, that the *anabolic* activity— i.e., *oxidative phosphorylation*—of the cell's *mitochondria* "captures" this energy and stores it in the chemical bonds of the human body's "battery," i.e., adenosine triphosphate, ATP. The energy thus stored in ATP is called *potential*, meaning that it is *available* to do work, such as driving the processes of metabolism, actively transporting various forms of mass, allowing muscles to contract, energizing biochemical synthesis, and so on. Availing ourselves of that energy means converting it from its *potential* form into a *kinetic* form. The former is energy *capable of being*—stored in the high-energy phosphate bonds of ATP, waiting to be released once these bonds are broken (hydrolyzed). The latter is energy embedded in *actual being*, which is *kinetic* (from the Greek *kīneîn*, meaning "to move"). Kinetic energy is derived (*transduced*) from potential energy; it is the *only* type of energy that we can perceive (Schneck 2011b). In the human body, the conversions from potential to kinetic energy progress from ATP (the "battery") to *action potentials* (nerve impulses, discussed in Chapter 4), that activate muscles (force generators)…that pull on bones (levers)…that rotate around joints (pivot points)…to create the desired motion. Moreover, as we shall see in the next chapter, these energy conversions are *digital*, based on *binary coding*.

> But before we get there, let's first make the point that: *All energy and material transformations that occur within living cells (i.e., metabolism) manifest themselves by generating forces that produce movement at various scales of perception.*

Indeed, our 639–656 *striated skeletal muscles*—the mechanical transducers that endow the human organism with the attribute of mobility—collectively constitute the single most abundant tissue in the body. Moreover, the 206 *bones*—the skeletal levers that give us a mechanical advantage—and *joints* (*articular system*)—the fulcra about which bones rotate—are part of an elaborate connective tissue system that also contributes significantly to body mass. If we add to these *cardiac* (heart) *muscle, smooth muscle tissue, tendons, ligaments,* supporting structures that keep these anatomical elements properly aligned and stable, and the *nervous systems* that innervate them, we will observe that at least 43 percent (women) to as many as 71 percent (men) of "us" exist to create *motion*—and for good reason! Think about it—there is no aspect of "life" at any level, from sub-microscopic to super-cosmic, that could survive without motion.

Major anatomical features of the muscular system

As was the case for blood cells, there are also three basic types of muscle cell: *cardiac, striated skeletal*, and *smooth*. The latter, along with cardiac muscle, are concerned mainly with maintaining the *internal* environment of the body. The former deal mostly with *external* locomotion of parts or all of the body. Because of these different functions, the three types of muscle tissue have different anatomical and physiological attributes (Schneck 1992). For example:

- Smooth muscle tissue consists of spindle-shaped, long, narrow fibers (cells) with a single nucleus located at about the middle of the cell. Within their cytoplasm, called *sarcoplasm* (from the Greek, *sarx*, meaning "flesh"), lie the contractile elements (*myofibrils*) of the tissue. These are organized into *myofilaments* that are innervated by efferent nerve fibers emanating from both divisions of the *autonomic nervous system* (see Chapter 4). Contraction of smooth muscle tissue is generally *involuntary*—not under conscious control. It acts to maintain the "tone" of structures such as blood vessels, as in *vascular smooth muscle tissue*, and the walls of various hollow organs, as in *visceral smooth muscle tissue* of, for example, the digestive tract, trachea, bronchi, urinary bladder, and gall bladder. It is also rather abundant in *multiunit* forms, contributing, for example, to the contractile properties of arterioles, the iris and ciliary body of the eye, the capsule of the spleen, precapillary sphincters, and the *piloerector muscles* attached to hair follicles (active when your "hair stands on end!").

- Skeletal muscle tissue consists of relatively large fibers (cells) grouped into bundles called *fasciculi* (from the Latin for "little bundles"). As is illustrated in Figure 3.1 on the following page, the fibers are multi-nucleated, appear striped (striated), have a polarized cell membrane (*sarcolemma*), and are innervated at the *myoneural junction* by efferent *alpha-moto neuron* fibers emanating from the ventral (stomach-side) root of the spinal cord. Muscle tissue also contains afferent nerve fibers that originate in *muscle spindles* and *Golgi tendon organs*, delivering sensory information to the central nervous system (Schneck 1992). More about that later.

The striated skeletal muscles of the human body are *voluntary*, i.e., they are under conscious control, and are attached to bones by strong cords called *muscle tendons*. When you want to move part of your body, your brain sends impulses via the efferent alpha-motor neurons to the muscles, "telling" them to contract (shorten). By virtue of their contractile properties, muscles, being *force transducers*, act via their tendons to pull on the bones to which they are attached, thus creating a lever-type rotation around the joints (pivot points) at which the bones articulate (Schneck 1992). The result is either a maintenance of postural balance and equilibrium, or locomotion of parts or all of the animal body. But, since muscles can only pull—they can't push— all of these activities are accomplished by them acting in pairs, while one muscle (the *agonist*) contracts to pull a bone one way, its partner (the *antagonist*) relaxes; and vice versa when the bone needs to be pulled the other way.

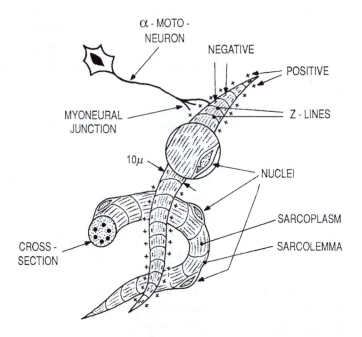

Figure 3.1 Polarized (inside negative relative to outside) striated skeletal muscle fibers. Each is a single, multi-nucleated cell, innervated at the myoneural junction by an alpha-moto neuron originating in the ventral (stomach-side) root of the spinal cord.

- Cardiac muscle is put in a class all by itself because: on the one hand, it has the anatomic/physiologic/mechanical attributes of striated skeletal muscles, yet, on the other hand, it shows electrical-stimulation/excitation-contraction behavior, and the involuntary characteristics more typical of smooth muscle tissue. This muscle is located in only one place—the heart—and serves only one function—to participate in the contractile phases 2 and 3 of the *cardiac cycle* described in Chapter 2.

Major anatomical features of the skeletal system

Actually, we have already said a good deal about this system. In Chapter 1 you were introduced to:

- *connective tissue*, to which category of tissue most of the skeletal system belongs
- the *synovial* fluid that lubricates human joints
- the *articular cartilage* (*chondrocyte* cells) or *gristle* that covers the articulating surfaces of bones, so that they can "slide" smoothly over one another

- *ligaments* (white, *fibrous cartilage*) that maintain the alignment among articulating bones and secure them to one another

- bone *marrow*, occupying the medullary cavity of bone tissue, and responsible for blood cell production (*hematopoiesis*)

- the various types of cells that are included in bone tissue, *osteocytes*, of which there are almost 100 billion in total, appearing as two basic types: (i) *osteoblasts* (germ cells from which bone is manufactured); (ii) *osteoclasts* (giant, multi-nucleated cells that *resorb* bone tissue by lysing and dissolving it)

- the *bones* themselves, which contain *osseous tissue* that comes in three basic types: (i) hard, *compact;* (ii) soft, *spongy;* (iii) *trabecular* ("little beams"). We also mentioned that there are 206 of them, which we now list specifically in Table 3.1.

Table 3.1 Major anatomical features of the skeletal system
ANATOMICAL STRUCTURE

• 206 bones:	• 1 sternum (breast bone)
° 29 skull bones:	• 64 upper extremity bones:
› 8 cranial bones:	› 2 clavicles (collar)
- 1 occipital (back of head)	› 2 scapulae (shoulder)
- 2 parietal (skull "wall")	› 2 humerus (upper arms)
- 1 frontal (forehead)	› 2 ulna (outer lower arm)
- 2 temporal (side of head)	› 2 radius (inner low arm)
- 1 sphenoid (base of skull)	› 16 wrist *carpals:*
- 1 ethmoid (contains sinuses)	- 2 navicular; 2 lunate;
° 14 facial bones:	- 2 trapezium; 2 hamate;
- 2 nasal (nose)	- 2 trapezoid; 2 pisiform;
- 2 maxillary (jaw bones)	- 2 triquetrum; and,
- 2 palatine (roof of mouth)	- 2 capitate
- 2 zygomatic (cheek)	› 38 bones of the hand:
- 1 mandible (lower jaw)	- 10 palmar *metacarpals*
- 2 lacrimal (eye orbits)	- 28 finger *ossa manus:*
- 1 vomer (nasal septum)	* 3 *phalanges* per digit
- 2 inferior nasal conchae (inner nasal "shells")	* 2 per *pollex* (thumb)
› 6 ear auditory ossicles:	• 62 lower extremity bones:
- 2 "hammers" (malleus)	› 2 pelvic (hip)
- 2 "anvils" (incus)	› 2 femurs (thigh)
- 2 "stirrups" (stapes)	› 2 patellas (knee caps)
› 1 hyoid (supports tongue)	› 2 tibias (shins)
	› 2 fibulas (calfs)
	› 14 ankle *tarsals:*

cont.

ANATOMICAL STRUCTURE	

• 26 movable vertebrae:
  › 7 cervical, neck, including: C-1: the atlas, and C-2: the axis
    - 12 thoracic, chest
    - 5 lumbar, lower back
    - 1 sacral (5 bones, fused)
    - 1 coccygeal (tail bone, 4 bones, fused)
• 24 (12 pairs) thoracic ribs:
  › 7 Pairs of *costae* are "true" attached to *sternum*
  › 3 pairs of *costae* are "false" attached to true ribs
  › 2 pair of *conchae* "float"
	- 2 calcaneus (heel)
	- 2 talus; 2 cuboid
	- 2 navicular (instep)
	- 2 primary cunneiform
	- 2 secondary cunneiform
	- 2 tertiary cunneiform
	› 38 bones of the feet:
	  - 10 plantar *metatarsals*
	  - 28 toe *ossa pedis:*
	    * 3 *phalanges* per toe
	    * 2 per *hallux* (big toe)
	    * 2 *longitudinal*, and
	› 1 *transverse* arch per foot
	• Bone marrow (blood cells)

In Chapter 2, we elaborated on:

- the *alimentary canal*, which includes skeletal structures such as the jaw, teeth, hard palate, and pharynx

- the *respiratory tract*, which includes skeletal structures such as the nose, ethmoid bone (contains the sinuses), various types of cartilage, larynx, and bony trachea

- the *circulatory system*, where we devoted a separate section to blood cell production (*hematopoiesis*) in bone marrow.

So…what is left to say about the skeletal system? Well, among other things, this system acts as a *mineral reservoir* for most body *ash*, which includes: phosphorus, magnesium, fluorine, chlorine, iron, and up to 99 percent of the organism's supply of calcium. In fact, that's why *osteoclasts* exist. That is to say, so important is calcium for the proper function of muscles, nerves, and cell metabolism, that no less that four tiny *parathyroid* glands of the endocrine system exist for the sole purpose of maintaining blood calcium levels at proper values. Part of the activity of these glands is manifest in the corresponding activity of osteoclasts.

The parathyroid glands straddle the thyroid gland (hence their name). Each is about the size of a pea, and each manufactures and secretes the hormone *parathormone*. Should blood calcium levels fall below "normal," 8.4–11.00 mg/dl plasma (mean, 9.7), the parathyroids go to work secreting parathormone, which does two things: (i) by itself, stimulates the biochemical dissolution of bone tissue; and, (ii) enhances the activity of osteoclasts to increase bone resorption. Both have the effect of increasing the concentration of blood calcium—as do, also, an increased rate of calcium absorption from the small intestine, and an increased rate of calcium reabsorption in the kidneys.

However, if blood calcium levels rise much above 11.00 mg/dl plasma, several things happen to bring it back down again, i.e., (i) calcium absorption from the small intestine drops; (ii) the rate of calcium reabsorption in the kidneys slows; (iii) the activity of osteoclasts is inhibited; (iv) the release of parathormone from the parathyroid glands is considerably reduced; and, (v) the thyroid gland kicks in to secrete the hormone *calcitonin* (or *thyrocalcitonin*), which blocks bone resorption and thus keeps the calcium safely tucked away in the bone matrix.

Evidence of *hypo-parathormone* release is a hyper-excitability of nerves and muscles (*tetany*), cataracts, teeth defects, bone lesions, and hair, nail and skin disturbances. Evidence of *hyper-parathormone* release is a generalized hypo-excitability of nerves and muscles (*laxity*), reduced muscle tone, increased bone fragility (due to resorption), and muscular weakness.

The skeletal system also provides structural support and shape to the body, as it:

- protects such vital organs as the brain, spine, lungs, and heart, and the very important bone marrow

- prevents us from being "crushed" by aerodynamic loading at sea level, and hydrodynamic loading down to certain ocean depths

- is constructed as a very sophisticated *composite material*—a meshwork of fibers and minerals that make it both strong and light. Because of this inherent strength, bones act as *compression load-bearing* structural elements in parallel with muscles, tendons, and ligaments acting as the *tensile load-bearing* elements of the physiologic system. Thus, we are able to assume certain complex anatomical *postures*, "carry our own weight," resist the pull of gravity, and otherwise tolerate the forces that we encounter as we go about performing our activities of daily living.

And finally of course, there's the role of bones as *levers* that give us a *mechanical advantage* to tolerate such internal and external forces, do meaningful work, and move about at will (when all is working properly!). Which brings us to the system of *joints*.

Major anatomical features of the articular system

The pivot points at which bones (*levers*) meet (*articulate*), and around which they rotate, are called *joints* (*fulcra*). In the body, joints are of three basic types: immovable (*syn-arthroses*), partially movable (*amphi-arthroses*), and freely movable (*di-arthroses*, or *synovial*).

- *Syn-arthroses:* the eight cranial bones, 14 facial bones, three fused bones of the hip—*ilium, ischium,* and *pubis* comprising the *innominate* ("un-named") bone of the *pelvic girdle*—and the five fused vertebrae that make up the triangular-shaped *sacrum* at the base of the vertebral column (see Table 3.1) are all examples of immovable joints. What they share in common is that the bones articulate at visible "seams," called *sutures*—and these are sealed so firmly (by a thin layer of dense fibrous connective tissue), that they allow no relative motion to take place at the articulating sites. End of story.

- *Amphi-arthroses:* these are joints that allow the articulating bones to *glide* smoothly over one another, but constrained—by cartilage, ligaments, and geometrical configurations—from having total freedom of motion relative to each other. Examples in the body are many, including the articulations between the:

  ○ vertebrae (fibro-*cartilage* connections) of the backbone that allow the trunk to twist and bend

  ○ radius and ulnar bones of the forearm that allow the wrist to be turned up (*supination*) or down *(pronation)*

  ○ tibia and fibular bones of the lower leg

  ○ chest bone (*sternum*) and rib cage (*sternocostal* joints)

  ○ heads, tubercles (bony eminences), and necks of the ribs at *costovertebral* (rib-vertebrae)*, costochondral* (rib-cartilage), and *sternoclavicular* (chest-collar bone) joints

  ○ small bones of the wrist (*carpals*) and ankle (*tarsals*)

  ○ collar bone *(clavicle)* and shoulder blade (*scapula*), at the *acriomioclavicular* joint that allows forward and backward movements of the shoulder

  ○ sacrum and coccyx (*sacrococcygeal* joint)

  ○ innominate (hip) bone and sacrum (*pubic* joint).

- These are just a few. Note that joints are *named* according to which bones articulate at that anatomical site, such as radio-ulnar, tibio-fibular, and so on. They are also classified by *type* (immovable, partially movable, freely movable) and *degrees of freedom* in motion, as we shall see below.

- *Di-arthroses (synovial):* these joints allow the most relative freedom of movement between bones, and they are further classified according to *how much* freedom that is. Thus, we have:

  ○ *trochoid* uniaxial motion (from the Greek *trochos*, meaning "a wheel"), akin to the rotation of a *motor* shaft around its center line, exemplified by the articulation of C-1 (the *atlas*) with C-2 (the *axis*), which allows you to pivot your head as if saying "No!" back and forth at the neck.

  ○ *ginglymus* uniaxial motion (from the Greek *gigglymos*, meaning "hinge"), akin to the rotation of the *spoke* of a wheel around its axis, exemplified by the jaw (*temporo-mandibular*), ankle (*talo-crural*), and elbow (*humero-ulnar*) joints.

- *condyloid* biaxial motion (from the Greek, *kondylos*, meaning "knuckle"), akin to moving along the two convex (oval), outside surfaces of an automobile tyre, exemplified by the wrist (*carpo-radial*) and knuckle (*metacarpophalangeal*) joints, and the articulation of the vertebral column (C-1, the *atlas*), with the occipital bone of the cranium, i.e., the *atlanto-occipital* joint, which allows you to (i) nod your head up and down as if declaring "Yes!" and (ii) tilt your head back and forth from shoulder to shoulder.

- *saddle* biaxial motion: convex in one direction but concave in the other, just like moving along the surface of a horse saddle, exemplified by the *pollar* (*carpo-metacarpal*) *joint* at the base of the thumb, where it articulates with the palm of the hand.

- *enarthrosis* tri-axial motion (from the Anglo-Saxon, *en*-meaning "on," and the Greek *arthron*, meaning "joint"), in the purest ball-and-socket sense— restricting action least of all and allowing three-dimensional rotation around any axis in space...exemplified by the articulation of the head of the humerus with the *glenoid cavity* of the scapula, i.e., the *shoulder joint*, and the head of the femur with the *acetabulum* of the innominate (pelvic) bone, i.e., the *hip joint*, allowing movement of the arms and legs, respectively, in almost any direction.

All freely movable joints, regardless of how many degrees of freedom they allow, contain a joint cavity filled with a lubricating *synovial* fluid that has both the consistency and appearance of "egg whites"—hence its name: *syn*, meaning "like," and *ova*, meaning "eggs."

The architecture of the musculoskeletal system illustrates yet another basic anatomical design principle, one that can be appreciated only after we say a few words about levers and leverage.

Levers and principles of leverage

A *lever* is a device that consists of a "handle" (for example, a *bone*), that is attached along its length to some "pivot point," *fulcrum*, around which it rotates (e.g., an anatomical *joint*). Operating this lever is a force, called the "effort" such as one generated by a contracting *muscle*. The force pulls on the lever at some point along its length (e.g., where a muscle is attached, or *inserts* into a bone by a *tendon*). The distance from the pivot point (*fulcrum, joint*) to where the effort acts on the lever (muscle *insertion point*) is called the *lever arm*.

Now, the whole idea of the device is that the "effort" (muscle force), acting at the "lever arm," should be able to rotate the lever (bone) around its fulcrum (joint), and thus produce some desirable effect. But that's not as easy as it sounds because most often, such rotation is impeded by some *resistance* to moving. The resistance might derive from:

- *friction* in the joint (anatomically minimized by both cartilage and lubricating synovial fluid)

- the *weight* (*gravitational load*) of the bone (lever) involved (anatomically minimized by endowing bones with a high strength-to-weight ratio)

- some extraneous *counter-effort* (for example, the activity of *antagonist* muscles, or a mechanical loading on the bone over and above simple gravity) that works *against* the attempted action of the *agonist* muscle ("effort")

- *all of the above*, and perhaps more opposing influences.

But here's the point: the *effectiveness* of the "effort" in generating the desired rotation of the lever depends on how close it is to the fulcrum. If the effort acts far away from the fulcrum—i.e., has a *long lever arm* (as is the case, for example, for a wheelbarrow or crowbar)—then it is *very* effective at getting good results, especially if the net resistance against which it is acting is distributed *between* the fulcrum and the point of action of the effort. Technically, the latter situation defines what is known as a *second-class lever.*

The human body is endowed with very few second-class levers, the most notable of which is the jaw. Its second-class construction is why the jaw can generate such huge chewing power—being able to generate strong "bite forces" to crush things with its teeth. Rising up onto the balls of your feet—which generates large ground-reaction forces—also involves the powerful second-class lever action of the musculature acting on the calcaneus (heel bone) and other bones of the foot. But that's about it! With very few exceptions, the tendons of striated skeletal muscles insert into their respective bones very close to the joint around which they act—giving them very short lever arms, and thus compromising their ability to generate much power, i.e., have significant *leverage* action with which to rotate the lever.

In the latter case, if the fulcrum (joint) lies *between* the muscle insertion point and the resistance against which it acts—a "see-saw" arrangement, as is the case for the *triceps brachii* muscle acting to *extend* ("straighten") the forearm at the elbow joint—the lever is called *first class.*[2] On the other hand, if the muscle insertion point and the resistance against which it acts both lie on the *same side* of the fulcrum—a "sugar tongs" arrangement wherein the resistance is located further away from the fulcrum than is the effort, as is the case for the *biceps brachialis* muscle acting to *flex* ("bend") the forearm at the elbow joint—the lever is called *third class.* In either case, the *leverage* does *not* favor force, but it *does* favor speed. That is to say, given enough effort to get the lever to move, the resistance against which it acts will gain much speed, because that speed is directly proportional to how far the *resistance* is from the joint—which, for the first- and third-class levers of the human body, is much larger than is the point at which the muscle tendon inserts into the bone. Thus, we have:

---

2 The crowbar is actually a first-class lever, but, unlike the triceps, it has a *long* lever arm compared with that of the resistance against which it acts.

Anatomical design principle number 4: The human body is a machine built for speed, agility, and range of motion, at the expense of force (and power)—i.e., it is a *kinematic* body, at the expense of being a *kinetic* one. It can perform relatively easily, those tasks that involve *rapid movement with light objects.* We are, by design, *mobile* creatures, not particularly powerful ones. Thus, when faced with tasks that require heavy exertion, we either avoid them altogether, or invent machines (like crowbars and wheelbarrows) to do the work for us.

That having been said, we close this chapter by saying a few words about an issue that confronts many music therapists in their practice—one having to do with *balance and equilibrium.*

Principles of balance and equilibrium

Have you ever wondered why, under the influence of gravity, we don't walk around all day with our jaws hanging open, or our heads tilted downward, or how we are simply able to stand erect and maintain a vertical posture, working against gravity? Well, if the truth be told, we can't! Gravity is always there, trying to knock us down. So how do we resist that tendency? Answer: through anatomical structures called *muscle spindles, Golgi tendon organs, semi-circular canals, otolith organs,* and *Pacinian corpuscles.* Working together with the central and peripheral nervous systems (Chapter 4), and our senses of sight, sound, and touch (Chapter 5), these specialized sets of *kinesthetic sense organs* are intimately connected to postural reflexes that orient the body in space, and provide feedback information concerning its dynamic relationship to its environment…and vice versa. A few examples will suffice to make the point, beginning with our ability to resist gravity.

The myotatic (proprioceptive) reflex

So…how *do* we manage to stand erect? In fact, we don't! The process of standing straight up is the process of swaying back and forth imperceptibly. You see, embedded deep within the belly of certain postural striated skeletal muscle fibers are numerous tiny "stretch receptors" called *muscle spindles* (Schneck 1992). Their purpose is to monitor by how much a muscle is being passively stretched. Should that stretch exceed certain prescribed values (*operating set points,* programmed into the spindle's frequency-response characteristics), the spindles signal the central nervous system to activate the respective muscle to contract, via what is called the *myotatic reflex* (also known as the *monosynaptic reflex arc* (MSR) the *stretch reflex,* the *myotactic reflex,* and the *proprioceptive reflex*—more commonly referred to as the "knee-jerk response"). The idea is to allow a muscle to maintain a relatively constant length by contracting in response to being stretched beyond that length.

The association of the myotatic reflex with the "knee-jerk" derives from the fact that if one crosses one's legs and then sharply "taps" the loose-hanging leg just below the knee cap, the lower leg suddenly extends outward, "jerking" at the knee in a kicking fashion. This happens because the *patella* (from the Latin for "a small pan") is a lens-shaped bone embedded in the tendon of the thigh muscle (*quadriceps*), which tendon inserts into the shank bone (*tibia*) via the *patellar tendon*. Thus, if this tendon is slightly stretched—by "tapping" it—that stretch is transmitted through the knee cap to the quadriceps muscle, which sets off the MSR. The quadriceps muscle thus spastically contracts, hence, the knee "jerk."

But we digress. Getting back to gravity…it is literally (and practically) impossible for anyone to stand perfectly erect in such a way that the body's center of gravity (c.g., located slightly above the "belly button") is: (i) *exactly* above, and (ii) *exactly* aligned with a point on the ground, located *between* the feet, through which a line drawn perpendicularly from the c.g. would pass. Thus, in "real life," the *actual* line drawn from the *actual* location of the c.g. through that *theoretical* point on the ground will invariably be "tilted" due to the influence of gravity. Suppose it tilts so that I am "leaning" slightly forward. Gravity tries to pull me down on my stomach. Postural muscles in the back of my legs, abdomen, and thorax are stretched by this "leaning forward" response to the gravitational pull. The muscle stretch triggers the myotatic reflex and the postural muscles contract, pulling me back to keep me from falling forward.

But inertia and instability now cause me to "overshoot," tilting me backward. Gravity again tries to knock me down, this time, on my back. Now postural muscles in the *front* of my legs, abdomen and thorax are being stretched, again triggering the MSR. Thus, *these* muscles contract, pulling me forward and starting the cycle all over again. Back and forth, back and forth, on it goes. In other words, maintaining a vertical posture is just the process of periodically rocking back and forth in response to alternating activation of the monosynaptic reflex arc, in response to the influence of gravity.

So why don't you "see" me rocking back and forth when I stand erect? Because, thankfully, *my* myotatic reflex is working properly—so fast (on the order of milliseconds or less) that the *amplitude* of the periodicity (i.e., how "far" I tilt in either direction) is so tiny, and its *frequency* (i.e., how many times per second the "back and forth" motion fluctuates) is so high, that the movements are totally unnoticeable to you, and imperceptible to me. I "think" I am standing perfectly still and upright. Notice I said "thankfully," because neurological disorders can affect and impede this reflex pathway. Such afflictions manifest themselves by increased and *very* noticeable postural sway when one attempts to "stand still." Such sway, which, if serious enough can actually cause one to lose one's balance, thus becomes a valuable, quantifiable clinical variable for assessing the extent of neurological damage in any given patient.

Of particular interest to the music therapist, one might add that the *sensitivity* to stretch of muscle spindles is controlled by the brain (Schneck 1992). This makes them particularly irritable during periods of extreme emotional stress, such as perceived threats to survival, fear, distasteful or hostile environments, anger, and so on. In turn, irritable muscle spindles cause the musculature of the body to be supersensitive— preparing it to mobilize in order to "flee or fight," as the situation dictates. That's the good news. The bad news is that hyper-sensitive muscle spindles cause one to become "jumpy" when nervous. The knees start shaking; one develops tics and twitches; begins to tremble; becomes hyper-reflexive; cries at the slightest provocation, and so on—all because the muscle spindles themselves have been mobilized to action by the central nervous system. As a music therapist, be especially cognizant of this aspect of musculoskeletal function, and be prepared to deal with it—perhaps by using *music* to calm the spindles.

Labyrinthine reflexes

Note the use of the word "proprioceptive" to describe the myotatic reflex. Derived from the Latin *proprius*, meaning "one's own," and *ceptus* from *capere*, meaning "to take," *proprioception* refers to our awareness (without "looking") of our "own" body position/posture, movement (and *resistances* to same), disequilibrating forces, spatial orientation of the limbs, and weight, in relation to the body. There are numerous proprioceptive reflexes in the body, one of which was described earlier. Others derive from muscle tendon receptors (*Golgi tendon organs*), joint receptors (*Pacinian corpuscles, Ruffini endings, Meissner's nerve endings, Golgi endings*), and from two of the three major divisions of the inner ear—the *semicircular canals*, and the *vestibule* (the third, *cochlea*, will be addressed in Chapter 5). In fact, proprioceptive reflexes are *too* numerous and complex to be described here (for details, see Schneck 1990, 1992), but a couple of the ones known as *labyrinthine reflexes* are worthy of consideration.

The *labyrinth* refers to two anatomical regions in each ear, illustrated in Figure 3.2 on the following page: the *semicircular canals*, of which there are three (inter-connected) on either side of the head, oriented mutually perpendicular to one another, and the *otolith organs*, of which there are two on either side of the head: the *saccule*, and the *utricle* (*note*: the otolith organs lie behind the cochlea and in front of the semicircular canals, forming the middle part of the inner ear, called the *vestibule*).

The labyrinth contains a specialized set of *kinesthetic* sense organs that are responsive to *linear* (vestibule) and *angular* (semicircular canals) movement, acceleration and velocity of the organism, as well as vibration and impact. These sensory "transducers" are directly responsible for providing feedback information to the central nervous system about the kinematic state of the body; and they are instrumental in initiating postural reflexes that orient and stabilize the body in space. More importantly, from the point of view of the music therapist, because of the intimate anatomical connection between the labyrinth, which is concerned with balance and equilibrium, and the cochlea, which is concerned with hearing, there is an inherent symbiotic relationship between the structures of the inner ear and music!

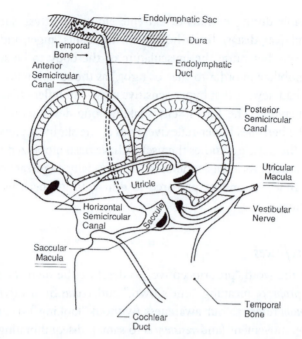

Figure 3.2 Schematic representation of the architecture of the labyrinth
of the inner ear (semicircular canals and vestibule)

So…briefly…the semicircular canals are derived from hollowed-out portions at the base of the temporal bones on both sides of the skull. They have a common origin at the utricle, and the interior of the canals contains a fluid called *endolymph* that bathes a weblike, gelatinous material called the *cupula*. Embedded in the cupula are the ends of hair-like sensory-receptor cells which emanate from the temporal bone, and hence move with the head when it rotates. At their base, these cells are attached to sensory nerve fibers located in the *crista acustica*. These eventually communicate with nerve fibers that ultimately combine to form the *vestibular branch* of the *eighth cranial nerve* (see Table 4.1 in Chapter 4), which carries sensory information to the *vestibular nuclei* situated at the boundary of the *medulla* and *pons* of the brain.

To experience how the semicircular canals work, do the following experiment: hold either hand about 10–12 inches in front of your face, with your palm directly in front of and turned toward your eyes. Keeping your head perfectly still, move your hand rapidly back and forth, left to right to left several times and try to keep your eyes fixed on your hand as it moves—*without moving your head!* Not too easy, is it? Now, instead, keeping your hand perfectly still, rotate your head rapidly, back and forth, left to right to left several times, keeping your eyes fixed on your hand. Much easier? It should be!

That's because, in the latter case, the *motion* of your head—and the semicircular canals that move with it—deforms (bends) the sensory hair cells that are embedded in the cupula/endolymph, which, because of its own stagnant inertia, *lags* the head motion. Deformation of the hair cells activates the *tracking reflex*, which is to say, through the eighth cranial nerve, the semicircular canals transmit the motion of your head to the brain, which promptly responds by sending motor signals to the musculature of your eyes. These motor signals are synchronized with the movement of the head so that, when your head is rotating one way, your eyes are being rotated the other way *at exactly the same angular speed at which your head is turning!* Thus, via this tracking reflex, you are able easily to fix your gaze on your hand. In the first case, when your head is *not* moving, that reflex action is not activated, and so, you have great difficulty keeping your eyes fixed on the moving hand, tracking and staying focused on the movement. But, again, we emphasize that this experiment works *because your tracking reflex is working properly!* As a music therapist, be on the lookout for neurological impairments that can upset postural reflexes, causing balance and equilibrium problems that need to be appreciated.

Signals transmitted by the vestibular system are also important for maintaining the tone of antigravity muscles and for supporting one's balance and equilibrium as the body *falls* to one side, forward, or backward. For example, most of us have experienced the tendency to "grab" for support after tripping or inadvertently starting to fall, or as you doze off to sleep in a sitting position, suddenly "jerking" your head up and becoming erect in the chair to avoid collapsing if your body "slumps" too far from an equilibrated, balanced position. This is an illustration of the *righting reflex.*

There are many more that, as I said, are too numerous to explore here, but the interested reader might wish to see Schneck (1992) and other musculoskeletal anatomy books for further details. I think for our purposes in this book, we've made the point. Thus having said a great deal so far about nerves, nerve impulses, and nerve networks, let's take a closer look!

CHAPTER 4

The *Digital* Living Engine/Instrument

Like the flashing yellow lights that warn of a red traffic signal ahead, or those that capture our attention on the marquee of a theatre—on/off, on/off—the essence of physiologic information processing through the activity of action potentials in *excitable* tissues is coded into the binary digits: on and off, i.e., *whether* ("on") or *not* ("off") the *anatomical* unit of information processing is "firing." *Firing* means electrically *discharging* from a polarized, "resting" state (see Figure 3.1 on page 94 and Schneck 1990, 1992; Schneck and Berger 2006). This anatomical unit is the "charged-up" *neuron*, or nerve cell, to which we were introduced in Chapters 1 and 2, and which is illustrated in Figure 4.1.

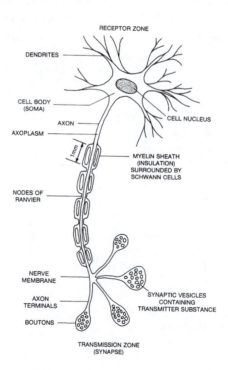

Figure 4.1 Schematic illustration showing the essential
features of a "typical," myelinated, motor neuron

The anatomical unit of information processing: the polarized neuron

All neurons have four basic components:

1. One or more input elements, called *dendrites.*

2. An integrative cell body, called a *soma.*

3. An active transmission line, or *axon,* which may (*myelinated*) or may not (*unmyelinated*) have a fatty material insulation.

4. One or more output elements called *terminals,* the ends of which flare out into bulb-like swellings called *boutons.* These contain up to 300,000 tiny *synaptic vesicles,* within which are stored active chemical substances called *neurotransmitters.*

"Charged up" means, literally, an axon actively *polarized*—inside negative relative to outside—to a net trans-membrane voltage, called the *resting potential* that makes the nerve "ready-to-fire," like a row of upright dominoes ready to be knocked over. "Fire" means turned "on," which corresponds to a *total depolarization* from its resting state of the *entire* nerve—*all* the dominoes are sequentially knocked down, front to back. The latter is an "all-or-none" response to an *adequate stimulus* of sufficient strength, i.e., the nerve either "fires" or it doesn't, like flipping a light switch. Depolarization begins when the dendrites are sufficiently provoked, i.e., the "lead domino" is knocked over *far enough,* hit with enough force to strike the next one down the line and thus start a chain reaction. This provocation initiates a cascading sequence of events—a *depolarization wave* called an *action potential*—that travels down the axon at a specific speed, all the way to its terminal branches. The propagation of an action potential is strictly a one-way event: input dendrites to output boutons.

The physiologic units of information processing: neurotransmitters

The *physiological* units of information processing are quantized packets of *neurotransmitters* that are released from synaptic vesicles in response to action potentials—acetylcholine and norepinephrine being two of the more than 50 that have been identified (Siegel *et al.* 1981). Each time a nerve "fires," the impulse reaching its terminal branches causes a *quantum amount* of the neurotransmitter contained in its synaptic vesicles (*terminal boutons*) to be discharged ("squirted") into a very tiny region called a *synapse*—from the Greek *syn-,* meaning "with," and *aptein,* meaning "to touch."

The higher the *firing frequency* of a nerve—i.e., the greater the number of action potentials reaching the axon's terminal branches—the more neurotransmitter is "squirted" into the synaptic region. Thus, although *each* action potential is an all-or-none response, action potentials can "add up" in the synaptic region, depending on the strength and persistence of the adequate stimulus. This is called a *graded response*. Moreover, since the synaptic junction is a gap between the terminal branches of the firing neuron and the downstream receptor sites of its targets, it, too, can act as a summation region where contributions arriving from many nerve terminals that empty into that particular synapse can be integrated to create a *net* signal (*compound action potential*) that is transmitted to (i.e., "touches") another nerve, muscle, or secretory gland.

Why the gaps?

- *Anatomical design principle(s) number 5:* One obvious reason is *precision* and *control* in information processing. That is to say, as mentioned above, the creation of synaptic junctions allows more than just one cell to influence the next one. Thus, *neural networks* are established that can:

    - mix and match signals, generating *integrated impulses* or *compound action potentials*

    - *modulate* them

    - combine information coming in from different sources, responding to different *adequate stimuli*, thus allowing for *cross-referencing* and checking for *self-consistency* in a process called *sensory integration*, to be described further in Chapter 6

    - short-circuit (*inhibit*) some impulses

    - enhance (amplify, or *excite*) others

    - reroute still others (like switching tracks in a railroad yard)

    - *recruit* additional neural networks as necessary to elicit an appropriate *graded response* to a stimulus…and so on…thus *organizing* the nerve paths to achieve and optimize a desired result.

Various estimates suggest that synaptic junctions associated with any given neural network can accommodate the outputs of some 1000 to as many as 30,000 terminal nerve branches that empty into them. The higher end of this range is typical of the α-motoneuron networks that service the major muscles of the body—part of some 20 billion somatic motor nerves contained in an "average" individual. At the other extreme, the estimated 100 billion neurons contained in the human brain each synapse with some 1000–10,000 other neurons, so that there are huge numbers of possible combinations.

And again, although *each* individual neuron has only two possible all-or-nothing states—on and off—each *synapse*, and the neural network with which it is associated, has many more than that, depending on (i) how many (and which ones) of the neurons feeding into and out of it are "on;" (ii) their firing frequency; and (iii) how many are "off." Thus, neural *networks*, too, can have their own type of "on/off" responsive state wherein their integrated, net output sends an "on" signal—*sometimes*—in response to a given adequate stimulus, yet, at other times, it transmits an "off" signal in response to that *same* stimulus! Furthermore, with 100 different neuroactive chemicals in the brain, some excitatory, others inhibitory, all of the above results in neural network outputs that yield Morse-Code-like *pulse trains*—the body's version of barcodes on product labels. The brain and body understand and "speak" *only* this digital, barcode language, using very sophisticated pattern-recognition algorithms to decipher this binary syntax in order to elicit very specific physiologic function. Therefore, anatomic transducers—sense organs included—serve to *convert* the various types of adequate stimuli to which the organism responds, into this digital syntax "language" before the incoming signals can be processed further. Let's probe some more.

The "language" of the human body

As we said, action potentials are coded into a unique physiologic syntax that target organs and tissues understand and respond to—it is the "language" by which all parts of the body communicate with one another (Deutsch and Micheli-Tzanakou 1987). To understand this better, consider the analogs that follow.

In *verbal* (frequency-based *sonic* energy) and *written* forms of communication, the "language" starts with "sound pictures"—alphabet characters or letters. These are combined to form words, which are spaced apart and strung together into sentences that express a thought or an idea. Sentences are expressed verbally with a certain prosody that conveys the emotion attached to the thought. In writing, we use punctuations—question marks, exclamation points, etc.—to do the same thing. We also organize sentences into paragraphs, which are often assembled into chapters that, perhaps, create a book such as this one. The reader "transduces" the written word to recreate what the author had in mind.

In *music*, the analog of alphabetical "sound pictures" are *notes*, written on a musical staff to define both their sonic frequency (*pitch*) and their temporal value (*duration*). *Words*, separated by "spaces," become in music *measures* separated by "bar lines;" *sentences* become *melodic contours* and *phrases*; *paragraphs* become *sections*; and *chapters* become the *movements* of a piece of music. Finally, the "book" becomes a completed *musical composition*, written in a specific *form*. *Prosody*—"getting the idea across"—in music, is embedded into *rhythmic patterns*, sound intensity (*dynamics*), sound quality (*timbre*), *harmonic sonority*, and *musical articulation* (Schneck and Berger 2006). Thus, performers "transduce" the written composition to recreate what the composer had in mind, and, it is hoped, to express that to an audience.

Note that both these types of communication—written/spoken and composed/ performed—share in common concepts related to *frequency, frequency patterns, intensity, duration, articulation,* and so on. Indeed, there is a basic communication principle illustrated here and one that carries over directly into *physiological syntax*, as well, where now we are dealing with the "language" embedded in action potentials—

our body's "alphabet" or "notes." The specifics of how action potentials are actually generated are beyond the scope of this book (see Deutsch and Micheli-Tzanakou 1987; Junge 1981; Schneck 1990, 1992, and Schneck and Berger 2006 for details). Suffice it to say for our purposes, that coded into this action-potential language are:

1. *which* nerve (or nerve *network*) is firing, to wit:

   a) depending on the nerve/nerve-network that is active, a corresponding *specific* part of the body is represented. If you think of your brain as a "satellite monitoring station," and nerves/nerve networks as having unobstructed "lines of sight" (sensory nerve pathways) to this station, then, effectively, your body has its own *global positioning system* (GPS) that provides location and time information to the GPS base. Your brain, then, is essentially a topographic "map" of the body—knowing *from where* information is coming (i.e., *sensory*) and *to where* it wants to send information (i.e., *motor*). Moreover,

   b) also depending on which nerve/nerve network is activated, a corresponding *specific* type of adequate stimulus, and hence, form of energy, is identified. The type of energy (*sensory modality*) that can excite nerve dendrites—i.e., generate *receptor potentials*—depends on its *frequency of vibration*, which classifies it as being: (i) electromagnetic (e.g., light, electricity); (ii) mechanical (e.g., tactile vibrations, sound); (iii) thermal (e.g., heat, infrared); (iv) chemical (e.g., taste and smell sensations); and so on. If strong enough (see (c) below), these stimuli can cause the *receptor potential* to reach *threshold* values, at which *action potentials* are triggered—the nerve "fires." Different nerves respond to *different* adequate stimuli, so one now knows not only the *part of the body* involved, but also the *type of stimulus* that is exciting it. Finally, we note that:

   c) there is a mathematical difference between the *threshold* potential at which a nerve will "fire"—say, -55 millivolts, mV—and its electrical *resting* potential—say, -90 mV. That difference is called the *depolarization potential* (from resting to threshold) of the nerve, which, in this case is 35 mV (i.e., -90 + 35 = -55). Highly sensitive nerves have very small depolarization potentials, such that a weak stimulus will easily cause them to fire, and vice versa. Thus, again, since *different* nerves have *different* depolarization potentials—that are directly proportional to the *strength* of the stimulus—*which* nerve/nerve network is firing also tells us something about the *intensity* of any given stimulus.[1]

---

1 Hyper- or hypo-polarizing the resting state of a nerve can *bias* its sensitivity to being driven to threshold. That is what allows *sensory* nerves to *adapt*—giving them the ability to "ignore" persistent, but benign stimuli; and *motor* nerves to *skew* muscle spindles—making muscles super sensitive to stretch (as in the discussion in Chapter 3 of both the "knee-jerk" response, and the effects on the musculoskeletal system of emotional stress).

2.   at what *frequency* (action potentials per second) the nerve/nerve network is firing, to wit:

    a)   all depolarized nerves display a brief *refractory period* during which the nerve is "recharging"—*repolarizing* ("setting the dominoes, or bowling pins back up")—while the neurotransmitter is also being enzymatically purged from the synapse. Only then is the nerve ready to fire again…and again…and again, generating a *firing frequency* that can hypothetically reach 2000 impulses/second (although it rarely gets that high, see Schneck 1990, 1992).[2]

    b)   the highest firing frequencies are associated with nerves that have the shortest refractory periods; thus, these are especially responsive to *instantaneous values* of an adequate stimulus. That makes them good measures of its *rate of change* and *persistence* (i.e., how often it repeats itself and how long it lasts).

    c)   nerves that have longer refractory periods fire at slower frequencies and thus, are more accurate measures of the *average value* of an adequate stimulus. *Which* nerve/nerve-network is firing tells us, then:

        i)   the part of the body involved

        ii)   the type of adequate stimulus generating the response

        iii)   its intensity

        iv)   its time-dependence.

But that's not all! Also embedded in this action potential "body language" is information coded into:

3.   the *firing pattern* of the excitation (recall our discussion of *pulse trains, graded responses* and "barcodes"):

4.   how far apart the patterns are *spaced*—a further measure of persistence and periodicity, as is

5.   the *duration* of each action potential burst, and how *continuously active* the nerve (or nerve network) is in a longer-term sense

6.   the *speed* at which the action potentials are racing down the axon, and at which the net compound action potentials propagate away from any given nerve network, or combinations of networks, to wit:

---

2 The frequency range of 0-2000 cycles per second (cps) for nerves is in the seven-octave range of musical note frequencies from 16 to 2048 cps—about four octaves below, to three octaves above "middle C" at 256 cps. This should be of particular interest to music therapists.

a) two-thirds of all nerve fibers in the human body are *unmyelinated*, i.e., they don't have a protective insulation. These thin (down to 0.30 μmD) fibers conduct impulses rather slowly (down to 0.5 m/sec) and are responsible primarily for "housekeeping duties," where speed of propagation is not an issue.

b) one-third of nerve fibers are *myelinated* (insulated), making them thicker (up to 22 μmD) and able to conduct impulses at very high speeds (up to 130 m/sec). This allows them to respond effectively to adequate stimuli that signal dangerous situations, where response speed is of the essence.

c) in general, there is an inverse relationship between velocity and action potential threshold: the more rapidly conducting axons are more easily excited (i.e., have a lower threshold) than are the slower ones.

d) compound nerve networks fire progressively in sequence—from their lowest-threshold, fastest (usually motor) fibers to their highest-threshold, slowest (usually sensory) fibers—so, again, a great deal of information is coded into which axons are active in any nerve network

e) moreover, *afferent* (sensory) neurons sending information *to* the central nervous system, CNS, outnumber by three to one *efferent* (motor) neurons delivering information *from* the CNS.

In summary, the brain is a "GPS, anatomical map" containing a topographic representation of every corresponding region of the body. From each such region, it knows *which* nerve/*nerve network* is firing, at *what frequency*, delivering what type of Morse-Code-like *pulse trains*, containing *what* information, for *how long*, under *what circumstances*, etc. How much information can the brain handle, and what does it do with it? Stay tuned.

Anatomical features of the three nervous systems

The central nervous system: brain and spinal cord

THE TRIUNE BRAIN (ENCEPHALON)

Nearly 25 years ago, the neurologist Paul MacLean (1990) proposed that we actually have *three* brains, nested within one another in order of evolutionary development. The oldest—and predecessor of the cerebral cortex—dates back some 500 million years or more. It is the primitive *archipallium* (literally, "principal cover"), also called the "reptilian" brain because it has remained virtually unchanged in our evolutionary progression from reptiles to mammals to humans. The archipallium includes the *brainstem, cerebellum, globus pallidus*, and *rhinencephalon*. Moving up from the top of the spinal cord, the *brainstem* includes the:

- *Medulla oblongata* (oblong "marrow"), also called the *myel-encephalon*—an enlarged region where are represented all afferent and efferent pathways to and from the spine, and through which *pyramidal tracts* initiate skillful movements of skeletal muscles. The medulla also has a number of vital regulatory and reflex centers that control circulation, breathing, swallowing, vomiting, coughing, and sneezing.

- *Pons varolii* ("bridge")—an intervening pathway from the medulla to the midbrain and cerebellum, containing important motor and sensory nuclei of cranial nerves V, VI, VII, and VIII (see Table 4.1).

- *Reticular* ("netlike") *formation*—extending from the top of the spinal cord, through the brainstem, into the *mesencephalon*, or *midbrain* and *diencephalon* ("through" brain). This formation consists of small, widely scattered areas of gray matter, including centers that coordinate visual tracking reflexes, hearing, postural reflex patterns, and motor movements. We shall have more to say about the reticular formation in Part II. For now, we note that it, together with the *medulla, pons varolii*, 12 *cranial nerves*, a *rhombencephalic cerebral ventricle* (the fourth of five brain cavities that are continuous with the central canal of the spinal cord), and the *cerebellum*, all constitute what is called the *hindbrain*, or *rhombencephalon*.

The tri-lobed, bilateral *cerebellum* ("small brain") is attached to the upper rear of the brainstem, behind the pons and medulla but overhanging the latter. It is the largest part of the rhombencephalon, being involved in control of skeletal muscles, and playing an important role in the coordination of voluntary muscular movements. It is endowed with what is known as "skill memory," and, together with the pons varolii, forms the *metencephalic* portion of the brain.

The *globus pallidus*, or *paleostriatum* is an ancient mass of gray matter containing the earliest basal nerve cells. And finally, since primitive reptiles roamed planet Earth relying for survival primarily on their sense of smell, the archipallium includes as well, the *rhinencephalon*, or "smell brain," or bilateral *olfactory bulbs*. Indeed, this reptilian (or R-) complex of tissues is concerned *purely* with survival functions—so-called *paw-to-jaw* reflexes, including: musculoskeletal balance and equilibrium (posture, locomotion, coordination of muscular activity, etc.), autonomic functions such as breathing and heart rate, levels of alertness (an "early-warning" system for threatening sensory inputs), and primitive types of survival behavior (often aggressive, mean, and self-serving—traits that prevail even in 21st-century Homo sapiens!).

Fast-forwarding about 200–300 million years, we start to evolve the second in this *triune brain* paradigm—the *limbic system*, so-called because it comprises a group of interconnected neural structures arranged in "border-like" fashion (*limbus* is Latin for "a border") surrounding the midline surfaces of the left and right *cerebral hemispheres* at the top of the brainstem. Together with the *archicortex*, this *limbic cortex* forms the *paleocortex* (the "ancient bark"), or *paleoencephalon* ("ancient brain"), and it connects with the brainstem.

The limbic system starts its anatomical journey around the brainstem at the front (anterior), stomach-side (ventral) surface of the cerebral *frontal lobe*, under the *septum pellucidum*—a "translucent partition" that encloses the *fifth cerebral ventricle*. It continues rearward as the *cingulate gyrus* (a "cerebral convolution"), up and over the *corpus callosum*, a bundle of nerve fibers that connect the left and right sides of the brain. Finally, it ends as the *parahippocampal gyrus*, at the medial (toward the midline of the body) surface of the *temporal lobe*.

The limbic system includes the:

- *Hippocampus* ("sea horse," because of its appearance), a ridge along the extension of each *lateral ventricle* (the first, or right; and the second, or left) of the brain. There are two of them—one on each side of the brain, under the *cerebral cortex*, in the *medial temporal lobe*. As we shall see in Part II, the hippocampus plays an important role in tagging and consolidating cognitive information from short-term to long-term memory, and in spatial navigation.

- *Thalamus* ("inner room"), there are also two of these ovoid bodies on either side of the brain, in the lateral wall of the *third (diencephalic) ventricle*. They consist of several *thalamic nuclei* that are "reception centers," receiving all incoming sensory information (except olfactory—smell—which goes directly to the rhinencephalon), and distributing it to appropriate cortical areas for further processing.

- *Amygdala* ("almond," because the amygdaloid bodies are shaped like one)—a group of cerebral nuclei adjacent to the hippocampus. They are commonly referred to as the *emotional brain* because of their ability to arouse pleasant or unpleasant feelings, and generate sentient responses to perceived threats or agreeable stimulation. When the amygdala is active, it suppresses the activity of the hippocampus...but not vice versa.

- *Parolfactory area*, also known as "Broca's area" on the left side of the brain, controlling movements of the tongue, lips, vocal cords, and motor speech area. The music therapist should be especially aware of this area in dealing with non-verbal clients.

- *Mammillary body*, a pair of small, "nipple-shaped," round bodies located on the underside of the brain that play an important role in recollective memory, especially spatial and feeding reflexes.

- *Fornix* (Latin for "arch"), a fibrous band connecting the cerebral lobes.

- *Hypothalamus* ("beneath the thalamus"). Being the chief subcortical region for the integration of sympathetic and parasympathetic nerve activities, it is also important in controlling visceral functions, such as the maintenance of water balance, sugar, and fat metabolism, and the regulation of body temperature and endocrine gland secretions.

The hypothalamus, together with the thalamus and sub-thalamus, form the *diencephalon* ("through brain") or *thalamencephalon*, which includes an uppermost portion—the *epithalamus*—a lowermost portion—the *hypothalamus*—and a rear (posterior) portion—the *metathalamus*.

The limbic system is concerned more generally with *homeostasis*: the maintenance within an acceptable window of physiologic variables critical to life, such as body temperature, heart rate, respiration rate, blood pressure, blood sugar levels, acid-base balance, sleep-wake cycles, etc. This system also adds *fight-or-flight* reflexes to the *paw-to-jaw* reflexes mentioned earlier. That is to say, it moderates behavior related to survival of the individual and the species, such as thirst/hunger reflexes, the drive for sexual fulfillment, and competitive confrontations. Closely connected to the latter are emotional instincts, reactions, and memories, which, again, is why the limbic system is also called the "emotional brain." Indeed, damage to parts of this system can affect our ability to react to situations that require making life-and-death decisions (*any* decisions, for that matter), confirming still further that we are, in fact, creatures of emotion, not reason. Our cerebral ability to reason comes much later—we need to fast-forward again, some 100–150 million years.

At this point in time, we start to develop a *cerebrum*, covered by a one-eighth inch-thin "new mantle" (*neopallium*), or "new bark" (the *cerebral cortex*, or *neocortex*). This convoluted, four-lobed cerebrum is called the *telencephalon*, or "*endbrain*," which, together with the diencephalon, forms the *forebrain*, or *prosencephalon*. For whatever reason(s)—and there are many theories, none proven—we are now endowed with an organ the size of a grapefruit, weighing about as much as a head of cabbage, endowed with a convoluted cortex that, if laid out flat, would stretch across an area 5.5 feet long by 3 feet wide (remember *Anatomical design principle number 1* from Chapter 2?), and wired with more internal connections than there are atoms in the universe! Our brain is divided into approximately equal-sized right and left *cerebral hemispheres*, connected by the *corpus callosum*. In accordance with *Anatomical design principle number 1*, the cerebral cortex is folded into four principal convolutions, called *lobes*, that allow it to fit into the cramped cranial cavity. The lobes—frontal, parietal, occipital, and temporal—are named after the skull bones beneath which they lie (see Table 3.1), and they envelope the cerebral ventricles. A few of their many functions are as follows:

- *Parietal lobe:* receives and processes—via the *somatosensory cortex* (again, a "map" representing the entire organism)—sensory information from various parts of the body, especially related to the special senses of taste and proprioception, and the general sense of taction. It responds to these inputs via the *motor cortex*.

- *Frontal lobe:* is primarily involved in planning, "rational" decision making, and following those with "purposeful" behavior. It is richly and intimately connected to the limbic system.

- *Temporal lobe:* gives us the ability to *perceive*—especially through the special sense of *hearing,* via the *auditory cortex*—and *interpret* what we experience in life, and commit some of those experiences to *memory.*

- *Occipital lobe:* also gives us the ability to *perceive*—this time through our special sense of *sight,* via the *visual cortex*—our world of existence.

Moreover, because we have a neocortex, we can communicate, think, understand, organize, appreciate, create, learn, manipulate symbols (as in mathematical and alphabetical), formulate theories, and deal with "cognitive" functions. Much of the latter we began to develop some four to five million years ago, long after we parted company with the chimpanzees! It progressed in stages that seem to have reached a temporary plateau dating back about one million years—with the lateralization of the brain into right/left specialization. That is to say, although it is not without controversy, a popular belief today is that the *left* brain seems to deal better with temporal/rational/cognitive/linear/verbal types of information processing, whereas the *right* brain appears to be more comfortable with spatial/creative/integrative/ abstract/visual types of activities—but the jury is still out (Edwards 1989; Ornstein and Thompson 1984; Springer and Deutsch 1981). Fortunately for the music therapist, *music* can access *both* sides of the brain with equal facility!

THE CRANIAL NERVES AND SPINAL CORD

There are 12 pairs of *cranial nerves* that originate in the brain and emanate from there *directly* to their respective target organs, without first passing down through the spinal cord. These, and their target organs, are listed in Table 4.1.

Table 4.1 Major anatomical features of both the cerebrospinal and peripheral nervous systems	
ANATOMICAL STRUCTURE	

• Cerebrospinal nervous system:
  ◦ 12 pairs of cranial nerves
    › I: Olfactory (smell sense)
    › II: Optic (sight sense)
    › III: Oculomotor (eyes)
    › IV: Trochlear (proprioception)
    › V: Trigeminal: 3 branches
      - Ophthalmic (cornea)
      - Maxillary (nose, face, scalp)
      - Mandibular (tongue, mastication, chin, teeth, mouth)
	• Peripheral nervous system:
	  ◦ 8 pairs of cervical branches
	  ◦ 12 pairs of thoracic branches
	  ◦ 5 pairs of lumbar branches
	  ◦ 5 pairs of sacral branches
	  ◦ 1 pair of coccygeal branches
	• Intercostal thoracic nerves
	• Major plexuses of central nervous system:

> VI: Abducens (to lateral rectus muscle of the eye)
> VII: Facial (facial expressions, gustation, taste sense)
> VIII: Vestibulocochlear
  - Auditory branch (hearing sense)
  - Vestibular branch (balance and equilibrium)
> IX: Glossopharyngeal
  - Sinus nerve of Hering
  - Tympanic branch (ear)
  - Lingual branch (tongue)
  - Pharyngeal branch (pharynx)
  - Carotid branch
  - Tonsillar branch (tonsils)
> X: Vagus/parasympathetic
> XI: Accessory to trapezius and sternomastoid muscles
> XII: Hypoglossal (tongue)
• Central nervous system:
  ° Brain
  ° Spinal cord
  ° Gray matter (nerve bodies)
  ° White matter (nerve axons)
  ° Connects to autonomic

° Brachial (lower neck to axilla)
  > Musculospiral nerves
  > Rhomboid nerve
  > Radial nerve (forearm)
  > Ulnar nerve (forearm)
  > Median nerve (arm)
  > Infracavicular
  > Posterior thoracic
  > Musculothoracic
  > Circumflex nerves
° Cervical (from C1 to C4)
  - Occipital nerves
  - Auricular nerves
  - Cutaneous nerves
  - Supraclavicular
  - Phrenic (diaphragm)
° Coccygeal (S4 to Co1)
  > Anococcygeal nerves
° Lumbar (L1–L4; psoas muscle)
  > Hypogastric nerves
  > Femoral (crural) nerves
  > Inguinal nerves
  > Lumbar nerves
  > Iliac nerves
° Sacral (front of sacrum; legs)
  > Saphenous nerves
  > Peroneal nerves
  > Popliteal nerves
  > Sciatic nerves
  > Gluteal nerves

The names of cranial nerves I (smell), II (sight), III (oculomotor, innervating five of the seven eye muscles), IV (involved in proprioception and innervating the superior oblique muscle of the eye), VI (another eye muscle), VII (facial), VIII (hearing, balance, and equilibrium), IX (taste), X (vagus), XI (joins the vagus), and XII (tongue), make it a fairly straightforward process to deduce their respective function. The fifth cranial nerve—trigeminal—deserves a bit more explanation. It has three branches (hence its name) that supply the central nervous system with most of the sensory information originating in the head and face. The first branch (ophthalmic) innervates the eyeballs, conjunctiva, lacrimal glands, cornea, eyelids, mucous membranes of the nose, and forehead. The second branch (maxillary) innervates the cheek, tongue, teeth, ear, muscles of mastication, face, scalp, and tonsils. The third branch (mandibular) also innervates muscles of mastication, the tongue, chin, teeth, mouth, taste buds, ears, and cheek. Note further that, in addition to several other functions, nerves III, VII, IX, and X also branch out to become the parallel-to-the-spine *cranial portion* of the *parasympathetic division* of the *autonomic nervous system,* to be described later.

Thirty-one pairs of *spinal nerves* emanate from the *intervertebral spaces* between the bony (vertebral) segments of the *spinal column,* within whose *spinal canal* lies the *spinal cord.* The latter is a 45–46 cm-long (~1.5 ft) ovoid column of nervous tissue extending in the *canal* from the medulla oblongata of the brain to the second lumbar vertebra. It is surrounded by a *pia mater* ("tender," or *pious* "mother") membrane, bathed in *cerebrospinal fluid* (CSF) and fused to the inner surface of the vertebrae by a *dura mater* ("hard mother"). Most notable about this structure are two things:

1. Its vertical, fore-aft, "double S-shaped" curvature that results from assuming an erect posture against the influence of gravity.

2. The fact that it also gives rise to both the *peripheral* and *autonomic* nervous systems.

Moving vertically downward from the head, the spine bends slightly forward (anterior curvature) through the neck. As we continue downward to about the middle of the thorax, this curvature reverses direction, bending slightly backward (posterior curvature) to complete the first backward-facing S-shape. Again the curvature reverses, becoming anteriorly directed as we continue down through the thorax to about the middle of the lumbar region, where it then completes a second—this time forward-facing S-shape—as we end our journey down through the lumbar region into the sacrum. The two anteriorly directed curves in the neck and thoraco-lumbar region are called *secondary curves;* the oppositely directed curves in the thorax and lumbo-sacral regions are called *primary curves.* All of these are normal. *Lateral* (left to right) curvature of the spine—called *scoliosis*—is not! Nor is exaggerated backward curvature in the upper thorax—called *kyphosis* (from the Greek word for "hunchback"), or accentuated forward curvature in the lumbar region—called *lordosis* (from the Greek for "to bend"). These can all result from poor body posture, congenital abnormalities, injury, spinal compression, disease (tuberculosis, syphilis, malignancies), and osteo and/or rheumatoid arthritis.

The peripheral nervous system

The 31 pairs of *spinal nerves* that originate in the *spinal cord* are attached to it by two roots—a *dorsal* (toward the back) *sensory* root carrying *afferent* nerve impulses *to* the CNS, and a *ventral* (toward the stomach) *motor* root discharging *efferent* nerve signals *from* the CNS *to* target organs and tissues. On leaving the spine, the nerves distribute themselves among six basic nerve networks, each called a *plexus* (from the Latin for "a braid"; see Table 4.1).

- The first four pairs of the eight *cervical* (neck) spinal branches give rise to the *cervical plexus.*

- The next four pairs spawn the *brachial* (arm) *plexus.*

- Moving down the spine, 12 pairs of *thoracic branches* yield a network of *rami* (Latin for "a branch") forming a *thoracic plexus* that innervates the *intercostal* ("between the ribs") regions of the chest.

- Next, the first four (out of five) pairs of lumbar spinal branches give rise to the *lumbar* (lower back) *plexus.*

- The remaining pair emanating from the last two of the lumbar branches, plus the first four (of five) pairs of sacral branches, yield the *sacral plexus.*

- To complete the peripheral nervous system, we have the *coccygeal plexus* that issues forth from the last pair of sacral branches and the remaining pair of *coccygeal branches.*

Action potentials carried by the peripheral nervous system:

- activate all moving parts of the organism

- stimulate glandular function

- regulate and coordinate all body activities

- bring about specific responses by which the organism adjusts to *changes* in both its internal and external environments; and, more importantly, *allow* for such adjustments by

- keeping the organism constantly in contact with and aware of its environment, both internal and external.

Again, the first four activities above are collectively referred to as the *motor* function of the nervous system; the last one, its *sensory* function, which we will address in Chapter 5. Recall, also, that *sensory* (afferent) nerve pathways outnumber *motor* (efferent) tracts by about three to one, and *unmyelinated* nerves outnumber *mylenated* (insulated) nerves by about two to one. An important, complementary nervous system that helps the central and peripheral ones in both sensory and motor functions— i.e., "sympathizes" with them—is anatomically derived from both of them. It is the *autonomic* ("automatic") *nervous system,* that has two divisions—a *sympathetic* one and a *parasympathetic* one "alongside it." We already mentioned the role of cranial nerves III, VII, IX, and X of the central nervous system in contributing to the parasympathetic nervous system. Turning now to the role of the peripheral nervous system, we observe that, on entering the spine, nerves of this system further divide into two additional branches—a *white ramus communicans* and a *gray ramus communicans.* These pass—via short *preganglionic efferent nerve fibers*—from the spine to *ganglia* (masses of nerve cell bodies) of the *autonomic nervous system* that runs parallel to the spine.

The autonomic (or visceral) nervous system

The 12 thoracic branches emanating from the spinal cord give rise to the *thoracic portion* of the *sympathetic division* of the *autonomic nervous system*. The first three branches of the lumbar plexus spawn the *lumbar portion* of this system. Derived from the middle three branches of the sacral plexus is the *sacral portion* of the *parasympathetic division* of the *autonomic nervous system;* and, again, emanating from cranial nerves III, VII, IX, and X is the *cranial portion* of this system. Why two systems?

Well, first of all, the *overall* function of the autonomic nervous system (ANS) is to control and maintain the internal environment of our "instrument" *involuntarily*— so we don't have to think about breathing, keeping our heart beating, digesting a meal, etc.—it's *automatic* (thank goodness!). Thus, the ANS sends its own nerve fibers to smooth and cardiac muscle tissue, some exocrine and endocrine glands, and even some skeletal muscle tissue (which is usually under *voluntary* control). This *system*—through a variety of *ganglia* and *plexuses*—innervates primarily portions of the following systems: circulatory, digestive, excretory, respiratory, reproductive, portal, renal...and more!

Second, while not "etched in stone" nor valid without exception, the "rule of thumb" is that whatever the *sympathetic* nervous system does, the *parasympathetic* nervous system does exactly the opposite. Thus, if *sympathetic* nerve stimulation *raises* blood pressure, *parasympathetic* nerve stimulation lowers it. If the former *increases* heart rate, the latter *slows* it. While *sympathetic* stimulation *dilates* the pupils of the eyes, *parasympathetic* stimulation *contracts* them...and so on. We'll get back to this in Chapter 7.

And as is true for all nerves, here, again, the mechanism of action is through *neurotransmitters*—*acetylcholine* from post-ganglionic nerve endings of *parasympathetic* fibers; and *norepinephrine* (noradrenalin) from those of *sympathetic* nerve fibers. Tissue responses to the former derive from *cholinergic* receptor sites on cell membranes; responses to the latter result from the presence of *adrenergic* receptor sites on *target* tissues and organs. There are actually two types of adrenergic receptors: α-receptors that generate *excitatory* responses to norepinephrine stimulation (as well as adrenalin, secreted by the supra-renal glands)...and β-receptors that *inhibit* such responses. Various drugs and pharmaceutical agents can also "block" these receptor sites to "trump" the activity of neurotransmitters and hormones. For more information, see Jacob *et al.* (1982), Siegel *et al.* (1981), and Tortora and Grabowski (1993).

Some closing remarks

The music therapist sees the neuro-musculoskeletal output of this sophisticated engine/musical instrument as being both, mechanical, and emotional. Indeed, this living instrument emotes! As we shall see in Chapter 8, it *needs* to express itself. To reiterate, the human body is, first and foremost, a creature of emotion, not reason— being "reasonable" only when it is inclined to, and has the time and resources to be so—and this aspect of its basic function must be clearly understood by the practicing music therapist, as must *Feature 3* of our "engine," which is addressed in Chapter 5.

CHAPTER 5

The Sentient Living Engine/Instrument

Feature 3 in our developing model of the human body recognizes its ability to be vigilant—consciously or sub-consciously—of both itself and its environment. That ability derives from the fact that the organism can *perceive* ("sense"), and *respond to* ("react" to) *adequate stimuli*. The latter are various forms of *energy* to which the body is exposed, both:

- *internally—corporeal*, from the Latin, *corporeus*, pertaining to "the nature of the body"

- *externally—ambient*, from the Latin, *ambiens*, pertaining to the process of circulating, or "going around."

The "sensing" is accomplished by sets of anatomical *transducers*—organs that can *convert* the various forms of energy to which they respond into a syntax ("language") that the body understands—i.e., *sensory action potentials.* Operating through the *central, peripheral*, and *autonomic* nervous systems (see Chapters 3 and 4), sense organs *monitor* how well the body is doing in its attempts to satisfy its basic physiologic needs and drives. They do so by keeping the CNS continuously aware of what's going on "inside," and constantly cognizant of what's happening in the world "outside," through a *sensory system.*

The sensory system

This system includes two types of transducers:

- *Special senses*—organs of smell, taste, sight, hearing, and balance and equilibrium (*kinesthesis*)

- *General (visceral, corporeal) senses*, i.e.:

  ○ *Tactile* organs responsive to linear and angular acceleration, velocity, displacement, "jerk," impact, vibration, etc.

- *Proprioceptive* organs responsive to spatial orientation, posture, and locomotion of parts or all of the body—with possible adverse consequences related to feelings of disorientation, vertigo, and motion sickness (*note:* some of these, and a few kinesthetic senses of balance/equilibrium were described in Chapter 3; and so...enough for now).

- *Circadian* organs—e.g., the *suprachiasmatic nuclei* of the hypothalamus, responsible for "measuring" *time* and synchronizing the body's internal processes with the daily cyclical events characteristic of our external environment.

- *Homeostatic* organs and tissues responsible for maintaining within narrow, prescribed ranges (*operating set points*):

  › *vital signs*, such as *thermodynamic variables* (including body temperature, blood pressure and volume); respiration rate, heart rate, pulse, etc.

  › *chemical variables*, such as acidity/alkalinity ("pH"), blood glucose concentration, blood gases (O_2, CO_2), toxicity, etc.;

  › and, responding to these...generating corresponding feelings of thirst (in the limit, *dipsosis*), and hunger (in the limit, *limosis*).

- *Piezoelectric* ("pressure electric") tissues and organs that monitor *mechanical variables*, such as deformation, bending, twisting, squeezing, pulling, pushing, etc., and, in response to these generate corresponding sensations, such as pain (*nociception*), fatigue (*bradykinesia*), discomfort (*malaise*), nausea, motion sickness (*vertigo*), itching (*pruritus*), etc.

To the extent that people-to-people *communication skills* are a form of bodily interactions with the environment, one might put *verbal expression* in the category of *sensory perception*. That would then include organs responsible for *generating* sound (see *The larynx* in Chapter 2), amplifying it (*pharynx, sinuses*), and configuring it into a mode capable of being deciphered and interpreted by other human "engines." In fact, carrying this reasoning one step further, the human body's ability to make other "engines" just like it—i.e, *procreate* (*Feature 7* of our anatomic/physiologic paradigm)—can also be classified under *sensory perception*, to the extent that this feature, too, involves:

- male-female sensory *attraction* (through senses of smell, sight, touch, etc.), *stimulation* (through "arousal" senses), and courtship, culminating in copulation (bodily *contact, mating*) via *genital* organs

- thus fulfilling the second strongest of all human drives—i.e., *survival of the species* through *sexual fulfillment*—that results in pleasurable feelings of ecstasy and euphoria.

Various forms of energy, and the biological sensory receptors (ceptors) that respond to them

Energy "likes" to vibrate

The first thing to note is that all perceived reality derives from various types of energy that, in turn, are a product of the physics of our universe (Schneck 2011b). This energy exists in basically two forms—*potential* ("capable" of being, but not yet realized), and *kinetic* ("actually" realized; being; energy in *motion*). Thus, every type of energy *pulsates*—oscillates, *vibrates*—back and forth, back and forth, back and forth, between *potential* (the *source* from which it is derived) and *kinetic* (the *form* in which it is realized) states. Moreover, energy can be *perceived* only in its kinetic state, and only to the extent that its motion can stimulate some anatomical sense organ, and/or, excite some technological transducer. Such sense organs/transducers are called *ceptors*—from the Latin *capere*, meaning "to take." So here's the point: the number of times per second that energy pulsates back and forth between potential and kinetic states is called its vibration frequency, designated "f," and expressed in "cycles per second," *cps*, or *Hertz* (1 Hz = 1 cps); and,

> *that very frequency determines the* **type** *of energy that will be experienced (perceived)— as an "adequate stimulus"—by a corresponding ceptor that is responsive to it.*

For example:

- When a patient has a clinical *x-ray* taken, he or she is typically exposed to energy vibrating at about 700 million cps (700 *mega*hertz)—about a tenth of television frequencies.

- Vibration frequencies used in clinical *ultrasound* are usually in the range 0.5–10 (to as high as 15) megahertz.

- Your *microwave* oven is probably operating in the trillion cps range (about one *tera*hertz), that our body—through thermal, taste, and smell ceptors— experiences as both *heat* and *chemical* energy.

- Increase f about 100 times that amount—to 400–800 terahertz—and it becomes *light* energy, *visible* to us ($f > 800$ terahertz is *ultraviolet* energy; $f < 400$ terahertz is *infrared* energy).

- Slow the vibration frequency all the way down to 20,000 Hz, and we start to *hear* it as *acoustic* energy…down to 20 Hz ($f > 20,000$ Hz is *ultrasonic* energy; $f < 20$ Hz is *infrasonic* energy; musical frequencies lie between 16 Hz— four octaves below "middle C"—and about 8200 Hz—five octaves above middle C.

- Below that, we can still experience energy in *mechanical* forms—through *tactile* senses that range all the way from $f \sim 0$ to vibrational frequencies on the order of 2500 Hz.

Get the picture?

- The *realization* and *experiencing* of energy is all about its *frequency of vibration*.

- The *sensing* and *perceiving* of energy is all about *transduction*…the conversion of a given, *realized* form of energy—the *adequate stimulus*—into another form, electrochemical *action potentials*. That's what our *sensory system* does. Let's take a closer look.

Sensory nerves

A sensory nerve cell looks essentially the same as the motor neuron illustrated in Figure 4.1 of Chapter 4 (page 106), except that the large cell body in the receptor zone region is replaced by a much smaller appendage—the appropriate *ceptor* (transducer). It is anchored to the sensory nerve axon. Ceptors that respond to *external* types of energy—adequate stimuli such as sound, light, electromagnetism, heat, inertia, gravity, and so on—are called *exteroceptors*, and the corresponding perception of those types of energy is designated *exteroception*. Ceptors responding to the same types of stimuli, but derived from *within* the body are called *interoceptors*, and the corresponding perception of the internal milieu of the body is designated *interoception*.

All of these ceptors share in common the fact that the adequate stimulus to which they respond generates in them a *receptor potential*—a slight depolarization of the ceptor membrane at the site of stimulation. Should the intensity (not frequency) of the energy be strong enough, it will bring the receptor potential to *threshold*, and the sensory nerve will "fire," i.e., generate an *action potential* (see Chapter 4). By "strong enough," we mean *of sufficient intensity to generate a depolarization potential in the sensory nerve* (Chapter 4). For example, it is difficult to "see" if there is *light energy* present (i.e., of sufficient *frequency*), but it is too "dim" (i.e., of low *luminescent intensity*) for us to clearly identify exactly what it is we are "looking" at. Similarly, it is difficult to "hear" if there is *acoustic energy* present (i.e., $20 \leq f \leq 20,000$ cps), but so "quiet" (i.e., of low *sonic intensity*—like a soft "whisper"), that we can hardly interpret the exact information that is encoded into the sounds we are hearing.

The key, in all cases, is how close the *receptor potential* is to the *depolarization potential* of the nerve. If the two are not far apart, then a relatively "weak" adequate stimulus can get the nerve to "fire," i.e., bring it to threshold. If the two are not even close to one another, then it takes a stronger adequate stimulus to generate a sensory action potential. This, again, is the essence of the process of *sensory adaptation*, by which a nerve succeeds in "tuning out" persistent, but benign stimuli that it "can't be bothered with." And although, as also discussed in Chapter 4, different nerves exhibit different sensitivities to the strength of the adequate stimulus, they *all* require a *minimum* stimulus intensity before they will fire.

The above discussion should be of particular interest to the music therapist—especially one working with an autistic individual. One of the salient features of autism is the individual's acute sensitivity to the intensity of sensory inputs (Berger 2002; Schneck and Berger 2006). What to you and me might sound like the mere pitter-patter of rain drops softly tapping the roof of the house to an autistic child might sound like very loud shotgun blasts pounding on his/her ear drums. What we might perceive to be soft lighting in a dim room, might, to the autistic child be an annoying glare. What we smell as fragrant, aromatic, or taste as savory or delicious, the autistic child might perceive to be putrid and foul-smelling or having an unpleasant flavor, or being pungent. In other words, the autistic sensory system is *biased* toward very low depolarization potentials. There is not much "room to spare" between an incident receptor potential and that nerve's threshold potential. Result: hyperactive sensory nerves, "inverted" response characteristics, and reactions to stimulation that are counter-intuitive to what one might otherwise expect, given the adequate stimuli involved...including music! We shall have more to say about this in Part II, when we discuss cerebral information processing and the role of the central nervous system. But there is one more point that needs to be made here, which we shall call: *Anatomical design principle number 6:* The sensory system is simply a collection of *transducers* (sense organs) and information-*transmitting* networks that merely convey raw data—in the form of compound sensory action potentials—to specialized regions of the central nervous system, which is thus informed of the corresponding situation that prevails at the site of the sense organ (see Chapter 4). That is to say, *ceptors do just that—sense and transduce—nothing more.* They do not interpret, define, integrate, or give any *meaning* to the data they perceive and transport. That function is left to the CNS. So, your eyes do not "see"—your brain does! Your ears do not "hear," your brain does! Your thermal senses do not tell you if you are "hot" or "cold," your brain does! And so on. This realization has important implications in terms of the research, design, and development of totally implantable *artificial* sense organs. That is to say, in order to duplicate faithfully, the organ they are intending to replace, *synthetic* implants—in addition to being bio-compatible with the host—need only convert the corresponding adequate stimuli into the same physiologic *syntax* ("body language") that the original *anatomic* organs did. If the transduction is true to the original, and the syntax reliable, the brain is convinced, and the artificial implant will do its job as well (or better!) than the organ it replaced. (An amusing aside is that the artificial device can actually be implanted *anywhere* in the body, as long as it is ultimately connected to the appropriate sensory nerve network sending the information to the CNS. Thus, one can literally have "eyes in the back of one's head!")

As we shall discuss further in Part II, the CNS receives, processes, integrates, and evaluates all sensory data—and, *reacts*, if it sees fit to do so. That is, based on the results of the appraisal, the CNS may decide: (a) to do nothing; or, if it does not "like what it sees," or feels the need for a "mid-course correction," or has other reason(s) to process the sensory signals further, it might (b) call for an appropriate physiologic response through the motor portions of the various nervous systems (Berger and Schneck 2003; Schneck 1990; Schneck and Berger 1999, 2006).

Motor networks innervate *effector organs* and *tissues* that actually carry out the desired response (Schneck 1990), as we shall see in Chapter 6 and Part II. For now, we say a few words about the ceptors, themselves.

The special senses (exteroception)

The senses of smell (*olfaction*), taste (*gustation*), hearing (*audition*), seeing (*vision*), and equilibrium (*equilibrioception*) are called "special" because:

- they are associated with the 12 cranial nerves that originate and emanate directly from the brain (see Table 4.1), without passing through the spinal cord

- their respective ceptors (sensory receptors) are located in relatively large sense organs (transducers) located entirely in the head, i.e., the nose, mouth (tongue), ears, eyes, and vestibule.

Because of the close anatomic/physiologic association between hearing and balance and equilibrium (see Chapter 3), the two are often combined into one, and a "fifth, special sense of touch" (*taction*), is added to the other four. Keep in mind, however, that, technically, "touch" is not a *special* sense, but, rather, a *general* one—even though the skin is, indeed, the largest "sense" organ in the human body (in fact, the largest *organ*...period! See Chapter 1).

Table 5.1 Classification of sensory receptors for exteroception

TYPE OF ENERGY/CORRESPONDING SENSE CEPTORS RESPONSIVE TO IT

Mechanoreceptors: Mechanical energy:

- Touch: *taction*; skin tactile receptors in epidermis and dermis
  - 19% Ruffini corpuscles: slowly adapting; wide receptor field for steady, continuous, distributed shear and pressure forces
  - 25% Merkel tactile disks: faster adapting; narrower receptor field for grasping, gripping, feeling things; finger prints
  - 43% Meissner's corpuscles: still faster adapting; even narrower receptive field for kissing, fondling, diffuse loading
  - 3% Pacinian corpuscles: fastest adapting; narrowest receptor field; proprioception; vibration; largest tactile receptors
  - 6% Hair end organs: lever-type skin projections; wind, shear; adapt as rapidly as Meissner's corpuscles
  - 4% free nerve endings: simplest sensory receptors; crude touch, pain, heat, itch; slow, poorly adapting nerve fibers.
- Hearing: *audition;* middle and inner ear, cochlea, Organ of Corti; sound receptor cells on basilar membrane; *acoustic* energy.
- Balance and equilibrium:
  - *Proprioception*; Pacinian corpuscles
  - *Myesthesia*; muscle spindles
  - Load cells; Golgi tendon organs; muscle force.
- Inertia: *kinesthesia* (kinetic energy):
  - Angular motion: semi-circular canals; vestibular hair cells
  - Linear motion: otolith organs; saccule; utricle; vestibule.

Thermoreceptors: *thermodynamic* energy, heat:

- Krause's end bulbs: cool, cold
- Ruffini corpuscles: warm, hot.

Pain: *nociception*; undifferentiated free nerve endings.

Light receptors: *electromagnetic* (atomic) energy:

- Eyes, *vision*
- Rods of retina…shades of gray between white and black
- Cones of retina…color vision from red to violet.

Chemoreceptors: *chemical* (molecular, thermodynamic) energy:

- *Olfaction:* smell: olfactory receptor cells in neuroepithelium of nose; rhinencephalon of brain
- *Gustation:* taste: taste bud receptor cells in mouth.

The special sense of smell (olfaction)

"*Cogito, ergo sum,*" said the French philosopher and mathematician René Descartes (1596–1650)—"I think, therefore I am." If he had been a student of anatomy/physiology, Descartes probably would have said, "I *smell*, therefore I am!" You see, as the triune brain model developed in Chapter 4 clearly shows, we *smelled* long before we thought! Indeed, the *olfactory system* represents one of the oldest (if not *the* oldest) sensory modalities in the phylogenetic history of mammals. So old, that:

- the sense of smell sports its own special brain—the *rhinencephalon* in the ancient *archipallium* (see Chapter 4)

- olfactory inputs travel *directly* to the "smell brain," without passing through the thalamus, as do all other sensations

- the very *first cranial nerve* is the *olfactory nerve* (Chapter 4)

- our earliest survival as a species depended on our ability to distinguish among food odors and the scents of predators

- also related to survival of the species, sexual attraction between the male and female genders of many breeds of animal has evolved to rely quite heavily on the sense of *smell;* so much so, that in humans, that very attraction is enhanced by perfumes, after-shave lotions, and fragrances designed specifically to titillate one's sense of smell (Ackerman 1990). An entire industry has evolved around olfaction!

And the list goes on…

The anatomic organ that endows us with the ability to smell is the *nose*, within whose *nasal cavities* (nostrils) is contained an *olfactory membrane* that houses millions of specialized *olfactory, neuroepithelial receptor cells.* Located on the surface of these cells are *olfactory cilia* that terminate in genetically coded, stereo-specific, *osmophore-receiving protein sites*, or *olfactory vesicles*, that have unique geometric configurations. Osmophores—smell stimulants—are complementary-shaped atomic clusters that give a substance its characteristic scent. Groups of neuroepithelial cells converge into a network of *olfactory sensory neurons* that provide the brain with a "smell map." (Remember? The brain always knows *which* nerve is firing, and from where!) Olfactory nerve networks eventually become the aforementioned first cranial nerve, which enters the brain at the *olfactory bulb* resting above each nasal cavity, between, and just slightly above, the eye balls.[1] From there, "smell information" is transmitted through the midbrain to the limbic system and, eventually, the *orbito-frontal cortex* of the brain, where it reaches conscious perception.

Olfactory transduction thus involves the generation of sensory action potentials in response to the stimulation of neuroepithelium by inhaled chemical *odorants*—

---

1 The olfactory bulb is believed to be the evolutionary forerunner of our newer cerebral hemispheres—hence, again, "we originally smelled…therefore we think!"

small, volatile, fat-soluble molecules—that dissolve into the olfactory membrane. Some 400 types of odorant protein receptors, genetically expressed by this membrane, allow us to discriminate among over 10,000 scents. And whereas *each* olfactory neuron originates from a *single* receptor-type, *all* neurons derived from the *same* receptor-type—identifying a *particular* odor—are connected to the *same* spot in the brain, a specific *glomerulus* ("GPS location"). Moreover, despite their many composite, *isomeric* combinations and permutations, odors can generally be grouped into seven basic classes:

- *Minty*—as in, peppermint—an odor that seems to be characteristic of wedge-shaped osmophores.

- *Fruity* ("ethereal")—as in, the scent of pears—characterized by rod-shaped molecular clusters.

- *Musky*—as in, the strong, lasting aroma of some perfumes—typical of disc-shaped stimulants.

- *Floral*—as in, the smell of roses—usually associated with rod-shaped elements that have disc-like out-pocketings at their ends, i.e., some combination of fruity and musky.

- *Resinous*—as in, camphor—generally derived from spherically shaped molecular configurations.

- *Pungent* ("acrid")—as in, vinegar—the result of stimulation by positively-charged ionic species.

- *Putrid* ("foul-smelling")—as in, rotten eggs—the result of stimulation by negatively-charged ionic species.

Two final points about smell:

1. Olfactory "hair" cells are the most *exposed* nerve endings in the body, and in many ways, the most *sensitive*. But, although it takes as few as eight molecules of an odorant to elicit an olfactory action potential, it doesn't take many more than that to elicit a *maximum* response; and nerve cells *adapt* very quickly, which is why, when we smell something continuously for a minute or so, we soon stop "noticing" it. In other words, all the evidence points to the fact that our sense of smell is less concerned with identifying the *intensity* or *rate of change* of an odor, than it is with detecting its *presence, type* and potential *threat* to survival.

2. Unlike sensory cells receptive to light or sound, which the body cannot replace when damaged, individual neurons in the nose are replaced about every 30–60 days. They are among the only types of sensory neuroepithelial cells that are capable of regenerating.

The special sense of taste (gustation)

In a way, our sense of "taste" is a special case of our sense of "touch" the word *taste*, itself, being derived from the Latin *taxare*, which means "to touch sharply." In this case, the "touch" involves bringing into contact with the mucous membranes of the *mouth*—the anatomic organ that endows us with this sense—certain soluble substances that are *ingested* (see Chapter 2). Taste is the second of our two *chemical* senses, the other one being smell. It derives from the transduction into action potentials, of the *chemical energy* carried by *testants*—which are solid and/or liquid substances that enter the mouth. These stimulate long, nucleated, spindle-shaped *taste receptor cells* located in the oral cavity, principally on the *tongue*. Embedded in the mucous membrane of this freely movable, muscular organ are from as few as 2000 to as many as 10,000 gourd-shaped *taste buds*, each of which houses up to 100 *gustatory*, neuroepithelial, taste-receptor cells.

As is true for olfactory cells, gustatory ones, too, are endowed with *microvilli* (*gustatory cilia*), on the ends of which are located genetically coded, stereo-specific, *testant-receiving, protein-binding sites* that have unique geometric configurations. Each such configuration has an affinity for, and is congruent with, a corresponding, specific testant, *except* "salty" and "sour" ones; these gain access to the neuroepithelium through *ionic channels* in the taste-cell membrane.

Each cell is attached to one or two nerve axons that eventually merge into networks of *gustatory sensory neurons*. These networks supply the brain with a "taste map" (is this starting to sound familiar?). They all enter it at the *solitary tract* of *taste nuclei* in the medulla, but they get there via different routes, depending on where the action potentials originate:

- Those signals that come from the front two-thirds of the tongue travel to the *solitary tract* by means of the *mandibular branch* of the *fifth cranial nerve* (see Table 4.1), which eventually meets up with the *seventh cranial nerve*.

- Action potentials originating at the back of the tongue reach this tract by means of the *ninth cranial nerve*, especially its pharyngeal, lingual, and tonsillar branches.

- Impulses derived from the deepest regions of the throat and pharynx get to the solitary tract via the *tenth cranial nerve*—specifically, the sensory portions of the *vagus*.

Leaving the medulla, these signals work their way to the posterior thalamus, and from there, to the *parietal lobe* of the *cerebral cortex*, where they reach conscious perception. The different pathways to the brain reflect different taste sensations, and how, in turn they are intended to be processed. Indeed, although we can discriminate among thousands of different flavors—i.e., permutations and combinations of various testants—our taste receptor cells only respond to four types of "primary chemical stimulants," to wit:

- Taste buds located on the tip and anterior (front) surface of the tongue are especially receptive to, among others: the *sweet* taste of *organic* stimulants (such as various sugars); some alcohols and alcohol derivatives (such as chloroform); and amino acids (such as alanine).

- Taste buds located at the base and posterior (back) surface of the tongue are especially receptive to, among others: the *bitter* taste of nitrogen-containing testants (such as nicotine, quinine, strychnine, and caffeine); and many of the *drugs* commonly used in medicine. From this part of the tongue there also originates a *gag reflex*, by which undesirable, bitter-tasting toxins and naturally occurring poisons are actively prevented from getting past the throat, into the digestive system. Bitter-tasting substances tend to have high positive-to-negative-ion ratios. The reverse is true for salty-tasting substances...read on.

- Taste buds located along the front lateral border of the tongue are especially receptive to *salty* stimulants, such as ordinary table salt, and others. As mentioned earlier, these gain access to the taste receptor cells through ionic channels located along the cell membrane, as do sour stimulants.

- Finally, taste buds located along the middle lateral border of the tongue are especially sensitive to the *sour* taste that comes from ingesting hydrogen-containing (low "pH," acidic) testants such as (among others): vinegar (acetic acid), certain carbonated beverages (carbonic acid), and various citrus fruits (citric acid).

Two final points about taste:

1. In terms of sensory "sensitivity," taste comes nowhere near smell. Remember, it takes only eight molecules of an odorant to get a response from an olfactory cell. By contrast, about 200,000 molecules of a testant are required to "wake up" a taste receptor cell! And we can detect "sweet" testants least of all, at a threshold of one part testant per 200 parts solution. Our sensitivity to salty tastes is about twice that good; but we are a thousand times better at responding to sour-tasting testants. Best of all, however, is our ability to detect bitter-tasting testants, probably because of the potential threat that they pose to our survival. Thus a mere single part of testant diluted into two million parts of solution can still be detected by our taste buds. Any way one chooses to evaluate it, however, taste is probably the *least* sentient of all the body's captors—not only to the *intensity* of a stimulant, but also to its *persistence* and *rate of change*.

2. Taste buds "wear out" as often as every seven to ten days (to as much as two weeks); and the taste receptor cells are replaced regularly—at least every three days, although less frequently past the age of 45. Thus, our sense of taste becomes somewhat impaired as we grow older.

The special sense of hearing (audition)

And so, we come to another sense of "touch"—but this time, it is molecules of air pounding on an *outer ear drum*, illustrated in Figure 5.1. And instead of dealing with *chemical* energy, as we did when we talked about our senses of smell and taste, we now deal with *acoustic* energy, which we perceive in the frequency range from 20 to 20,000 cycles per second. Since all musical frequencies—referred to as *pitch*—fall within this frequency range, our sense of hearing is obviously of great interest to the music therapist (Berger and Schneck 2003; Schneck and Berger 1999, 2006).

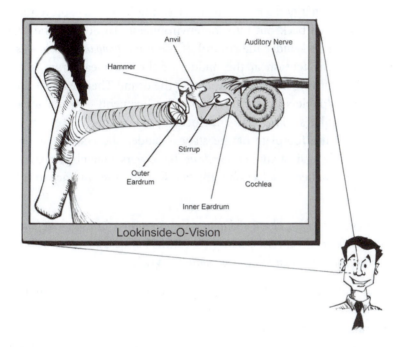

Figure 5.1 The human hearing apparatus from the receiving outer ear drum, through the ossicular chain of the middle ear, to the transmitting inner ear drum and cochlea of the inner ear, from which emanates the auditory nerve (shown schematically)

(Reprinted with the copyright permission of Geoffrey Rowland, from Figure 8.1 of *The Music Effect: Music Physiology and Clinical Applications,* by Daniel J. Schneck and Dorita S. Berger; Jessica Kingsley Publishers, London and Philadelphia, 2006.)

The outer ear drum, or *tympanic membrane* lies at the end of a one inch-long *auditory canal* (*external acoustic meatus*), that funnels pulsating masses of air collected by ear lobes (*auricles*) through this *external ear* region. Impinging against the tympanic membrane, the vibrating air molecules—like the mallets of a kettle drum—transfer their kinetic energy to the ear drum, setting it in motion at the frequency corresponding to that of the air. Were nothing else to happen, these vibrations would simply be *reflected* back out of the ear, and the story would end there!

But something else *does* happen...the outer ear drum is attached to a series of three tiny bones—the *auditory ossicles* (see Table 3.1 and Figure 5.1). Each about the size of a grain of rice, and named according to what they look like, the auditory ossicles—comprising the *middle ear (tympanic cavity)*—are the smallest bones in the human body, but they serve an enormous function, which is to establish a 20:1 *mechanical advantage* that serves two purposes: first, it *amplifies* otherwise inaudible sound signals by a factor of 17–22; and second, it establishes the means necessary to convert *gas* (external, air) molecular vibrations into *liquid* (internal, *perilymphatic/ endolymphatic* ECF) molecular vibrations, which, in turn, creates a direct path for *transmitting* acoustic energy from the outer ear to the inner ear—preventing it from being merely reflected back out into the environment. To do this, the "handle" of the *malleus* ("hammer")—under the control of the *tensor tympani* muscle—is attached to and modulates the tension at the middle of the outer ear drum, receiving its vibrations while adjusting its sensitivity, *biasing* the drum! The "head" of the hammer articulates—via a double-saddle joint secured by ligaments—to the *incus* ("anvil"), which, itself, articulates via a ball-and-socket joint with the stem of the *stapes* ("stirrup"). Finally, the footplate of the stapes—under the control of the *stapedius* muscle—seats firmly against an *inner ear drum* that covers a membranous *oval window*, lying just above a smaller *round window*, the two forming the entrance to the *inner ear*. To put it bluntly:

> *Absent the ossicular chain, absent audition! Absent the proper structure and function of the ossicular chain, absent corresponding transduction of acoustic energy into faithful reproduction and perception of incident auditory signals.*

Reaching the inner ear, amplified fluid oscillations now drive the motion of the *basilar membrane*—which originates between the bottom of the oval window and top of the round window, stretches across the interior walls of, and spans the entire length of the lumen of the previously mentioned (see Chapter 3 section on labyrinthine reflexes) *cochlea*. The latter (from the Greek *kochliās*, meaning "spiral") is shaped like a "snail shell"—a tapered bony tube wound two-and-a-half turns into a nested, truncated cone configuration ("spiral"), forming the terminal portion of the three divisions of the labyrinth (recall that the other two are the otolith organs and the semi-circular canals, not shown in Figure 5.1).

A closer look at the basilar membrane allows one to envision it as the body's version of a harp. That is to say, the "membrane" is actually made up of thousands of closely packed, tightly stretched fibers ("strings"). These are very short ("high" strings, 0.04–0.16 mm in length) and near the oval window, which allows them to resonate in response to the membrane being driven by high-frequency (up to 20,736 Hz) perilymph oscillations that derive from an equal number of inner-ear drum acoustic vibrations. Moving along the basilar membrane toward the apex of the cochlea (the *helicotrema*) the fibers gradually increase in length to 0.40–0.65 mm—becoming "low" strings that similarly resonate in response to low-frequency sonic vibrations (down to 16 Hz). These mechanical events bend, shear, and otherwise deform some 23,500 (on average) *neuroepithelial hair cell receptors* that project from the membrane into the surrounding pulsating fluid. Each hair cell is innervated by one or two (to as many as 20, depending on location) afferent sensory nerve fibers.

The neuroepithelial hair cell receptors, their supporting structures (including an additional *tectorial* membrane), and the sensory nerve endings with which all these structures are endowed, form a gelatinous prominence on the inner portion of the basilar membrane called the *Organ of Corti*, the *terminal auditory apparatus*, or, more simply, the "organ of hearing." This organ allows us to discriminate among some 400,000 different sounds, the direction from which the sounds are coming, and their potential "threat" to the individual who perceives them. And although its adequate stimulus is sound energy nominally in the 20–20,000 Hz acoustic-frequency range, the Organ of Corti is *most* acutely sensitive and responsive to frequencies in the 1000–4000 Hz range, which takes us along the basilar membrane from its origin at the oval window, through the first full cochlear turn, and part way into the second full turn. Compare this to:

- the range of the human singing voice (73–1175 Hz)
- maximum nerve firing frequencies (up to 2000 Hz, see Chapter 3)
- tactile mechanical vibration sensitivity (up to 2500 Hz)
- the range of an 88-key standard piano keyboard (27.5–4186 Hz)
- speech frequencies that generally range from 100 to 300 cps—with overtone series that can extend this range to 3 kilohertz, and even, at times, reach as high as 5 kilohertz
- "resonance" frequencies of various body tissues and organs, some of which—compared to corresponding musical pitches relative to concert "A" = 440 cycles/second—are illustrated in Table 5.2)
- musical frequencies that lie mostly between 30 and 8000 Hz

…and it does not take one very long to conclude that music *should* have a profound effect on physiologic function; and, indeed, it does, for reasons even beyond such "obvious" ones!

Table 5.2 Acoustic frequencies, f, in hertz; organs/tissues resonating at that frequency; and corresponding musical pitch based on A_4 = 440 hertz		
ACOUSTIC f, Hz	MUSICAL PITCH	RESONANANT BODY STRUCTURES
1 to 4	Not heard	Brain δ-waves (deep sleep)
4 to 8	Not heard	Brain θ-waves (drowsiness)
8 to 13	Not heard	Brain α-waves (tranquility)

cont.

ACOUSTIC f, Hz	MUSICAL PITCH	RESONANANT BODY STRUCTURES
12 to 15	Not heard	Brain spindle bursts; (Sensori-motor biorhythms)
13 to 30	C_0 to $A_0{}^{\#}$	Brain β-waves (wakefulness)
19.4454	$D_0{}^{\#}$ to $E_0{}^{b}$	Threshold of human hearing
30–to–80	$A_0{}^{\#}$ to $E_2{}^{b}$	Brain γ-waves (peak concentration)
110	A_2	Stomach
116.5 to 117.3	$A_2{}^{\#}$ to $B_2{}^{b}$	Pancreas
164.3	E_3	Gall bladder
174.3 to 176	F_3	Colon
220	A_3	Lungs
277.2 to 281.6	$C_4{}^{\#}$ to $D_4{}^{b}$	Small intestines
293.7 to 295.8	D_4	Adipose cells/tissue
311 to 315	$D_4{}^{\#}$ to $E_4{}^{b}$	Diaphragm
315.8	$E_4{}^{b}$	Brain cells/tissue/organ
317.83	$E_4{}^{b}$	Liver cells/tissue/organ
319.88 to 330	$E_4{}^{b}$ to E_4	Kidneys
321.9 to 330	$E_4{}^{b}$ to E_4	Blood (body fluids)
324 to 330	E_4	Muscle cells/tissue
341 to 349	F_4	Heart
352 to 370	$F_4{}^{\#}$	Bladder; thymus gland
384 to 392	G_4	Throat
415.3 to 418.3	$A_4{}^{b}$	Bone cells/tissue
492 to 494	B_4	Spleen; thyroid; adrenal; parathyroid glands
537.8	$C_5{}^{+}$	DNA base: cytosine
543.4	$C_5{}^{++}$	DNA base: thymine
545.6	$C_5{}^{\#--}$	DNA base: adenine
550	$C_5{}^{\#-}$	DNA base: guanine
586 to 588	D_5	Sex glands; blood vessels
21,100	E_{10}	Limit of human hearing
1 to 2500	Not heard to $D_7{}^{\#+}$	Vibrational tactile sense
73.4 to 1174.7	D_2 to D_6	Range of human voice
27.5 to 4186	A_0 to C_8	Piano 88-keyboard range
78 to 150,356	$D_2{}^{\#}$ to D_{13}	Porpoise hearing range
49 to 1109	G_1 to $C_6{}^{\#}$	Tuna fish hearing range

As illustrated in Figure 5.1 (page 133), sensory hair-cell vibrations generated as described above in the Organ of Corti of both ears are transduced by this organ into afferent (sensory) action potentials that ultimately converge on the left and right cochlear branches (i.e., the acoustic, or auditory nerves) of the eighth cranial nerve—the vestibulocochlear nerve (see Table 4.1, page 116)—en route to their ultimate destination: the auditory cortical area in the upper part of the temporal lobe of the brain. Interestingly, for reasons discussed elsewhere (Buser and Imbert 1992; Schneck 2009b), the bilateral input received by the auditory cortex from the two ears comes in *reversed*, which is to say, impulses originating in the right ear "cross over"—*decussate*—to enter the brain from the left, and vice versa.

The acoustic nerves contain both afferent sensory nerve fibers that deliver auditory information to the brain, and efferent motor neurons. The latter provide a means by which the central nervous system can "bias" the cochlea—primarily through the previously mentioned *tensor tympani* and *stapedius* muscles. And once again, your ears do not hear, your brain does. In the auditory cortex, specialized cells can locate:

- the *source* of a sound, i.e., the direction from which it is coming

- its fundamental "pitch," i.e., basic *frequency*, as determined by the *primary* part of the basilar membrane that is transmitting the *major* component of the generated auditory signal

- its "timbre," i.e., sound quality, as determined by how many *other* parts of the basilar membrane are being recruited in response to the incident sound waves, thus contributing *secondary*, harmonic *Fourier components* super-imposed onto the primary signal (Schneck and Berger 2006)

- its *intensity*—loudness (*dynamics*, in music) which is a function of the *amplitude* associated with the undulating basilar membrane as it responds to the amplitude of the corresponding acoustic vibrations.

Sound intensity is expressed in units called *decibels*, which is a logarithmic scale wherein a decibel level of zero is the threshold loudness for human hearing, and every ten decibels above that corresponds to a ten-fold ("ten times!") increase in perceived loudness. Thus, listed in Table 5.3 are various levels of sound intensity, expressed in decibels, and how they compare to corresponding musical experiences. Note, in particular, that exposure to a decibel level of 90 for extended periods of time can result in significant impairment of the hearing apparatus—and remember, as a music therapist, that:

> *Whereas you might be perceiving sound at a decibel level of, say, 20 or 25, someone else, such as an autistic child, could very well be experiencing it at a decibel level of 120–130, the threshold for pain! Be aware, and be alert!*

Table 5.3 Acoustic intensity, db, in decibels; "typical" sound sources generating such intensity; and corresponding "typical" musical experiences		
Acoustic Intensity, dB	**Sound Source**	**Musical Experience**
0	Threshold of human hearing	Nothing audible
10–20	Rustling of leaves; stream flow	Faint audible sounds
20	Gentle breeze; average whisper	Very soft; pianissimo
20–25	Purring cat at 3 ft	Soft; piano (p)
30	Turning the page of a newspaper Loud whisper at 3 ft; quiet street	Mezzo-piano (mp)
40	Residential neighborhood at night Quiet radio in home	Soft piano practice
50	Quiet automobile; low speech volume; average office/home sounds	Low voice volume
45–66	Normal conversation level between two people	Medium voice volume
60–70	Busy street traffic	Normal piano practice
65–70	Giving a speech; ordinary conversation at 1.67 ft	Forte singing at 3 ft
70	Busy street traffic	Fortissimo singer at 3 ft
75	Street noise in N.Y. City on 5th Ave. and 42nd Street; Automobile interior at 60 mph	"Average" string quartet
80	Vacuum cleaner; noisy restaurant; average car horn; loud radio music	Forte string quartet; Soft bass, cello sound
75–85	Loud argument	Chamber music in small auditorium
82–92	Electric shaver	Cello
85–95	Riveting at street level	Violin in lower strings
90	Water at foot of Niagara Falls; elevated/subway train; Very loud speech	Soft French horn; "subdued" rock concert
90–94	Yelling; screaming	Oboe range
92–95	Piercing, loud shrill	Fortissimo piano

95	Pneumatic drilling/riveting heard up-close; noisiest spot at Niagara Falls; loud car horn	Soft piccolo; medium clarinet; violin in upper strings
100	Siren at 30 m; jack hammer	Soft tympani
105	Gas-powered lawn mower	Soft bass drum
106	Pneumatic hammer at 15 ft	Tympani and bass drum rolls
84–103	Garbage disposal; dishwasher; Motorcycle at 25 ft; helicopter at 100 ft	Violin sound range
90–106	Boeing 737 or DC-9 aircraft about a mile out on approach to landing	French horn sound range
92–103	Newspaper presses; jet flyover at 1000 ft	Clarinet sound range
110	Pneumatic hammer at 5 ft; violent hammering on steel plate	Loud flute; piccolo; trombone
85–111	Steel mill	Flute sound range
85–114	Outboard motorboat	Trombone sound range
95–112	Jet take-off at 305 m	Piccolo sound range
90–120	Loud thunderclap; chain saw	Rock concert
120	*Lowest threshold of ear pain; severe discomfort;* oxygen torch	Typical dance clubs
125	Jet take-off from aircraft carrier	Severe ear pain
120–137	Aircraft carrier deck noise	Symphonic music Peak intensities
130	Close range machine gun fire *Limit of ear's endurance; highest tolerance for ear pain; threshold of feeling*	Loud rock concert
140	Jet plane at 30 m; shotgun blast at ear level; sonic boom	Serious ear damage
150	Jet take-off at 25 m	Intolerable ear pain Ear drum ruptures
160	Wind tunnel blast at close range	Hearing protection absolutely necessary
180	Rocket launch at 150 ft	Hearing protection required
188	Blue whales underwater	
194	Loudest decibel level ever measured	

Notes:

- *One decibel is the minimum difference in sound intensity that the human ear can discriminate.*
- *Every 10 decibels represents a ten-fold increase in sound intensity.*
- *The threshold for hearing damage is an exposure level of 90 dB for an extended period of time.*

A final word about how your brain locates the direction from which a sound is arriving at the ears. It is actually related to the same type of Morse-Code-like *pulse trains* and *barcoding* paradigms that we introduced when we talked about neurotransmitters early in Chapter 4. That is to say, the direction from which the sound entered the ear apparently stimulates only those auditory receptor cells that have as their *receptive field*—i.e., the spatial *zone of influence* toward which they are physically oriented—sound coming from *that particular direction*. All together then, there are enough receptor cells to cover the entire three-dimensional region in all directions around the head.

Thus, auditory hair cells are *selectively* stimulated as a function of sound direction, and that selectivity is encoded into a corresponding set of pulse trains that are relayed to the brain, which—you will recall—always knows *which* nerve is "firing." Moreover, because we have two ears spaced a finite distance apart, there is a measureable *timing pattern* that results from the fact that both ears do not receive incident sound waves at *exactly* the same time. There is a momentary delay between when the first ear—"closest" to the sound source—"hears" it and when the sound enters the second ear—"furthest" from the sound source. That delay, too, is encoded into the *timing sequence patterns* with which the brain receives auditory afferent signals. The combination of *selective excitation* and *delayed transmission* causes certain specific populations of brain cells in the auditory cortex to fire—in synchrony—when sound arrives from different directions, thus, again, endowing the brain with a topographic sound map, or a *cerebral GPS system!* And while we are on the subject of two ears and topographic *sound* maps…let's carry this reasoning one step further, to talk about two eyes and topographic *light* maps.

The special sense of sight (vision)

Take a look again at Figure 5.1 (page 143). What do you see? If you said, "I see a diagram of the hearing apparatus surrounded by a rectangular border, or type of 'frame'," you would be saying exactly what I would expect. But that's not what your *brain* "sees," it's what your brain *tells you* you *saw*, after it has *reconstructed* the image. This it does by instantaneously *recalling from working memory*, sorting out, and making sense of the digitized signals the *visual cortex* received from your organs of vision—the eyes. Indeed, like your hearing apparatus—whose *Organ of Corti* converts *acoustic* energy in the frequency range 20–20,000 Hz into *auditory* action potential pulse trains—your visual apparatus contains an *optic organ* (the eye) that converts *light* energy in the 390–790 *tera*hertz range of the electromagnetic spectrum into *ophthalmic* (from the Greek *ophthalmós*, meaning "eye") action potential pulse trains.

And what the *auditory basilar membrane* is to "hearing," the *retina* at the back of the eye is to "seeing." That is to say, like the former, which has *auditory receptive fields* that encode into *acoustic* pulse trains, direction-specific pitch, loudness, and timbre, the latter has *visual receptive fields* that encode into *light* pulse trains, corresponding direction-specific color (hue), brightness, spatial orientation, and motion—but these, as we shall see, are *not* delivered to the brain as fully assembled "motion pictures!"

The hearing apparatus communicates with the *temporal* lobe of the brain mainly through the eighth cranial nerve; the visual system accesses the *occipital* lobe of the brain mainly through the second (afferent, sensory optic) cranial nerve for vision, and the third, fifth, and sixth (efferent, motor) cranial nerves to affect eye movement. Let's take a closer "look" by first doing another simple experiment which might surprise you.

Take an 8.5 by 11-inch blank sheet of paper and, using a sharp implement (like a pencil tip), poke a small hole about one-eighth of an inch in the middle of it. Now, select any prominent, easily visible object in the room and, *keeping both eyes open*, position the sheet of paper in front of your face such that you locate the object in space by looking ("peeping") *only* through the hole (make sure your vision is otherwise completely blocked by the rest of the sheet of paper). Then, *without moving the paper*, close your right eye. Do you still see the object? Open both eyes. Now again, *without moving the paper*, close your left eye. Do you still see the object. If the experiment worked correctly, you should have been able to see the object with *one* eye closed, but not the other.

What you have thus determined is which one of your eyes is your *sighting* eye—the one that allows you to *locate* things in space. The other eye basically *triangulates* to give you bi-focal *depth perception*. That is, when you kept *both* eyes open, without consciously realizing it, you actually positioned the sheet of paper in front of your *sighting* eye, say it was your right one. Then, when you closed your right eye, the object disappeared from view because the paper was interfering with your left eye's "line of sight;" it blocked your vision because the hole was not positioned in front of your open, left eye. But when you closed your left eye, you continued to see the object because the hole was positioned in front of *that* eye to begin with! So far as we know, right or left *sightedness* does not appear to be related to right or left handedness, intelligence, etc., but take note, it *could* be affecting how your clients "see" things and judge distance.

Speaking of seeing things and judging distance, just as sound does not reach the basilar membrane directly, neither do incident rays of light from the environment reach the retina directly. First of all, they pass through a thin, curved (convex), transparent *cornea*, which "bends" the light beams toward one another in a process called *refraction*. Passing through the cornea, the bent light rays enter the *anterior chamber* of the eye—filled with a watery *aqueous humor*—and then continue on to reach the *pupil*. The pupil is the "black circle" one sees in the center of the eye. It is surrounded by the *iris*, which gives the eyes their characteristic color, and within which are contained *dilator* and *sphincter pupillae muscles* that act to widen or shrink its opening, respectively. Thus, the *amount* of light reaching the retina can be controlled: the pupils *dilate* to let more light in when the environment is dim or dark; they *contract* to prevent too much very bright light from reaching and possibly damaging the retina. You can actually see them do this by looking in a mirror—first in a bright place, then in a dim one. The *brightness* of light corresponds to the *loudness* of sound. The *color* of light energy—increasing in frequency from red to orange to yellow to green to blue to violet (the visible spectrum)—corresponds to the *pitch* of sound.

Like the outer and middle ears, the architecture of the exterior chambers of the eye is designed to prevent light from simply being reflected back out into the environment, while *biasing* anatomical structures that modulate the intensity of the energy that is allowed to pass through to the retina. That energy that makes it through the pupil is now processed by the crystalline *lens* of the eye. Here, light rays are bent further towards a common *focal point* that *should* (emphasis on the "should") lie right on the retina. If the focal point lies *in front of* the retina, the eyeball is too long from front to back, and the person is thus "near-sighted" (*myopic*), i.e., they can see things well up close, but have trouble visualizing things at a distance. If the focal point falls *behind* the retina, the eyeball is too short and the person is thus "far-sighted" (*hyperopic*), i.e., they see distant things more clearly than near ones. The extent to which a near or far-sighted person will need glasses to correct his or her vision depends on the ability of that person's lens to *accommodate. Accommodation* refers to the process by which the thickness of the lens can be adjusted to keep the focal point right on the retina when viewing objects that lie at variable distances in front of the eyeball. Thus, *longitudinal, radial,* and *circular smooth ciliary muscle fibers* function together (contract) to actively thicken the lens for *near vision;* they "relax," allowing the lens to get passively thinner for *far vision.* However, if the lens "clouds up," as happens in a condition called *cataracts,* vision is seriously impaired. Vision is also affected as the ciliary muscles age and their function is compromised, as happens in a common condition called *presbyopia* ("old eyes"). Moreover, past the age of 40, the eye's ability to recover from glare slows down, and one's peripheral vision also tends to decline.

Okay, so our eyes can *sight* a target, give us *depth perception* (by triangulation), *focus* it on the retina (by accommodation, with help, if necessary), and *track* its movement, as we discussed in Chapter 3 when we talked about labyrinthine reflexes. But what is this about *visual receptive fields* and *image reconstruction?* Well, continuing with our journey, electromagnetic photon energy is finally transformed into sensory nerve action potentials when the now-focused light rays reach light-sensitive *photoreceptor cells* called *rods* and *cones* located in the retina. Rods give us black-to-white-with-various-shades-of-gray-in-between light perception; cones give us color perception. In general, the ratio of rods to cones is about 18:1 (range: 10–20:1) in a "typical" retina. But…these photoreceptor cells are highly specialized! For example:

- Some detect only *horizontal* lines; others "fire" only when exposed to *vertical* lines.

- Neurons with a receptive field for horizontal lines will not fire signals when exposed to vertical lines, or diagonal ones, or any other type of geometry— *they are activated only by horizontal lines!*

- There are cells that specialize in specific colors, types of motion, physical location in space, and orientation in space, etc. Most people can identify between 150 and 200 shades of color that are various combinations and permutations of the red to violet spectrum. But:

     Of special interest to the music therapist, the color green appears to have a "restful," sedentary effect on the brain; and the color blue appears to "calm" it.

- Some receptors help to determine *what* an object is; others help to decide *where* it is (based on sighting information and the location of the eyeballs in the head), and *how far away* it is (based on triangulation).

- Still others help to *track* and to calculate the *trajectory* of a moving target (see labyrinthine reflexes).

- Different receptor cells respond to different *intensities* of light…

     but remember, again, that the physics definition of light intensity is often far different from one's subjective perception of such intensity—so what to you might seem very dim lighting, to an autistic child might be glaring, annoying brightness!

To summarize, all visual sensory inputs to the brain are digitized bits and pieces of information derived from the attributes of what is being observed—*not a complete, finished picture!* Moreover, the situation is further complicated by the fact that:

- the optic nerves carrying this information (as did the auditory nerves) *decussate* (cross over one another) en route to the brain

- the information they carry is *turned upside down* because, as the light rays are refracted and focused en route to the back of the eye, they, too, cross over one another, thus delivering an inverted signal to the retina

- the brain, itself, is constrained by *information-processing speeds.* Indeed, it takes about 100 milliseconds to establish a good image on the retina, and the light having thus been processed takes another fraction of a second to reach the visual cortex, traveling through the optic nerves at speeds on the order of 10–130 meters per second, depending on the information being carried by the nerve fibers (i.e., color, geometric attributes, etc.). (Note that 50–100 msec are required for the hearing apparatus to "lock onto" and identify an incident sound frequency.)

Then…the visual cortex is only capable of processing and reconstructing images at the rate of 50–60 per second—a fact exploited by cinematographers in making motion pictures. That is:

- digitizing "continuous" motion into a series of 50–60 "still frames" per second, that are

- projected onto the retina, which, in turn

- converts them into digitized action potentials that are

- transmitted to the visual cortex and reconstructed at this same rate of 50–60/ sec, will

- be translated by the brain to be, in fact, *continuous*—even though, in reality, the motion is being projected onto the retina in discrete time steps.

The lower limit of this discretization is around 24 frames/sec, the so-called "flicker speed." Below this speed, the brain "sees" each individual frame as a distinct "still shot," and thus, the movement is observed to be *jerky* and discontinuous. The same thing happens at very fast digitization speeds, where now, the visual cortex *loses* the in-between frames and thus, again, envisions the motion to be discontinuously changing from one configuration to another.

So, the interpretation by the visual cortex of transduced light sensations that are transmitted to it by the optic nerves is a complicated mess! But somehow, miraculously, the brain manages to sort through this plethora of data, *reconstruct* the outside world from which it came, turn the image back right side up, and allow us to construct by imagery a spatial representation of what we "saw!" As was the case for hearing, the specialized receptive fields to which the photosensitive cells respond allow the brain to "map" its environment into cognitive consciousness—we become *aware* that we are "seeing" something!

But, that awareness is not instantaneous. We don't experience life and the world around us in *real time*. No…we actually "see" something a split second later than we actually "looked" at it! What we "looked at" were just lines, geometric shapes, and colors projected onto the retina. The retina transduced these into electrochemical bits of data that the optic nerves transmitted as digitized attributes to a temporary, working memory. These attributes were expeditiously recalled and reconstructed by the visual cortex, delivered to your consciousness as a time-delayed image, and that's what you "saw!" Furthermore, during the time delay, before ever reaching consciousness, the reconstructed image might already have triggered a sub-conscious physiologic *response* to the perceived information, especially if it is deemed to be in some sense *threatening* (Schneck and Berger 2006). In fact, one can extrapolate and generalize this basic feature of vision—i.e., that our consciousness of any given experience is time delayed—into *Physiological optimization principle number 4*, by noting that, to guarantee a *timely, effective, instinctive* response to sensory inputs, all sensory information processing makes us consciously aware of adequate stimuli only after the brain has already processed them and, if necessary, initiated a response to them. Often, that response is totally sub-conscious and already in progress before we even become aware of "what happened!" (Schneck and Berger 2006).

Having established the above as a general physiologic principle, and using the special senses as a basic paradigm for *Feature 3* in our developing model of the human body (i.e., the idea of monitoring our internal and external environments), let's now examine some general senses (in somewhat less detail, since the pattern has already been set).

The general senses of extero and interoception

For virtually every one of the sense organs that allow us to perceive our *external,* ambient environment (*exteroception,* Table 5.1), there is a corresponding anatomic transducer that allows us to be in contact with and constantly monitor our *internal,* visceral environment (*interoception,* Table 5.4), to make sure that the body is functioning well within its intended operating set points. And, as described below and illustrated in Table 5.4, the general senses, too, are classified according to the type of energy (*adequate stimulus*) to which they respond, be it mechanical (force, pressure, tissue deformation, etc.), thermodynamic (heat, body core temperature, etc.), chemical (blood sugar, acidity/alkalinity, gases, toxins, etc.), electromagnetic (piezoelectricity, streaming potentials, etc.), and so on. Let's probe a bit deeper.

Mechanoreceptors accounting for some general senses

As the name implies, *mechanoreceptors* are responsive to adequate stimuli that take the form of *forces.* These tend to:

- *pull* and *stretch* (tension; tensile forces)
- *press* and *squeeze* (pressure, compression forces)
- *bend* (curl); and/or *twist* (torsion)
- *rip* and/or *shave* (shear; tangential forces)
- *shake* (vibration)
- physically *move* (by rotation, and/or translation)
- otherwise mechanically *distort* or *deform* the organs and tissues on which they act

in: (a) either concentrated ("sharp") or distributed ("diffuse") receptive fields; and (b) either continuous, persistent ("chronic") or occasional, temporary ("acute") fashion. Any or all of these cause the sensors to convert both the *amount* and *rate of deformation* into action potentials that correspond to the forces applied. We have already mentioned a few mechanical anatomic transducers when we talked in Chapter 3 about:

- *balance and equilibrium* (myotatic reflexes derived from the *tensile stretch* of muscle spindles)

- *proprioception* (articular feedback data derived from *compression* of Pacinian corpuscles)

- *kinesthesia* (labyrinthine reflexes derived from the *bending* and *deformation* of neuroepithelial hair cells embedded in the walls of the semicircular canals and otolith organs)

- *myesthesia* (neuromuscular reflexes derived from *stretching* muscle spindles and applying *tensile forces* to Golgi organs located in muscle tendons)

and, in this chapter, when we described hearing. Let's take a look at some more, starting with a general sense that is actually the *first* to develop *in utero*, and which is critical to the human experience, i.e., the sense of *touch!*

Table 5.4 Classification of sensory receptors for interoception
TYPE OF ENERGY/CORRESPONDING SENSE CEPTORS RESPONSIVE TO IT

Mechanoreceptors: *mechanical* energy:
• Somatoception: deep tissue sensibilities (see also Table 5.1)
  ○ Proprioception—encapsulated nerve endings; Pacinian corpuscles
  ○ Myesthesia—muscle spindles; Golgi tendon organs
  ○ Kinesthesia—balance and equilibrium; macroscopic kinetics
  ○ Free nerve endings and other mechanical receptors
• Baroreception: arterial blood pressure; tissue pressure
  ○ Carotid sinus baroreceptors (pressure → stretch)
  ○ Aortic sinus baroreceptors (pressure → stretch)
  ○ Pulmonary and systemic circulation baroreceptors
  ○ Post-capillary sphincters (contraction = ↑ pressure)
• Volume receptors
  ○ Auricular (cardiac) and vascular strain-gage-type ceptors
  ○ Visceral (mainly stomach) volume (stretch) receptors
  ○ Tissue stretch receptors and load cells
Thermoreceptors: *thermodynamic* energy, heat, body core temperature, *thermoesthesia*
• Visceral thermodetectors (thermistors)
• Spinal thermistors (heat-sensitive ceptors)
• Hypothalamic thermoreceptors

Pain: *nociception*
- Undifferentiated free nerve endings
- Deep tissue sensibilities

Electromagnetic (atomic) energy:
- Piezoelectricity ("pressure-electric" energy)
- Streaming potentials ("injury" potentials; healing)

Chemoreceptors: *chemical* (molecular, thermodynamic) energy:
- Hypothalamic osmoreceptors (sodium concentration; osmotic pressure; ionic distribution)
- Aortic bodies (arterial O_2; CO_2; pH)
- Carotid bodies (arterial O_2; CO_2; pH)
- Cerebral (medulla) chemoreceptors (acidity/alkalinity)
- Hypothalamic gluco-(sugar) amino-(protein) lipo-(fat) receptors
- Glucoreceptors of liver and caudal hindbrain (glucose, sugar)
- Nerve endings in the mouth and pharynx (water)
- Pre-capillary sphincters (relaxation = ↑ flow; lactic acid)

The general sense of touch (taction)

The embryo in the mother's womb actually begins to "feel" just before the eighth week of its gestational age. This is roughly four weeks before its sense of smell develops, six weeks prior to it being able to taste, eight weeks in advance of it being capable of responsive listening, and at least 16 weeks before it can focus on and track a moving target. Eventually, ceptors from which the sense of touch derives will be embedded primarily in the largest single organ of the body—the skin—and they will have the greatest number of sensory receptors in the adult body, responsive to the utmost variety—up to 100!—of different tactile sensations. These ceptors, as shown in Table 5.1, can be conveniently divided into six basic types, depending on:

- the *adequate stimulus* to which they respond, i.e., type of force (tensile, compressive, etc.), heat (Ruffini corpuscles), cold (Krause's end bulbs), pain (nociception), pressure, etc.

- the *intensity* of the stimulus (recall: each mechanoreceptor, as do *all* sensory receptors, has a different response threshold)

- their receptive field (narrow, concentrated; broad, distributed)

- their *spatial resolution* ability, which is commonly referred to as "two-point discrimination" (Ackerman 1990; Coren and Ward 1989). This is a measure of how close together two pointed probes can be used to simultaneously touch the skin of a blindfolded person, and still have that person perceive the stimulation to have derived from two, separate, distinguishable objects. The shorter the distance between the probes—at which the person still recognizes them to be two separate instruments—the better the resolution ability of the sensory organs involved

- their ability to *adapt*—loosely classified as being:
  - slowly adapting *tonic receptors*, such as Ruffini corpuscles and Merkel tactile disks that, together, account for about 44 percent of all mechanoreceptors. These are good continuous pressure and displacement transducers that are active when one is "feeling" things, grasping (a process called *prehension*), shaking hands, hugging, nudging, feeling one's clothes on the skin, etc.

  - rapidly adapting *phasic receptors*—including about an equal number (43%) of Meissner's corpuscles concentrated especially in *glabrous* (bald, smooth, hairless) skin such as that found in the palm of the hands, soles of the feet, lips, and erogenous zones of the body. Thus, they are active when one is kissing, fondling, licking, kneading, scratching, tickling, "finger tapping," and doing things that involve unsteady, time-dependent movements, since these are good velocity sensors.

  - a much smaller number (on the order of 3%), but the largest, and fastest-adapting of all *phasic receptors*, i.e., Pacinian corpuscles, that are especially adept at sensing acceleration and vibration. We've already mentioned their role in proprioception, but it is worth noting that they are also active in sensing vibrations as high as 2500 cycles/sec, although their maximum sensitivity is between 200 and 400 Hz (roughly the octave between G_3 and G_4 in the musical scale based on "concert A_4" = 440 Hz); those tactile vibrations in excess of 500 ($\sim B_4^+$-C_5^-) become "irritable."

All the sensory information from the skin receptors is passed on to the spinal cord through the dorsal roots of the afferent pathways in the 31 pairs of spinal nerves (see Table 4.1), one member of each pair for a corresponding, *ipsilateral* side of the body. Then, again, the signals *decussate* (cross over to the other, *contralateral* side of the spinal cord) en route up to the brainstem, and through it, to the thalamus. Leaving the thalamus, tactile data eventually terminates in the *somatosensory cortex* located in the upper central region of the *parietal lobe*.

"Paw-to-jaw" reflexes, additional general senses, and "vital signs"

One could write an entire book just about the body's mechanoreceptors. Indeed, they are many, they are varied, they respond to, and they are therefore measures of the body's:

- orientation in space (*proprioception*)
- blood and other tissue pressures (*baroreception*)

- various tissue and fluid volumes *(strain-gage transduction)*
- body movement *(kinesthesia)*
- stresses and strains *(myesthesia)*

and a long list of other *mechanical* variables that the body needs to *know about* and *carefully control* if it is going to survive! For example, many of the "paw-to-jaw" reflexes introduced in Chapter 4 ("The triune brain") and mentioned again earlier in this chapter ("The sensory system") are responses to feedback from mechanoreceptors, to wit:

- the need to *drink* ("thirst" reflex) is a response based partially on measurements of intra- and extracellular fluid volume
- the feeling of satiety after having satisfied the need to *eat* ("hunger" reflex) results from feedback received from the stomach's volume stretch receptors
- the need to *urinate* ("micturition" reflex) is triggered by stretch receptors responding to the increasing volume of the urinary bladder; and, by visceral volume receptors that sense excess ECF (such as occurs during "cold stress," when fluid accumulates in the torso due to peripheral vasoconstriction; Schneck 1990) and
- the need to have a *bowel movement* ("defecation" reflex), which derives from volume transducers located in the walls of the sigmoid colon, rectum, and anal canal.

Also:

- stretch receptors in arterial walls (e.g., the aortic and carotid sinuses) trigger responses that result from increased blood pressure, which dilates the walls of the artery
- *functional adaptation* in bone tissue is triggered by "pressure-electric" *(piezoelectric)* signals that derive from increased forces on the tissue. These stimulate the activity of bone-forming *osteo-blasts*, which inhibit *osteo-clasts*, while building additional bone tissue to reduce and redistribute the loading on the bone (see also Chapter 3 discussion of calcium metabolism, and Chapter 12, dealing with *adaptation*).
- *healing* is a process triggered in part by electrical "injury potentials" that, too, derive from increased tissue pressure due to inflammation of the injured tissue

and so on—the list, indeed, is very long!

But there are other variables, not necessarily *mechanical*, that, too, must be carefully monitored and controlled for the sake of *survival*. Several of these are handled by a category of general senses that monitor what are called *vital signs*—addressed in Table 5.5. For example, remember from Chapter 2 that we are an *isothermal* engine, so *body temperature* is among the *vital thermodynamic variables* that need attention. Note from Table 5.5 that we basically have only a degree-and-a-half Celsius temperature range, from 36°C to 37.5°C, to "play with," so we are in a very tight "window of opportunity."

Table 5.5 Vital sign ranges for a "typical" adult		
TEMPERATURE (FAHRENHEIT)	**PHYSIOLOGIC EFFECT**	**CENTIGRADE**
74.0	Lowest sustained body core temperature ever recorded in an individual who actually survived, but for only a very brief period of time	23.3
78.8	Death from hypothermia	26.0
89.6	Unconscious	32.0
95.0	Hypothermia	35.0
96.8	Lower limit of normal	36.0
98.6	Normal body temperature	37.0
99.5	Upper limit of normal	37.5
101.3	Febrile disease and hard exercise	38.5
102.2	Hyperthermia	39.0
104.0	Severe fever	40.0
105.8	Critical condition	41.0
107.6	Brain lesions	42.0
109.4	Heat stroke	43.0
111.2	Death from hyperthermia	44.0
114.0	Highest recorded limit at which an individual could actually survive, but for only a very brief period of time	45.6
ACID-BASE BALANCE pH	**CONCENTRATION OF HYDROGEN IONS IN NANOEQUIVALENTS PER LITER**	
<6.80	Death from acidosis	160
6.8–6.9	Comatose	127–160
<7.00	Critical condition	100
7.0–7.1	Disorientation	80–100
<7.20	Central nervous system depression	63

7.35	Lower limit of normal	45
7.40 ....General normal body alkalinity.....................40 (blood plasma; extracellular fluid; glomerular filtrate)		
7.45	Upper limit of normal	35
>7.60	Overexcitability of central and peripheral nervous systems	25
7.6–7.7	Severe anxiety and nervousness	20–25
7.7–7.8	Muscle spasms; critical condition	16–20
>7.80	Convulsions	16
>7.90	Death from alkalosis	10–12

RESPIRATION

8 to 18 breaths per minute at rest

HEART RATE

- 60–100 beats per minute at rest; "2+ pulse"
- Range, 39–129; mean = 80
- >100 beats per minute = tachycardia; "3+ 'bounding' pulse"
- <60 beats per minute = bradycardia; "1+ 'weak' pulse"
- 0 beats per minute = cardiac arrest; "absent pulse, 0"

BLOOD PRESSURE IN MILLIMETERS OF MERCURY:

SYSTOLIC	PHYSIOLOGIC EFFECT	DIASTOLIC
<90	Hypotension resulting in shock	< 60
90	Lower limit of normal	60
120 .... "Normal" blood pressure 70–80		
140	Upper limit of normal	90
140–160	Borderline hypertension	90–95
>140	Isolated systolic hypertension	~90
140–150	Mild high blood pressure	90–104
150–160	Moderate high blood pressure	105–114
>160	Serious high blood pressure	>115
.... Hypertension with danger of pulmonary edema and stroke...............		
160–200	Likelihood of severe heart disease and cardiac compromise; kidney failure; irreversible stroke	

cont.

pH RANGES FOR VARIOUS BODY FLUIDS		
Blood plasma	7.35–7.45	
Interstitial fluid	7.4	
Intracellular fluids:		
• Muscle	6.1	
• Liver	6.9	
Gastric juices	1.20–3.00 (highly acidic)	
Urine	5.50–7.00 (neutral, water)	
Saliva	6.35–6.85	
Pancreatic juice	7.80–8.00	
Bile	7.80–8.60 (highly alkaline)	

Also, take a look at how critical acid/base balance—involving *chemical variables*—is to the *vital* welfare of the organism. Not much "wiggle room" here, either, from an acidic lower limit of pH = 6.8 to an alkaline upper limit of pH = 7.9. That's a mere 1.1 range in pH level—for blood plasma and interstitial fluids, that is. Elsewhere in the body, especially in the alimentary canal, pH levels can vary considerably. Thus, as also shown in Table 5.5, stomach acid and gastric juices have highly acidic pH values down to 1.20 (or even as low as 1.00); and pancreatic juices and liver bile can be highly alkaline at pH values up to 8.6 (or even as high as 8.9).

As shown in Table 5.5, other vital signs include respiration rate (hyperventilating can lead to alkalosis due to excessive carbon dioxide depletion); heart rate (note, especially, the dangers of excessively high heart rates—*tachycardia*, and excessively low ones—*bradycardia*); and blood pressure.

And that's all we are going to say, for now, about *Feature 3* of our developing paradigm…except to emphasize that the music therapist must be especially aware of what can happen if one's sensory system is not "hitting on all cylinders!" It can result from anatomical issues that have to do with *structural* problems, or physiological issues that result from information-processing networks that have gone awry. One such "affliction"—not all that uncommon—is called *synesthesia*.

Synesthesia

Scene 1: There, lying in front of you is a luscious red apple. You can "see" it, and, suddenly, you can "taste" it, even though you haven't taken a bite!

Scene 2: You have a bad cold, seriously impeding your sense of "smell," which seems perfectly logical, since you can't breathe either, but suddenly, your sense of "taste" disappears as well! People speak of "hearing" or "tasting" *colors!* What's going on here?

What's going on is what we technically define to be *synesthesia*, from the Greek prefix *syn-*, meaning "together," plus *aisthanesthai*, which is Greek for "to perceive." Thus, to "perceive together" is to experience a situation wherein stimulation of *one* sense excites *another*. One may think of this as physiology's version of "checks and balances." Anatomically/physiologically, this form of sensory perception is attributed to afferent nerve pathways that "mingle" in the limbic system of the brain—which, you will recall, is one of the most primitive parts of this organ—rather than in the more specialized, more sophisticated, and more recently evolved sensory cortex. Indeed, long before we developed *cognitive* perceptive skills, we operated purely according to our *instinctive* sensory guidance, which was crucial to our survival. This guidance derived in part from "cross-talk" and *sensory integration;* from assembling into a "whole self-consistent picture," the digitized inputs from *all* sensory modalities—not relying entirely on any one, specific sense, to the exclusion of, or independent of, any other.

The *collective* input of *all* of the senses was relied on for survival; and interdisciplinary communication among *all* of the senses allowed one to develop associations that, perhaps, were even the earliest forms of what was later to become intellectual cognition. Thus, certain *sounds* are often associated with certain *shapes*. In music, for example, one speaks of soft "round tones," or shrilly "pointed" notes. Low-pitched sounds are often associated with "dark colors," and higher-pitched sounds, with "bright" ones. Certain perfumes stimulate in some people a corresponding sense of sound; and in others, a particular "vision." Taste and smell are perhaps the most salient example of synesthesia—they "go together" like the proverbial "love and marriage;" and so on.

The point of recognizing that synesthesia is an important aspect of sensory function—not an "abnormal enigma," that is unfairly considered to be an "affliction"—is, again, to emphasize that the human body functions as a *whole*, as the integrated sum of *all* of its parts, and not as an assemblage of pieces that merely *happen* to be put together a certain way. We don't *just* have "eyes" that respond to a certain portion of the electromagnetic spectrum to give us a sense of vision, and that's that! We don't *just* have "ears" that perceive certain forms of vibrational molecular kinetic energy, and thus, allow us to hear, and that's that! We don't *just* have thermal sensors for hot and cold; chemical sensors for sour and sweet; and tactile sensors for hard and soft. We make *connections* between hot and sour, cold and hard, sweet and red, and so on. We *perceive*, and we *check*, and we *cross-check*, and we *integrate*, and we *interpret*, and we *respond accordingly*, and we do all that we need to do to function optimally, and to survive. Thus, in Chapter 6 we shall examine this business of "survival" and of the control that is necessary to achieve and maintain it! We have identified this as *Feature 4* of our "living engine."

CHAPTER 6

The *Responsive* but *Stationary* Living Engine/Instrument

Feature 4 in our developing paradigm of the body recognizes that our "living engine/ instrument" must be able to *respond* to sensory stimulation if it is to succeed in meeting its most fundamental need (and drive), which is *survival of the self!* Indeed, that very attribute of living systems, i.e., their ability to respond to adequate stimuli, is one of seven that actually *classify* the human organism as being "alive" (Schneck 2005a). The other six include its ability to:

- metabolize—recall from Chapter 3, that this word derives from the Greek, *metabolē*, which means "change," as in *convert* the biochemical potential energy stored in food (which, in turn, originated as solar energy), into the kinetic energy associated with the transport and utilization of mass, energy, and momentum in all *living* systems (Schneck 1990). Again, this aspect of life includes enzymatically catalyzed biochemical reactions that either *build up (anabolism)*, or *break down (catabolism)* the protoplasmic constituents of living cells. We examined the essential features of *metabolism* in Chapters 1–3.

- *move*—i.e., as also discussed in Chapter 3, *movement* (kinetic energy) is the very essence of *reality*, in general, and *life* in particular. Indeed, *the* fundamental attribute of all living systems is *motion:* "*if movement ceases…life ceases!*" (Schneck 2005a and Chapter 3).

- *grow* and *develop* ("mature")—to the point of being able to

- *reproduce*—which is *Feature 7* in our model of the human body, representing the second strongest of all human needs: *survival of the species*, manifest in the drive for "sexual fulfillment." Indeed, *living engines have the ability to procreate… to make new engines (progeny) derived from their predecessors (parents)*, with one important caveat: they rely on evolutionary modifications to be introduced as necessary in order to ensure that the species *will* survive. In other words, *survival of the species* leads invariably to *survival of the most adaptable of the species* ("Thank you, Mr. Darwin"). That is, such modifications derive from *Feature 6* of our developing model, i.e., the living organism's ability to

- *adapt!*—this is an important attribute of living systems, about which we shall have much more to say in Part II, because of its particular relevance to how music therapy is applied clinically (see also Schneck and Berger 2006; Berger 2015).

Finally, living systems have the ability to *maintain* and *control* their internal environment in a process that goes by the name of *homeostasis*. We have alluded to this process before, but shall discuss it further below because—while it is true that in order to survive, living systems must be *responsive* to adequate stimuli—that response must be taken one step further, to include an effort to maintain *stationarity*.

Stationarity

The human body is an *ecosystem*. Allow me to explain: the word, *ecology* derives from the Greek *oîkos*, meaning "house." In everyday usage, at the *macroscopic*, so-called "continuum" scale of perception, "ecology" is most commonly associated with that aspect of *sociology* that addresses the relations between human beings— the populace; residents of the "house," which is planet Earth—and the environment that "houses" them. However, more generally—and more technically accurate at *any* scale of perception—*ecology* is that branch of *biology* that deals with the relation of *all* living things to both each other and the surroundings in which they exist and thrive. Thus, rather than the term *ecology*, which is "traditionally" used to study this relation, I prefer to use the more descriptive term, *bionomics*. Literally, *bionomics* refers to the "management" (Greek, *némein*) of "living things" (Greek, *bíos*) in relation to themselves and to their environment. Thus, an *ecosystem* is composed of all *bionomic* relationships on which the life of any particular living organism is based, in a *symbiotic*, as opposed to *parasitic* sense. The ecosystem includes such elements as food supply and distribution, waste management, weather, natural enemies, synthetic threats to survival, and so on.

At the *microscopic* scale of perception then, by definition, the *interior* of the human body fits the description of a bionomic ecosystem. The residents of this "house" (i.e., fats, proteins, carbohydrates, nucleic acids, etc.) dwell in the basic functional unit of the body, which is the *cell*, a type of microscopic *"village"* (see Chapter 1). Collectively, these "residents" constitute a self-contained populace living in regions surrounded by protective barriers, or "retaining walls"—*cell membranes*—that separate them from: (a) their surroundings; (b) *interstitial* environment; and (c) other "villages." However, these tiny villages attempt to *survive* by co-existing in symbiotic fashion with each other and with their environment (*Aside:* we humans could benefit a great deal by structuring our *social* and *political* systems the same way!). Each village (cell) is part of a buffered (see Table 5.5 and Chapter 5), isothermal (Chapters 2 and 5) ecosystem that depends for its survival on:

1. what is going on in all of the other cells of the body (*intercellular dynamics*)

2. what is going on *inside* the cell, itself (*intracellular* metabolic processes)

3. what is going on in the environment immediately *outside* the individual cell (*extracellular, interstitial* activity)

4. a very delicate balance among all three of the above, including movement across the cell membrane (*transmembrane* transport). This balance goes by the umbrella term *homeostasis*, although I consider that to be a misnomer for reasons on which I shall elaborate below.

From the Greek *hómoios*, meaning "like" (as in "the same") and *stásis*, meaning "position," *homeostasis* means, literally, "the same position" (the operative word here, which I object to, is "same"). In physiology, the term *homeostasis* connotes the condition wherein certain variables critical to life—such as temperature, pH, blood pressure, heart and respiration rate, etc.—are maintained within narrow limits (see Chapter 5). The term also includes those finely tuned feedback-feedforward physiological control mechanisms that are responsible for sustaining this *dynamically* balanced state of affairs. *Notice* I said, "*dynamically balanced* state of affairs," not "static," as implied by *stasis!* That's why I prefer the more accurate and descriptive term, *stationary* (defined below), rather than *homeostasis.* The latter suggests an unchanging, equilibrated state, a continuous "like position" wherein regulatory bodily processes insure that *nothing is happening*, as opposed to a *dynamic* state wherein a great deal *is* happening! Indeed, the human body is anything *but* equilibrated, for if it were, life-sustaining metabolism would cease completely and the organism would be dead! *Without movement…life ceases!*

In real life, the human body is in a constant state of flux—things coming in; things going out; things within the organism undergoing life-sustaining metabolic transformations. The "village gates" (membrane *pores*), spaced regularly along the retaining wall (cell membrane) constantly allow traffic to pass through them. Inbound traffic (*influx*) delivers to the village crucial supplies—oxygen, nutrients, and other life-sustaining biochemical raw materials. Outbound traffic (*efflux*) removes from the cell both toxic wastes—i.e., carbon dioxide, nitrogenous and non-nitrogenous products of metabolism, etc.—and those manufactured products, such as hormones and other biochemical compounds, that are intended to be delivered to neighboring villages for the purpose of serving specific functions there.

Often, *trucks* (*carrier molecules*) are used to transport certain substances more effectively—especially when those substances might otherwise not be able to make it through the village gates on their own—or, if it is necessary for them to pass directly *through* the walls of the village (effectively "jumping over the walls"), rather than accessing it through its gates. The study of cellular influx/efflux processes falls into the general category of *physiologic transport;* such transport is affected/controlled by the *permeability* of the cell membrane to the substances involved (Schneck 1990). One may think of cell-membrane *permeability* as the body's version of an "Immigration and Naturalization Services" branch of government, and *control* of permeability as being the anatomical analogue of "border patrol."

When all is said and done, however, *on average*, the ratio of conditions inside the cell to those outside remains relatively constant and stable. That constancy results from the fact that metabolic function subscribes to what, in the language of feedback control theory, is called, "operating set-points" (see Table 5.5, for example). And whereas one might argue that the relative constancy of these operating set-points justifies the use of a word like *homeostatis*, I consider a more appropriate description of this state of affairs to be one that is *stationary*—from the Latin *stāre*, meaning "to stand"—rather than *static* (i.e., unchanging).

In a statistical sense, a system is said to be *stationary*, or to possess the attribute of *stationarity*, when—even though all of the attributes/variables used to describe its state at any given time can deviate ("vary," dynamically) from rigidly fixed values—the *averages* over time of these "variables" do not wander very far from the fixed operating set-points of the system (e.g., 37°C body core temperature, 7.4 pH alkalinity, etc.). In other words, although the system is constantly changing dynamically, the variables that define its instantaneous state of affairs "wander" within only a very narrow neighborhood of prescribed reference quantities, and the statistical set of all their relevant *mean* values, averaged over time, do not change significantly, barring disease, trauma, or other serious disturbing influences. Thus, given all of the possible realized states of the system, i.e., the entire set of states that it can both exist in and shift into and out of dynamically without consequence:

- *if* anatomical feedback/feedforward control mechanisms exist (and in our body, they do when not otherwise impaired)

- *if* these are able, when working properly, to maintain reasonably time-invariant and stable, the respective *averages* of *all* the statistical variables used to describe these realizations

- *if* those averages conform to prescribed operating set-points for the system, within acceptable limited ranges

- *then*, the system is said to be *strongly stationary*.

That, to me, is a more accurate description of how the human body operates than is the misleading term *homeostasis*. I prefer to think of the human body as a *strongly stationary ecosystem* (Schneck 2006b).

To illustrate these concepts, consider the stationarity and control of, for example:

- *the balanced distribution of fluids inside and outside cells.* Recall from our discussion in Chapter 1 of body fluid compartments that, to avoid metabolic complications, the ICF/ECF ratio must be maintained in the narrow range between 2.0 and 3.0. Thus, control of: (i) cell-membrane *permeability;* (ii) transmembrane physiologic *transport;* (iii) daily *influx* of fluids; and (iv) daily *efflux* of fluids are all critical for survival. Should the proper distribution of fluids across the cell membrane be significantly disrupted, chemical-concentration gradients and other processes that drive transport into and out of the "village" can be so adversely affected that the quick and untimely demise of the individual involved would be imminent and quite inevitable! Upset the proper transport across a cell membrane—especially the *efflux* of metabolic waste products—and the physiologic system just plain shuts down! More to the point: you will die quicker from an accumulation of "garbage" in the system than from an absence of nutrients, because the accumulation of metabolic wastes "feeds back" through biochemical pathways to completely block the forward progression of the very life-sustaining reactions that created the waste products to begin with. The feedback—intended to prevent the production of more wastes—has dire adverse, life-threatening consequences! That's reason enough to require ICF/ECF fluid volumes and distribution to be among the "homeostatic" variables most carefully controlled, such control going by the name *compartmental kinetics*, and being one of the main functions of the kidney.

Recall further from our discussion in Chapter 2 that almost *all*—up to 99.75 percent—of the water contained in tubular urine is *reabsorbed* as it travels through the kidney nephron. However, depending on whether there is an excess or deficiency of ECF, the kidney maintains fluid balance by correspondingly regulating its output of urine—increasing that output (and stimulating micturition) to accommodate increased ECF, and decreasing the output (to a virtual urinary trickle, if necessary) when the opposite is true. In any case, for health reasons, a *minimum* of 300–400 milliliters of urine per day *should* be excreted to rid the body of nitrogenous wastes, which, as already mentioned, is probably why we even have a kidney to begin with! Note, too that one of our "paw-to-jaw" reflexes—thirst—kicks in if ECF volume drops by as little as one percent from a "desired" operating set-point.

The kidney's response to fluctuations in ECF derives from the activity of previously described *mechanoreceptors* (see Chapter 5)—physiological stretch receptors ("strain gauges") that are positioned at several strategic anatomical locations. These sensory receptors essentially monitor total fluid volume, being stretched as ECF increases, and vice versa. They relay this information to vasomotor centers in the brain which, in turn, modulate renal function. Such control is accomplished via sympathetic pathways (*renal plexuses*), and parasympathetic nerve fibers (*vagus nerve*) that richly innervate the blood vessels of the kidney. If ECF drops, the decreased volume lowers the firing rate of the stretch receptors, causing kidney urinary output to drop accordingly; if ECF rises, the increased volume stimulates the stretch receptors to fire at a higher frequency, causing kidney urinary output to increase by a corresponding amount.

This very neat feedback-control system can backfire, however, if the signals received are misleading or misinterpreted. For instance, we already talked about (see Chapter 2) the pooling of blood in the core of the body, due to reduced flow to the periphery during cold stress. This gives a *false* "ECF overload" alarm to the *core* stretch receptors, which triggers a tendency towards excessive urination without a compensating thirst response, and hence, a consequent danger of dehydration (again, both Napoleon's and Hitler's troops suffered severe dehydration in the Russian winter, see Chapter 3).

Similarly, the pooling of blood in the periphery of the body (mostly the head and neck), due to impaired venous return during exposure to a sub-gravity environment, gives a false ECF overload alarm to the *peripheral* stretch receptors, with similar results. So regrettably, the body can, indeed, be fooled, leading to some not-so-nice consequences!

But continuing, stationarity also involves control of:

- *body core temperature.* We have already talked a great deal about our body's need to function as an *isothermal* engine, at 37°C ± 1°C, so not much more needs to be said here.

- *blood chemistry*, in particular:

  ○ calcium levels (see Chapter 3, the skeletal system and the role of the parathyroid glands)

  ○ glucose concentration (we talked in Chapter 2 about the role of the liver in glycogen metabolism and we shall address later how the pancreas and its secretion of insulin affect blood sugar levels)

  ○ electrolytes (here, again, through selective reabsorption in the nephron, the kidneys have a first-order influence on the concentration of bicarbonate, potassium, sodium, and chlorine ions in blood plasma, not to mention glucose, too)

- *balance and equilibrium* (see discussion in Chapter 3)

- *vital signs* (see discussion in Chapter 5 and Table 5.5)

and so on; the list, again, is long and impressive! But when all is said and done, when we speak of the organism's ability to respond to adequate stimuli, in order to maintain stationarity, four key questions come immediately to mind, namely:

1. Exactly *what is it* the organism is responding *to?*

2. *Why* is it responding, i.e., what *needs/drives* is it trying to satisfy?

3. *How* is it responding, i.e., what *principles* govern the response mechanisms?

4. What anatomical architecture (organs and systems) is available to accomplish this response?

To answer these questions, we must develop our paradigm a bit further.

What the organism is responding to: the concepts of error signals and sensory integration

Error signals

Technically—again in the language of feedback/feedforward control theory—the body is responding to *error signals*. One may think of these as quantifying the gap between, on the one hand, the state in which the body *actually* finds itself at any given time, and, on the other hand, the state in which it would *prefer* to be at that time. The former is established by *intero- and exteroception*, as discussed in Chapter 5. The latter is in the form of *operating set-points*, some of which are hardwired (encoded) into one's genetic blueprint—*nature*. In fact, we have been addressing *nature's* physiologic operating set-points throughout this book, e.g., those related to vital signs (Chapter 5: Table 5.5, body core temperature, pH, blood pressure, respiration rate, etc.), balance and equilibrium issues (Chapter 3), enzyme and compartmental kinetics (Chapters 1, 2, 6), and so on. Moreover, we have emphasized the fact that these set-points are established in order to satisfy two fundamental human needs, to wit: *survival of the self*, and *survival of the species* (sexual fulfillment).

In Chapters 8 and 9 of Part II, we will add to this list of operating set-points additional human drives that may be classified as having been derived from *nurture*, i.e., one's *anthropocentric* (egocentric?) ambitions, experiences, stage of life, societal influences, and other contributing "intangibles." These will help to answer question 2 above, i.e., *why* the body is responding to error signals. The quick answer, of course, is that the body responds to error signals in an effort to be in a preferred state, which is the one in which its fundamental needs are being optimally met, and its drives to satisfy desired operating set-points are being adequately fulfilled.

As for the error signals themselves, they are generated in the body's central processing unit (CPU), which is the central nervous system, i.e., the brain and spinal cord (see Chapter 4). Operating set-points are stored there in permanent memory. Intero-extero-ceptive input signals are received there in temporary memory. The two are then "compared" to see how well they agree with one another. The comparison is made after all afferent signals are first *integrated*, which partially addresses question 3 above.

Sensory integration

We encountered the concept of sensory integration at the end of Chapter 5, when we talked about *synesthesia*. The word *integration* derives from the Latin, *in-*, meaning "not," and the word-root, *teg-*, meaning "to touch" (the same word-root that gives us *taste*). Hence, to *integrate* is "not to touch," in the sense of breaking something up into its parts. *Sensory integration*, then, connotes taking *all* sensory inputs—from *all* modalities (sight, sound, taste, smell, touch, etc.)—and "assembling them into a whole, not to be touched," which is to say, *integrating* them, as opposed to considering them separately and independent of one another. But…"whole" what?

Answer: the *whole* state of affairs—the *entire* intero-extero-ceptive situation that prevails, as encoded into *all* sensory modalities taken together; the *total* scenario of what's going on, to the extent that a response may or may not be necessary; a self-consistent, stable "portrait," in its entirety, perceived through all sensory modalities; a scene intended to affect a meaningful, optimal response to what the body is experiencing, based on an accurate, comprehensive assessment of that experience.

Since each sensory modality provides the CNS with only a *piece* of what the *entire* body is experiencing, i.e., a *particular* type of energy to which the corresponding ceptor is "tuned," what the CNS then receives are the individual *pieces* of a "jigsaw" puzzle. The CNS must assemble these pieces in order to "visualize the whole puzzle," and that's what sensory integration is all about. There are those (see, for example, Edwards 1989, and Springer and Deutsch 1981) who claim that this "assembly" takes place on the *right* side of the brain, the *left* side providing the "pieces" of the jigsaw puzzle. Thus, in the vast majority of humans, the "left brain" is presumed to be the rational, language-based, temporal, symbolic, cognitive side that handles the "details"—i.e., the "pieces" of the puzzle—while the "right brain" is supposedly the creative, intuitive-based, spatial, holistic, integrative side that "puts all the pieces together." In fact, the brain is probably not that *laterally specific*—and *both* sides handle *both* functions to varying degrees. But if we put all of these observations in context, another physiological optimization principle surfaces—one that is directly applicable to the subject of music therapy.

Remember in Chapter 2, when we spoke about the alimentary (digestive) system—how it breaks foodstuffs down into their *fundamental elements*, i.e., amino acids (for proteins), fatty acids (for lipids), simple sugars (for carbohydrates), etc.; how most of these are then absorbed as such, to be stored as *ingredients*, from which the body is able to manufacture ("assemble") its needed products, in accordance with *recipes* housed in its basic "cook book" (the genome)?

Remember in Chapter 5, when we spoke about the senses—how the brain "assembles" a *visual image* from the digitized information encoded into the optic nerve, or an *acoustic expression* from the digitized information encoded into the auditory nerve, and so on?

Well…in a cumulative sense, in the process of sensory integration we have yet another example of what is developing into a basic principle of physiologic function. Observe in this case, that the brain first processes *separately*, the digitized data encoded into *each* modality as it "reports in" to the CNS. Then it processes *collectively, all of these results*, from *all modalities taken together*, to arrive at a *net, compound, state-of-the-system* signal that it can compare to its stored operating set-points. In general, the two will not be equal, and so, there results *error signals* that derive from *all* of the information, encoded cumulatively, into *all* of the afferent nerves that feed into the CNS. Thus, we have:

Physiological Optimization Principle Number 5: The body synthesizes products from stored ingredients, such as digested food elements stocked in the cell's pantry; and digitized sensory signals deposited to its working memory. The organism breaks things down (catabolism) and builds them up (anabolism), as necessary, to meet its various needs. It thus economizes on both space and time; and optimizes its use of limited resources.

This principle is actually a special case of a generic paradigm for the formulation of an integrated body of knowledge in any area of study (Schneck 2001b, 2011b). The paradigm describes a seven-step process that is precisely applicable to how the body processes information on which to make life-and-death decisions.

The elements of knowledge embedded in principles of physiologic information processing and sensory integration

Interestingly, the etymology of the word, *know*, is of physiologic origin and has come to mean what it does today via a rather devious route, whereby the absorption of food was equated to the absorption of information. Back in ancient Aryan times (perhaps 3500 years ago), words beginning with kn- or gn- were used to describe a swelling or biting. The reference to swelling is obvious in such derived words as "knot, knee," or "knuckle," while the reference to biting shows up in words such as "gnawing," and "gnashing."

Corresponding to the idea of biting and swelling were the related concepts of eating (chewing food), which is followed by the associated distension of the stomach (bloating), which precedes the absorption of food there from (see Chapter 2). Thus, by extrapolation, if one "eats" *facts* (as opposed to food), the *brain* (as opposed to the stomach) will swell; and, if one then *absorbs* these facts and attaches some meaning to them, one becomes *aware* of whatever information was contained in those facts—nourishing the mind just as food nourishes the body. So, we have the Greek "gnostikos," followed by the Latin "gnoscere," which evolved into the Anglo-Saxon "cnawan," which later became "knawen," then "knowen," and finally, the shortened version, "know," which has survived to date.

Therefore, to "know" is to have absorbed information that endows us with an intellectual awareness of the meaning inherent in facts, figures, and sensory inputs. And that meaning can be considered to have derived from seven "pillars," if you will, that are the foundation for all we call "knowledge," and the brain calls *sensory integration*. These seven elements of knowledge are: frame of reference, scale of perception, resolution, structure, order, relation, and synthesis.

1. Frame of reference

As was formalized by Einstein in his Theory of Relativity, no observation or measurement is absolute and totally objective. Quite to the contrary, it is impossible to separate the measure*ment* from the measur*er*—the observer, and the frame of reference in which the observation is being made. All knowledge is, in fact, dependent on "who's doing the looking;" there is really no such thing as an "absolute reality"— *perception is reality!* As noted by the famous American writer, Anaïs Nin, "We don't see things as they are, we see them as we are" (Nin 1961). In other words, *we* are the ultimate instrument of knowing, the ultimate observers, the frames of reference to which all perceptions are referred; and "All our knowledge has its origins in our perceptions," in the words of Leonardo da Vinci. Diane Ackerman (1990) explains it this way, "When scientists, philosophers, and other commentators speak of the real world, they're talking about a myth, a convenient fiction. The world is a construct the brain builds based on the sensory information it's given, and the information is only a small part of all that's available." Continuing, "Evolution didn't overload us with unnecessary abilities,"…"We're given only the sensory information crucial to our survival," although, "we can modify our sense and broaden that sensory horizon with technological amplifying devices." Bottom line:

> *As a music therapist, you must understand, first and foremost, that your client is the one doing the "sensing." He or she is the "frame of reference" to which all sensory inputs are ascribed. Perception is client specific and thus, what is real to him/her is what you must deal with!*

2. Scale of perception

Going one step further, what we sense in our space/time experiences—*adequate stimuli*—depends entirely on the level at which we are looking. As we discussed in Chapters 1 and 3, that level or *scale of perception*, can range in *space* from sub-nuclear dimensions theoretically approaching zero length, to super-cosmic expanses hypothetically reaching out to infinity; and in *time*, from miniscule fractions of a second, approaching zero duration, to huge time scales also approaching infinity. We operate primarily in the electromagnetic (light), thermodynamic (heat), chemical (smell, taste), and mechanical (hearing, touch) regions of this spectrum, expanding it modestly by microscopic and telescopic technologies. However, at each level of perception, we are constrained in our ability to "know" by resolution.

3. Resolution

We can narrow down our observations and perceptions—fine-tune them—only to the extent that we can discriminate as being *separate* and *distinctly different*, two adequate stimuli that are delivered to our various sensory receptors close together in space and/or in time. This fact is embedded in the concept of *resolution*—the ability that an anatomical sense organ or technological transducer has to distinguish among individual pieces of information that arrive extremely close to one another, either spatially or temporally. We spoke briefly in Chapter 5 about our senses' ability to resolve adequate stimuli and this issue is addressed in much greater detail by Ackerman (1990), Coren and Ward (1989), and Tortora and Grabowski (1993), among others.

4. Structure

This element of knowledge deals with the *attributes* that *characterize* a particular manifestation of reality that we want to know about and interpret. As previously mentioned, one may think of "structure" as the individual pieces of a jigsaw puzzle, or, alternatively, the raw ingredients of a cake—flour, water, yeast, eggs, milk, and so on. The process of "knowing"—within the constraints imposed by frame of reference, scale of perception, and resolution—generally begins by impregnating ("swelling") the brain with pieces of information that, collectively, presumably define the elements ("ingredients") that make up the whole of anything we want to know about. To the brain, *structure* takes the form of afferent nerve pathways that bombard it with *action potentials* emanating from the body's various sense organs. Now it has to "go to work," ordering, defining relationships, and synthesizing—integrating this plethora of data into a comprehensive interpretation of "what's going on;" putting the jigsaw puzzle together into a final picture; "baking the cake!"

5. Order

In this phase of sensory integration, the brain seeks to *arrange* structure into some logical groupings, i.e., layer the data into some meaningful *sequence* that gives it *temporal* significance, look for similarities in shape, color, etc., that give the data common attributes; unique features that distinguish them from one another, and thus, create an array of data *sorted* according to these common features. Again using the jigsaw puzzle analogy, after one has collected all of the pieces to the puzzle (*structure*), one sorts them, separating them according to shape, color, "edge pieces," and so on, *ordering* them into some logical sets for further, *inductive* processing. Order deals with converting *raw data* into *temporal/spatial information*, from which one can eventually extract *meaning*. Remember back in Chapter 4, when we spoke about the language of the human body and drew a parallel to verbal communication, wherein alphabetical letters (structure) are arranged (ordered) to form words, which are put together (ordered) into sentences, which are assembled into paragraphs, which, collectively, make up chapters and…eventually…a book (the entire jigsaw puzzle)? Well, what we are talking about here is quite analogous. But the brain takes it one step further by extracting *meaning* from this *ordered* set of *structure*.

6. Relation

In establishing relationships, we are actually going through the process of *assembling* our jigsaw puzzle. We are attempting to extract meaning from information, which is the essence of *perception*. For example, when ordered:

- *if* individual elements of an adequate stimulus are found to be in close proximity to one another—spatially or temporally—even *if* we can resolve them as two separate inputs, *then* they are perceived to belong to a single unit or figure, i.e., have that *relationship* in common with one another; and *then* they are *assembled* accordingly (e.g., we put all of the "edge pieces" together to form the border of our jigsaw puzzle). This is known as *cerebral sensory grouping* and *assembling.*

Going one step further:

- *if* consecutive individual elements of an adequate stimulus are perceived to follow one another in the same direction, *then* they tend also to be grouped together, i.e., to share *directionality* in common with one another. This has directly to do with *sensory tracking.*

Moreover:

- *if* sensory data suggests that a physical space or region is enclosed by, or otherwise bounded by a continuous closed curve, *then* that region tends to be perceived as being entirely self-contained. In fact, as a complement to the previous bullet of *directionality*, if your brain senses that a region it perceives *should* be self-contained (i.e., the region *should* be closed), actually has gaps in its enclosing boundary, it (your brain) automatically "fills in the gaps," thus closing the perceived perimeter of the region!

The bottom line is that "relation" deals with how well the brain can extract connections and/or affiliations from among the ordered data so that, once "assembled," it can tell what the jigsaw puzzle is all about. This element of knowledge also deals with spatially *coordinating* structure, and temporally *synchronizing* the ordered elements, so that their ability to perform in one's mind, the functions for which they were intended in "real life" is clear, and the brain is thus (at least hypothetically) able to define those functions uniquely. Finally, having gone through the cognitive processes of structuring, ordering and extracting relations, as constrained by frame of reference, scale of perception, and ability to resolve sensory inputs, the last step in "knowing" is *synthesis.*

7. Synthesis

Derived from the Greek *syn-*, meaning "alike, together with," and *thesis*, meaning "a proposition," *synthesis* deals with an ability to combine into a "whole," everything hitherto known only in bits and pieces; how well the entire body of processed information can be *organized* and *assembled* into a self-consistent, meaningful, reproducible, logical entity—the entire jigsaw puzzle! Moreover, it connotes how well we *understand* this body of information; how well we can, by deductive reasoning, derive meaningful conclusions from it; and how well the body of information, and the conclusions drawn from it stand up to the test of time. If we can *identify* what the assembled jigsaw puzzle tells us—what the puzzle is a picture of, and how accurate our interpretation of it is—then the processes of sensory integration and synthesis have worked to perfection. Similarly, with respect to "knowing," if there is a coherency and consistency to the information accumulated and processed, then we can truly call it a "body of knowledge."

So, how does this all relate to music? Well, recall that *music*, as a *whole*, is also composed of fundamental elements: rhythm (pulse, pace, pattern), melody (pitch—see Table 5.2, prosody, phrasing, profile), harmony (intervals, consonance, dissonance), timbre (sound quality), dynamics (loudness/softness—see Table 5.3), form, and so on (Schneck and Berger 2006). Thus, the music therapist must be especially conscious of how the body handles these in terms of *physiological optimization principle number 5*. For example, how is *rhythm* "broken down" and processed (Berger 2015)? How does the brain handle dissonant intervals and how are error signals generated in response to dissonance? How does melody track through cerebral pathways? And so on. And, how can I, as a music therapist, exploit these aspects of physiologic information processing in order to optimize how I use music in the management of my clients?

Moreover, the music therapist must be especially aware that everything we have been saying assumes that the anatomical systems involved in sensory integration are all working properly. In diagnosed populations, something may have gone awry—error signals might be generated when they *shouldn't* have been, leading to *fear responses* to *perceived* threats, real or imagined (Schneck and Berger 2006; Berger 2002, 2015). But also, these might not be generated when they *should* have been, resulting in *pathological responses* (Berger 2002), such as occurs in cold stress, when the body dehydrates without triggering a thirst reflex. The error signals, themselves, might be flawed (Schneck 1990, 1992), and so on. In other words, be aware, alert, and on the look out for such possibilities as you formulate a music therapy approach to managing such populations. Be also aware that:

Error signals often manifest themselves as symptoms!

Thus, through physiologic mechanisms that result in, for example, discomfort, fatigue, pain, signs of over-exertion, thirst, hunger, fever, cardiac arrhythmias, high blood pressure, anxiety, depression, behavioral issues, unexplained mood swings, crying, sleeplessness, and, yes, even clinical issues such as autism, attention deficit hyperactivity disorders (ADHD), and a long list of diagnosed ailments…

The body is trying to tell you that something is wrong…listen!

One last point: there is a complementary anatomical design principle that follows directly from this physiological optimization principle. We shall address the *anatomical design principle* in Chapter 13 of Part II, when we talk about the body in space. For now, we note that the seven-point paradigm outlined above is described in more detail in Schneck and Berger (2006), and Coren and Ward (1989). It goes by the more formal name of the *Gestalt Laws* that govern the perceptual organization and management of sensory data. Briefly, these laws define our instinct to minimize confusion, make order out of chaos, and create the most stable, consistent, and meaningful interpretation of sensory stimuli, so that we can respond most effectively to the error signals that those stimuli might be generating. And how does that response come about? Through *Feature 5* of our developing paradigm: that is to say, as necessary, error signals can stimulate the release by the CNS of *control* (efferent, motor) signals. These act to mobilize target, *effector* organs and tissues, as described in the next chapter.

CHAPTER 7

The *Controlled* Living Engine/Instrument

As mentioned in Chapter 6, *sensory integration* only partially answers the third question posed, i.e., "*How* does the body respond to error signals generated by the central nervous system?" A second part of that answer is embedded in *Feature 5* of our developing paradigm, i.e., the concept of *control signals*. Again in the language of feedback/feedforward control theory, *control signals* are those messages delivered to *controlling systems*—composed in this case of specialized organs and tissues that allow them to either totally eliminate, or at least reduce significantly (to acceptable levels), the error signals generated by the CNS. The objective is to bring the errant *controlled systems*—i.e., those found to be suffering from disturbed function (hence the error signals)—back to within a reasonable neighborhood of their operating set-points.

> *As a music therapist, this is precisely your objective, too, i.e., to control the body using music as your "control signal." By thus eliciting profound responses from controlling systems (the subject of this chapter), music is capable of driving controlled anatomical systems gone awry back toward a state of optimal function.*

Physiologic control signals

When the CNS concludes that the body is not functioning within an acceptable neighborhood of its desired operating set-points, based on:

- an *accurate* intero-extero-ceptive result derived from "proper" sensory integration; or real or imagined
- a *misinterpreted*, "perceived" state of disarray

it documents that perceived deviation by generating *error signals*, within which are embedded information about:

- how *far* the organism has "wandered off course" from the prescribed operating set-points, i.e., the *amount of deviation*
- the *rate of deviation*, i.e., how *fast* it has been "going off track"

- the *history of deviation*, i.e., the extent to which the disruption has *persisted;* how *frequently* it has occurred; and for *how long* the problem has been going on.

This last consideration actually takes us to *Feature 6* of our developing model, i.e. in a "long-term" sense, addressing *survival of the species, evolutionary* anatomical design changes necessary to satisfy this objective; in a (relatively) "short-term" sense, to satisfy the drive for *survival of the self;* and of more immediate interest to the music therapist, *physiologic accommodation,* the discussion of which we reserve for Part II. For now, we note that:

- the body's attempt to correct for *amount of deviation* is called *proportional control*
- *rate of deviation* is handled by *differential control*
- *history of deviation,* including *adaptation,* is managed by *integral control* mechanisms.

In all three cases, the *control signals,* themselves, take the form of:

- specific *hormones.* Recall from Chapter 1 that these are chemical substances released into the blood, to be carried to "target organs" that have hormone-specific *receptor sites* for them. These organs are thus stimulated to increased functional activity. In particular, because:
  - hormones need first, to be *manufactured*…then
  - *transported* to their respective target organs, by the bloodstream—which travels to *all* regions of the body…and finally
  - cleared from the body once they have accomplished their intended mission.

They tend to be used when responses to error signals can:

  - be *momentarily* (on the order of milliseconds) *delayed*
  - *recruit* more than one target organ to the rescue (leading to a generalized, systemic response)
  - *persist* for an extended period (up to a few seconds or more) of time until the hormone is eventually *cleared.* Thus, as a general rule, *hormones are most effective for proportional control.*

This is as opposed to

- specific *neurotransmitters,* described in Chapters 1 and 4. Because these:
  - *already exist* (manufactured in advance and stored in the synaptic vesicles of axon terminals)
  - have *direct synaptic connections* with the respective organs and tissues that they innervate, thus limiting their influence to *just* those nerve-network-specific anatomical regions

    ◦ are cleared almost *immediately* (on the order of *micro*seconds),

They tend to be used when responses to error signals need to be:

    ◦ *virtually instantaneous* (much faster than hormones)

    ◦ *localized* to specific anatomical regions ("first responders")

    ◦ *not* expected to persist, i.e., be immediate, but short lived.

Thus, as a general rule, because of their ability to respond very quickly, *neurotransmitters are most effective for differential control.*

Going one step further, important contributors to *integral control* are:

- specific *antibodies*, described later in this chapter. These are substances that incite immune responses to invading organisms and "foreign" proteins (see related discussion of food allergies in Chapter 2); and their association with integral control has to do with their ability to "remember" previous encounters with these invaders, and be "ready for them" the next time they strike. In their function, antibodies resemble:

- *enzymes*, in that they are associated with and often derived from serum proteins. Recall that enzymes are critical for all metabolic function—control included— in that they catalyze the manufacture of any biochemical constituents that are required to maintain stationarity.

In summary, the living engine is thus "fine tuned" by feedback/feedforward, proportional, differential, and integral control signals that operate on systems that respond to them. This partially answers question 4 posed in the previous chapter, i.e., "What anatomical architecture is available to generate responses to error signals?" Let's finish the answer by noting that, following the above reasoning regarding hormones, neurotransmitters, and antibodies/enzymes, the *controling* systems that actually *generate control signals* in response to CNS-generated *error signals* are, respectively, the: endocrine (hormones), autonomic (neurotransmitters) and, immune (antibodies) systems. Let's take a closer look.

The endocrine system of ductless glands

The endocrine system is a diverse group of glands that produce and release (Greek *krinein*, meaning "to secrete," or "to separate")—in response to error signals—*directly* (as opposed to via connecting ductwork) into the bloodstream some 40–50 *hormones* that remain *inside* ("endo-") the body to perform a variety of regulatory (control) functions. As mentioned earlier, because of their distribution by the bloodstream, hormones can deliver a *systemic, proportional,* "global" response to error signals, permitting different, more anatomically widespread tissue/organ groups to act in concert to effect a desired outcome. Such an outcome, although temporally delayed, can also persist for a "relatively" long period of time—compared, that is, to autonomic responses. (While it is true that response times on the order of *milli*seconds are 1000 times slower than are those on the order of *micro*seconds, they are both still pretty fast! Moreover, most endocrine glands, in turn, are actually under the direct control of the autonomic nervous system).

Table 7.1 Ductless endocrine glands and their respective hormone secretions	
GLAND	**HORMONES**
H-P-A Axis:	
• Hypothalamus:	Oxytocin, OT (pitocin; manufactured)
	Thyrotrophin-releasing hormone, TRH
	Corticotrophin-releasing factor, CRF
	Growth hormone-releasing factor, GHRF (somatocrinin)
	Growth hormone-release inhibiting hormone, GHRIH (somatostatin)
	Antidiuretic hormone, ADH (vasopressin; pitressin)
	Gonadotrophin-releasing hormone, GnRH
	Prolactin-releasing factor, PRF or PRH
	Prolactin-release inhibiting factor, PIH (dopamine)
	Melanocyte-stimulating hormone-releasing factor, MRF
	Melanocyte-stimulating hormone-release inhibiting factor, MIF
• Pituitary (Hypophysis):	Oxytocin/pitocin stored/released
	Thyroid-stimulating hormone, TSH (thyrotrophin, TTH)
	Adreno-cortico-trophic hormone, ACTH (adrenotrophin)
	Growth hormone, GH (somatotrophin, STH)
	Antidiuretic hormone, ADH (vasopressin; pitressin)
	Follicle-stimulating hormone, FSH (gonadotrophin-1)
	Luteinizing (lactogenic) hormone, LH (gonadotrophin-2-Type-I; Luteotrophic hormone, LTH)
	Interstitial-cell-stimulating hormone, ICSH (gonadotrophin-2-Type-II)
	Prolactin/Lactogenic, PRL
	Melanocyte-stimulating hormone, MSH

cont.

GLAND	HORMONES
H-P-A Axis:	
• Adrenal (Suprarenal)	
° Gluco-(Oxy-)Corticoids:	Cortisone; cortisol; corticosterone-A; corticosterone-B
° Deoxy-(Gluco-)Corticoids:	Deoxy-cortisol; deoxy-corticosterone
° Mineralocorticoids:	Aldosterone; dehydro-epiandro-sterone
° Gonadocorticoids:	Androgens; estrogen; progesterone
° Medullary Hormones:	Epinephrine (adrenalin) norepinephrine (noradrenaline) dopamine
Thyroid	Thyroxin (T4) Tri-IodoThyronine (T3) Thyrocalcitonin (Calcitonin)
Pancreatic Islets of Langerhans	Insulin Pancreatic polypeptide Glucagon (pancreatic glycogenolytic factor) Somatostatin (growth hormone-release inhibiting hormone)
Parathyroids (4)	Parathormone
Pineal (Epiphysis Cerebri) ("Third Eye")	Melatonin Adrenoglomerulotropin
Thymus	Thymosin
	Thymic humoral factor, THF
	Thymic factor, TF
	Thymopoietin
Kidneys Endocrine Function	Erythropoietin (bone marrow) Renal erythropoietic factor, REF
Male Testes (Androgens)	Adrenosterone Androsterone Isoandrosterone Testosterone
Female Ovaries	Estrogens Estradiol Estrone Estriol
Progesterones	α-and-β-progesterones
Other	Relaxin Inhibin
Female Placenta	Human chorionic gonadotropin, HCG Human chorionic somatomammotropin, HCS (Human placental lactogen, HPL)
Some Paraganglia	Various

Listed in Table 7.1 are most of the ductless endocrine glands, together with their respective major hormone secretions. Although, technically, the hypothalamus is not part of the endocrine system, for purposes of discussion, it is listed among these glands because it:

- actually *manufactures* several of the hormones—e.g., pitocin and vasopressin—that are then *stored* in an endocrine organ and subsequently *released* from it

- actually *controls* endocrine glands such as the pituitary and kidney, by the use of "releasing hormones and factors," and their opposites, "release-inhibiting hormones and factors

- is at the head of the *hypothalamic-pituitary-adrenal* (or "H-P-A") *axis* of organs that is so crucial to the body's response to *stress!*

As we learned in Chapter 4, the hypothalamus is an important cerebral center for regulating and integrating many vital body functions, among them:

- body temperature (thermoregulation)

- the timing and synchronization of internal physiologic processes with natural, external *circadian* and *circannual* cycles

- cardiovascular activity

- the maintenance of body fluid balance (osmoregulation)

- control of sugar and fat metabolism, hunger, gastric acid secretions, thirst, digestion, etc.

- the activity of the autonomic nervous system

- the activity of the endocrine system

- emotional feelings of "rage," "fight-or-flight" mechanisms, and other behavioral responses to adequate stimuli

- control of the pituitary gland via the *hypothalamo-hypophyseal-portal system.*

The hypothalamus does all of this via the hormones that it manufactures and releases, as listed in Table 7.2. Despite accounting for a mere one-three-hundredth of the total mass of the brain, it lies at the very center of the limbic system, just below and behind the frontal lobe of the cerebrum, and it is linked by many complex neural pathways to almost all of the other regions of the brain, giving it a disproportionate share of cerebral responsibilities. The hypothalamus is physically attached to the posterior lobe of—and thus communicates *neurologically* with—the pituitary gland (hypophysis, or "master gland") by the *infundibular hypophyseal stalk.* Otherwise, it communicates with the latter via *vascular* channels, as described below.

The pituitary gland

The "P" portion of the *H-P-A axis* is the pituitary gland. It is second only to the "H" portion—the hypothalamus—in its hormone function, but *first* in its endocrine importance. "Officially" designated to be the *hypophysis* (from the Greek for "an undergrowth," as in "growing below") *cerebri* ("the brain"), this gland lies just below the hypothalamus, at the base of the brain, as a downward extension of the floor of the third ventricle. Like the hypothalamus, the hypophysis is also quite small in proportion to its physiologic importance, having just 15 percent of the mass of the former. However, through its secretion of so-called *tropic* hormones (from the Greek prefix *trop-*, connoting "to turn on"), this tiny gland controls virtually all of the functional integrity of the other major endocrine glands, as well as their morphological development. That's why it is often called the "master gland."

The word *pituitary* derives from the Latin *pituita*, meaning "phlegm." This "phlegmatic" gland has two readily identifiable anatomic divisions—an *anterior* (front) *lobe*, or glandular portion called the *adenohypophysis;* and a *posterior* (rear) *lobe*, or neural portion called the *neurohypophysis.* The latter is where the hypophysis shares *neural* pathways with the hypothalamus, through the hypophyseal stalk. Only two hormones—antidiuretic (ADH), and lactogenic oxytocin (OT), both synthesized in the hypothalamus—are stored and released from here in response to direct *nervous* stimulation from the latter. The other pituitary hormones listed in Table 7.1 are produced, stored, and secreted from the adenohypophysis in response to various "release," and/or, "release-inhibiting" hormones and factors. These are manufactured and secreted by the hypothalamus (see Table 7.1) and delivered to the glandular portion of the pituitary by communicating *blood vessels* and capillary networks. Among the many organs controlled by the pituitary are the: adrenal cortex, thyroid gland, gonads, mammary glands, and kidneys. Let's take a look at the adrenal gland(s), the "A" portion of the *H-P-A axis.*

The adrenal glands

Like the pituitary gland, the two adrenal glands—located above (*superior*) and lying on each kidney (hence their more formal designation as *suprarenal glands*)—also have two identifiable anatomic divisions: a larger, glandular *adrenal cortex*, and a smaller, neural *adrenal medulla*. The cortex of these triangular-shaped organs—in response to having its blood supply deliver to it adrenocorticotrophic hormone (ACTH) from the pituitary adenohypophysis—manufactures and secretes at least 11 *adrenocortical hormones*—*corticoids*, which are *steroids* made from cholesterol precursors (another important use for cholesterol!). Steroids are distinguished chemically from three other types of hormones:

- *Biogenic amines* (e.g., the thyroid gland's T_3 and T_4; the "tissue damage hormone," histamine; the brain's serotonin; the pineal gland's melatonin; and the adrenal medulla's *catecholamines:* epinephrine and norepinephrine).

- *Peptides/proteins* (e.g., TSH and glyco-protein chains of amino acids with attached carbohydrate side chains.

- *Eicosanoids* (e.g., prostaglandins and leukotrienes).

Adrenal steroids deal with the proper metabolism of electrolytes, carbohydrates, and proteins; and in the maintenance of the functional integrity of the membranes of many types of cells. But here's a very important point:

Any and all types of stress promptly activate the adrenal cortex to "do its thing!"

Thus, responses of the H-P-A axis play a critical role in regulating the systems that help to protect the body from *perceived* (that's the operative word) danger and/or environmental hazards.

Major secretions of the adrenal cortex are listed in Table 7.1. The major hormones involved in the body's *resistance reaction* to stress are listed in Table 7.2 (more about that in Part II).

Table 7.2 Major stress hormones (resistance reaction)	
ORGANS/GLANDS INVOLVED	HORMONES SECRETED
Hypothalamus	Corticotrophin releasing factor, CRF Growth hormone-releasing factor, GHRF Thyrotrophin-releasing hormone, TRH
Anterior Pituitary	Adreno-cortico-trophic-hormone, ACTH Thyroid-stimulating hormone, TSH Human growth hormone, GH (to the liver)
Adrenal Cortex	Gluco-corticoids (mainly cortisol) Mineralo-corticoids (to the kidneys) Aldosterone
Thyroid Gland	Tri-Iodo-Thyronine (T3) Thyroxin (T4)

In response to receiving impulses from the nerve fibers of the sympathetic division of the autonomic nervous system, the *adrenal medulla* manufactures and secretes three major *adrenomedullary hormones:*

- Epinephrine (adrenalin, or adrenine—the principal adreno-medullary secretion)

- Norepinephrine (noradrenalin, or arterenol)

- Dopamine (a precursor of adrenalin, derived in equal amounts from the adrenal medulla and the hypothalamus).

As mentioned earlier, these hormones are *catecholamines*, made from amino acid precursors (principally tyrosine). Their major physiologic influence is on metabolic regulation and cardiovascular function, specifically in response to various emotional and anticipatory states, and to "fight-or-flight" reactions to emergency situations or *perceived* threats. Thus, again, we note that:

> *any and all perceived threats to one's well-being immediately activate the adrenal medulla to mobilize the body, in an effort to "fight or flee!"*

Moreover, in the body's response to perceived threats, adrenal catecholamines "enjoy" a synergistic relationship with hormones secreted by another endocrine organ—the thyroid gland—such that the responses of the organism to the hormone secretions of the former, are elaborated upon, enhanced, and augmented by the complementary hormone secretions of the latter.

The thyroid gland

We have already said a great deal about the thyroid gland, so not much more needs to be said here. Recall from Chapter 3, that this endocrine organ straddles the trachea and secretes three major hormones: (i) *thyroxin* (T_4), secreted in response to TSH-stimulation (being delivered by vascular networks emanating from the pituitary gland); (ii) *tri-iodo-thyronine* (T_3, also manufactured in the liver and striated skeletal muscles), synthesized by "de-iodinating" thyroxin; and (iii) *thyrocalcitonin* (or calcitonin), secreted in response to plasma circulating levels of gastrin and calcium.

Recall further that thyroxin, acting via the *calorigenic effect*, plays a major role in thermoregulation, allowing the thyroid gland to be the body's *thermostat*. Calcitonin is intimately involved, together with the four *parathyroid glands*, in regulating blood calcium levels. Thyroid hormones also stimulate respiration, protein synthesis, fat metabolism, and ATP-utilization, and they have varying effects on mineral balance. And speaking of the parathyroids…

The four parathyroid glands

These, too, were discussed in Chapter 3, when we talked about the importance of calcium for the proper function of muscles, nerves, and cell metabolism. Indeed, calcium may very well be *the* most important electrolyte in the human organism, playing a major role in, at least:

- neuromuscular excitability and contractile processes
- cell membrane permeability
- tissue secretory processes
- the activity of enzyme systems
- blood clotting (calcium is clotting *Factor IV*)
- neural network synaptic transmission

- the activity of hormones
- bone and teeth growth, development, metabolism, and mechanical behavior
- acid-base (pH) balance
- photoreception and, more generally, the proper transduction behavior of sensory mechanisms

...to name just a few! Thus, it is not surprising to learn that a drop in serum calcium concentration of as little as 3 percent from the desired "operating set point" range of 8.4–11.0 mg/dl, will cause these disk-like endocrine glands that straddle the posterior (back) sides of the thyroid to "go to work," secreting the hormone *parathormone* to "do its thing" as described in the aforementioned chapter.

Further to our consideration of endocrine organs that we have mentioned and discussed previously, let's say a few more words about the kidneys.

Endocrine function of the kidneys

The kidney's contribution to the endocrine system involves the manufacture and secretion of the hormone *erythropoietin*, EPO, under conditions of *hypoxia* (a lack of oxygen). This hormone acts on bone marrow to increase the production of oxygen-carrying red blood cells (*erythrocytes*). It does so by exploiting the fact that *all blood cells derive from the same precursor—a hemocytoblast—by a process called cellular differentiation.* Depending on the body's needs at the time, the hemocytoblast will mature into a red blood cell, white blood cell, or platelet. However, under the influence of EPO—essentially acting as a critical enzyme in the differentiation pathway (a "track-switch," so to speak)—this process is *biased* toward the production of erythrocytes, as opposed to any other type of blood cell. This is contrary to the activity of yet another endocrine organ: the *thymus gland*, which promotes the maturation of *white* blood cells.

The thymus gland

As already introduced in Chapters 1 and 2, the thymus gland is a bi-lobed lymphatic organ located behind the chest bone (*sternum*), between the lungs. As shown in Table 7.1, this gland secretes four hormones, all of which promote the maturation of white blood cells *(leukocytes)* called *T-cells*, which are a type of *lymphocyte*. These destroy foreign microbes and substances in the body. Although relatively large in youngsters, the thymus gland gradually atrophies, so that by adulthood, it is replaced almost entirely, but not completely, by fat and connective tissue. Be that as it may, what's left of this endocrine gland in the elderly *does* seem, still, to play a vital role in the organism's immune processes; and, apparently, its hormone secretions might even contribute to retarding the aging process. We need to learn more...so let's now move from blood *cells* to blood *chemistry*.

Endocrine function of the pancreas

We alluded to the pancreas's endocrine function in Chapter 2, when we introduced its *Islets Of Langerhans*. These manufacture and secrete directly into the bloodstream the four hormones listed in Table 7.1. Of these, perhaps the most important is *insulin*, secreted in response to increasing concentrations of blood glucose. Insulin is basically a *carrier molecule* for glucose, as is *hemoglobin* for oxygen. Left to its own devices, glucose has great difficulty leaving the blood to pass through cell membranes. Thus, in the absence (or impaired manufacture and release) of this hormone, digested carbohydrates "pile up" in the bloodstream, increasing blood (and urinated) sugar levels in a clinical condition called *diabetes mellitus* (from the Greek prefix *dia-*, meaning "through," *bainein*, meaning "to go, " and *melit-*, a word-root connoting "honey" or "sweet"), and its associated *melituria* ("sweet urine") as the "excess" sugar is excreted. Insulin is also important for the proper metabolism and utilization of glucose by the cells themselves, and for optimizing the storage of body fuels.

By contrast, in response to decreasing blood glucose levels (compared to what the body "needs" at the time), and acting in concert with epinephrine, glucagon stimulates the liver to both: (i) start *releasing* glucose into the bloodstream—as a result of the hormone's catalysis of the breakdown of stored glycogen, in a process called *glycogenolysis*; and (ii) start *manufacturing* glucose de novo—"new, from scratch," as a result of the hormone's catalysis of *gluconeogenesis*. Glucagon and insulin, then, comprise a *reciprocally inhibiting system of pancreatic hormones* that together regulate blood glucose levels and control carbohydrate metabolism.

As we move down Table 7.1, we come next to a set of endocrine glands that are intimately associated with *Feature 7* of our developing paradigm, i.e., the living engine's ability to *procreate* as a means for ensuring *survival of the species*. Procreation involves satisfying the need for *sexual fulfillment*…and so, we have the *pineal gland* and the *gonads* (male testes and female ovaries).

The pineal gland

The pineal gland, or body—more technically called the *epiphysis cerebri*—derives its name from its pine-cone-like shape. This small endocrine gland hangs like a wasp's nest from the roof of the third ventricle of the brain, its "pinealocyte" cells manufacturing and secreting two hormones. One of them—*adrenoglomerulotropin*—may assist in stimulating the adrenal cortex to secrete *aldosterone*. The other one—*melatonin*—is believed to exert an inhibitory effect on the gonads. The pineal gland is often referred to as the body's "third eye," because it apparently functions only in the dark, i.e., it is a *nocturnal* gland, turning off when light hits the retina of the eye. The organ is also (apparently) intimately involved with our sense of well-being, the onset of puberty, the amount of testosterone (male) and estrogen (female) that is produced, and our "sense of season." The latter is associated in particular with *subtle* seasonal behavior, especially as it relates to sexual drives and "seasonal" urges to reproduce, which brings us to *Feature 7* and the sexual function of the endocrine glands.

Endocrine functions of the sex organs (genital glands)

As shown in Table 7.1, the male *testes* manufacture and secrete four *androgens*, of which the major one is *testosterone*. This hormone enhances normal sexual development and behavior; and it also stimulates and promotes the growth of secondary sexual characteristics, such as deepening of the voice at puberty. The female *ovaries* manufacture and secrete three *estrogens*, two *progesterones, relaxin* (which helps to prevent premature labor), and *inhibin* (which inhibits the secretion of *follicle stimulation hormone*, FSH). The female estrogens function in basically the same way as the male androgens, but have the additional responsibility for the development of an *ovum* (egg cell), and for cyclically preparing the uterus for an impending pregnancy during the first half of the (approximately) 28-day *menstrual cycle* ("period"). The progesterones take over for the estrogens during the second half of the menstrual cycle, preparing the uterus for the expected implantation of a fertilized egg cell (*blastula*). They are also responsible for the development of both the maternal placenta and the mammary glands, following which placental hormones take over during the ensuing pregnancy (if there is one). The placental hormones, in addition to increasing the subsequent production of more estrogens, progerones, and relaxin, also prepare the mother's breast tissue for lactation and reduce her utilization of glucose (making more available for the growing *fetus*).

Although details of the human *reproductive system* are "beyond the scope of this book" (for more, see, Goss 1966; Jacob *et al.* 1982, and Tortora and Grabowski 1993), suffice it to say here that this system is a collection of organs and tissues by which the organism can propagate the species by giving birth to offspring. *Sexual* reproduction requires systems that include:

- *male organs:* scrotum and penis; testes; seminal vesicles; prostate gland; and bulbourethral (*Cowper's*) glands

- *female organs:* vulva; vagina; uterus; uterine tubes (*fallopian*); ovaries; and mammary glands (*breasts*).

Thanks to your biological parents' drive for sexual fulfillment, and the success of their efforts, "you" started out as a *zygote* (Greek *zygōtós*, meaning "yoked," as in fastened together). You were a single cell, derived from the fusion of your mother's mature egg cell (*oocyte*), with your father's mature sperm cell (*spermatocyte*).

Not too long thereafter, the zygote began to divide over and over again, becoming specialized in a poorly understood process called *cellular differentiation*. Such specialization allowed *you* to grow from one fertilized egg to, eventually (some nine months later), a mature baby. The process of *cellular differentiation* resulted in the development of some 210 different types of cells (see Chapter 1), in such a way that the 100 trillion *total* cells that are now the adult "you" can perform all of the functions necessary to keep themselves, and, therefore *you*, alive.

The vast majority of these cells can also procreate, with the notable exception of red blood cells, which have no nucleus, and a few others. The architecture for accomplishing this was mentioned in Chapter 1 (see Figure 1.1); it includes "centrally located," cellular *centrosomes*, which contain *centrioles*, surrounded by *centrosphere* protoplasm that allows for cell division:

- *reduction* division (*meiosis*)—generating gametes that have half the chromosomes of each parent; and/or, otherwise:

- *reproductive* division (*mitosis*) that effectively *clones* the parent cell.

As was pointed out in the Preface, we defer further discussion to anatomy and physiology references, as we close this section on the endocrine system with a few words about the paraganglia and exocrine glands.

The paraganglia and exocrine glands

As the name suggests, *paraganglia*—from the Greek prefix *para-*, meaning "along side of," and *ganglia*, describing "a mass of nervous tissue"—are groups of secretory cells associated anatomically ("along side of") and embryologically with the neurological pathways ("ganglia") of the sympathetic nervous system. They are located in various organs and parts of the body including, for example:

- where the stomach empties into the duodenum (*pyloric gland*)

- in the first portion of the small intestine (*duodenal glands*)

- at the level of the coccyx (*coccygeal gland*)

- in the region of the inferior mesenteric artery (*aortic bodies*)

- in the atria (*cardiac muscle fiber glands*)

- in the liver (*chromaffin bodies*)

- near the celiac, renal, supra-renal, aortic, hypogastric, and abdominal ganglia of the sympathetic nervous system.

In all cases, these paraganglia have a variety of both—endocrine *and* exocrine functions. *Exocrine* refers to glands whose secretions *leave* the body as a result of being transported directly, or through a duct, to an epithelial surface. There are dozens of such glands scattered throughout the body, including:

- sudoriferous, sweat-secreting glands of the skin

- Bartholin's glands that secrete a vaginal lubricant

- various salivary glands
- Bowman's olfactory glands in the nose
- Brunner's glands in the duodenum
- Cowper's semen-secreting bulbourethral glands at the penis' base
- Ciacrio's tear-secreting lacrimal glands in the eye
- ceruminous wax-secreting glands in the ear
- sebaceous oil-secreting glands of the skin
- Frankel's glands below the edge of the vocal cords
- semen-secreting male prostate gland
- Theil's glands in the gall bladder
- pancreatic exocrine glands
- goblet cells of the digestive, respiratory and urinary systems
- crypts of Lieberkuhn glands in the intestinal mucosa
- milk-secreting mammary glands in the female breast

...to name just a few! These, in fact the entire endocrine/exocrine systems, work to generate *hormonal physiologic control signals* that complement (and are even, themselves, controlled by) *neurotransmitter physiologic control signals* generated by the *autonomic nervous system.*

The autonomic nervous system revisited

The title of this section says, "revisited" because we already "visited" the autonomic nervous system in Chapter 4. Recall that it is the responsibility of this system to control *involuntary* (not under conscious control) bodily functions (including the activity of many glands); and that it consists of two divisions: a *sympathetic* (thoraco-lumbar) and a *parasympathetic* (cranio-sacral) one. Recall further that, although not etched in stone, whatever the sympathetic nervous system does, the parasympathetic nervous system does just the opposite. We gave a few examples in Chapter 4; Table 7.3 goes into some more detail.

Table 7.3 Major effects of the autonomic nervous system

SYMPATHETIC DIVISION	ORGANS/TISSUES AFFECTED	PARASYMPATHETIC DIVISION
Norephinephrine	MAJOR NEUROTRANSMITTER	Acetycholine
Rate increased (chronotropic effect)	HEART	Rate decreased
Ejection force increased (inotropic effect)	HEART	Very little effect
Constriction	ARTERIOLES	No significant effect
Diminished viscous secretion	SALIVARY GLANDS	Copious watery secretions
General vasoconstriction	STOMACH	Very little effect
Increased alkaline juice secretion	STOMACH	Increased acidic juice secretion
Inhibited (Decreased motility)	G.I. TRACT	Stimulated (Increased motility and tone)
Contraction	ANAL SPHINCTER	Inhibition
Diminished secretion	PANCREAS	Enhanced secretion
Wall inhibited	URINARY BLADDER	Wall excited; contracted
Sphincter excited	URINARY BLADDER	Sphincter inhibited
Pupils dilated	EYES	Pupils constricted
Lens weakly flattened	EYES	Lens strongly bulges
No significant effect	LACRIMAL GLANDS	Stimulates secretion
Dilated bronchi	LUNGS	Constricted bronchi
Glycogenolysis	LIVER	No significant effect
Free fatty acid release	ADIPOSE	No significant effect
Stimulated to secrete epinephrine	ADRENAL MEDULLA	No significant effect
Stimulated (copious sweating)	SWEAT GLANDS	No significant effect
Contracted	SPLEEN CAPSULES	No significant effect
Contracted	PILOMOTOR MUSCLES	No significant effect
Contracted	URINARY SPHINCTERS	Relaxed
Variable	UTERUS	Variable
Ejaculation	PENIS	Erection
Energy mobilized	HOMEOSTASIS	Excretion; protection; Conservation and restoration of resources

Note from the Table that the *parasympathetic* nervous system—operating through its neurotransmitter, *acetylcholine*—conserves and restores energy, and maintains *routine* daily functions of the body, such as salivation, digestion, excretion, and homeostasis. It has little or no effect on blood pressure, arterioles, the adrenal gland, and several other organs and tissues that are not involved to a great extent in fight-or-flight stress responses. By contrast, the sympathetic nervous system—operating through *its* neurotransmitter, the catecholamine, *norepinephrine* (noradrenalin)—mobilizes the body to react to stressful situations or emergencies, such as fear or anger. Both divisions operate through numerous *ganglia* (nerve masses) and pre- and post-ganglionic nerve fibers that eventually innervate the corresponding receptor sites of *target, controlled* organs and tissues to effect a desired response. Target receptor sites for *acetycholine* are called *cholinergic receptor sites;* those for *noradrenalin, adrenergic receptor sites.* The latter are of two types: α- (eliciting an *excitatory* response); and β- (eliciting an *inhibitory* response). There is one notable exception to this "rule:" stimulation of the β-receptors of *heart muscle*—designated "β-1 receptors"—is *excitatory, increasing heart rate and strengthening the force of contraction.* Hence, one hears, in pharmaceutical jargon, of "beta-blocker" drugs intended to suppress this excitatory response.

Finally, stimulation by the sympathetic nervous system of α-receptors in blood vessel walls (i.e., arteriolar smooth muscle tissue) evokes *active* excitatory responses that cause constriction of the vessels leading to the periphery, compromising flow to the extremities. This is important in the body's response to cold stress, which we explored in Chapters 2 and 3. The reverse happens during heat stress, i.e., sympathetic stimulation of the β-2-receptor sites in these blood vessel walls (and in bronchioles, as well) evokes an inhibitory response, causing the smooth muscle tissue to relax. This allows blood pressure to *passively* dilate the artery and hence increase flow to the periphery in order to dissipate the heat (Chapters 2 and 3). And so…we come last (but certainly not least) to the immune system.

The immune system

We spoke in Chapters 1 and 2 of how our body has developed sophisticated mechanisms to distinguish its own anatomical constituents from foreign, potentially toxic, harmful, destructive or damaging substances. Thus, we have an *immune system:* a collection of biochemical factors, cells, tissues, and organs responsible for the body's resistance to, or recovery from, invasion by microbes and foreign matter. This system includes several sub-systems, among them: (i) skin and a variety of mucous membranes that present external barriers to microbial invasion; (ii) bone marrow, where most invasion-and-infection-fighting white blood cells are produced; (iii) the previously discussed thymus gland; (iv) blood, itself; and (v) lymph nodes, also previously discussed.

Special white blood cells—called *lymphocytes*—are "trained" to recognize the unique, one-of-a-kind, chemical and structural (geometric) identity of cellular polypeptide chains that distinguish the genetically coded configuration of one "engine," from that of another, or of a different species altogether. As mentioned in Chapter 1, these unique chains are called *human leukocyte antigens* (HLAs), part of the *histocompatibility complex* (MHC), or, clinically, "transplantation antigens." The mechanism of identification is actually quite straightforward, and exploits *Anatomical design principle number 7:* a geometric property of *organic* compounds, called *chirality.*

Chirality

Recall that the human body is "written mainly in the key of C," i.e., we are *organic engines,* biochemically configured around the carbon atom (Schneck 2007a). Why? Because, to create complex, life-giving molecules requires an attribute that *only* the carbon atom possesses, i.e., the unique ability to *share* electrons with other atoms. This attribute allows carbon to form, at once, *covalent* (as opposed to *ionic*) bonds with as many as four other, either individual, or groups of, atoms. When these are four *different* atoms (or groups) the resulting molecular configuration lacks a plane of symmetry, i.e., it is not of "even parity." Such a lack of symmetry—called "odd parity"—allows for the existence of two *geometrically* (spatially) distinct, although *chemically* identical arrangements of molecules—configurations that are *exact in every way, except that they are non-super-imposable mirror images of one another.* This condition is designated *chirality*—a term borrowed from the Greek *cheir,* meaning "hand," as in, your right and left hands are *chiral* or non-super-imposable mirror images of each other. Thus, carbon atoms sharing electrons with four *different* groups are called *chiral centers.*

Now, the significance of chirality is that in biological systems, such stereo-chemical specificity is the rule, rather than the exception, because:

- it allows for the type of *substrate-specific,* geometric molecular congruence that is the basic mechanism exploited by such processes as metabolic catalysis, active transport, and cell-membrane receptor-site activation. That is to say

- typically, only *one* of the two stereo-isomers of a chiral substance has the preferred orientation required for the rigid "lock-and-key" compatibility criterion exploited by the above bullet, e.g., your right foot has difficulty fitting into your left shoe; your left hand does not fit easily or comfortably into a "right" glove, etc. In other words

- it makes sense for the all-important catalysts, enzymes, carrier molecules, cell-membrane markers, etc., and most of the compounds they work on, to have the *desirable* property of chirality.

It is "desirable," in the sense that, among other advantages, asymmetric specificity in molecular structure guarantees the *uniqueness* of the *only* configuration required to ensure proper physiologic function. That is, the opposite of chirality, i.e., symmetry or *isometry,* by definition *precludes* there being any *preferred* configuration or molecular

THE *CONTROLLED* LIVING ENGINE/INSTRUMENT

orientation, so *specificity* cannot be guaranteed. However, by applying this anatomical design principle that imposes *geometric constraints—forcing* molecular "building blocks" to have asymmetric configurations, such that they can *only* be assembled in *one unique* way—one effectively minimizes the possibility of winding up with undesirable alterations in patterns of assembly, alterations that might lead to non-functional (even potentially harmful) end-products. Thus:

> *Anatomical design principle number 7: Molecular chirality, helps to minimize the element of chance, resulting in the same geometric structure—the same product—time after time, with no exceptions; and so, it guarantees biochemical success, while optimizing both structural efficiency and functional effectiveness.*

Due to the existence of carbonic chiral centers, organic substances also exhibit the property of *optical activity*. This term derives from the fact that a purified ("resolved"), homogeneous (*homochiral*) solution of only one, but not both, of the two possible mirror images of the material, can rotate the plane of polarized light passed through it. It does so because the homogeneous arrangement of its molecules is *not* random, but rather, uniform and highly organized.

That is, if plane-polarized light passes through a *heterogeneous* chiral substance composed of huge numbers of randomly oriented, highly disorganized molecules that have *no* preferred orientation, for every "right-handed" molecule that acts to rotate the light clockwise, there is another "left-handed" one that rotates it counter-clockwise. The *net* result is *optical inactivity*—all rotations are neutralized and the light passes clear through the material, totally unaffected.

On the other hand, if the substance is purified to ensure that all of its chiral molecules are oriented in the *same* direction, individual rotations of the plane of polarized light do *not* cancel…they *add!* Thus, there is *optical activity*—the plane of polarized light experiences a net rotation. If the rotation is to the right—clockwise viewed along the light-beam axis toward its origin—the substance is said to be *dextrorotatory* (from the Latin *dexter*, meaning "right") and it is designated by a prefix (+)-, or D- attached to the name of the substance. If the rotation of the polarized plane of light is to the left (counter-clockwise), the substance is said to be *levorotatory* (from the Latin *laevus*, meaning "left") and it is designated by attaching a prefix (-)-, or L- to the name of the substance.

At this point, I'll bet you're wondering what all of this has to do with the immune system and human anatomy. It will become clearer if you persist to read on—I promise! So…continuing…

Substances that have identical chemistries, but differ in at least one physical attribute, are called *isomers* (from the Greek *isos*, meaning "equal," and *méros*, meaning "part"). If the physical attribute involved happens to be *chirality*, the isomers are called *enantiomers* (from the Greek *enantios*, meaning "opposite," and *méros*). (*Note:* Those isomers whose molecular configurations are not necessarily mirror images of one another are called *diastereomers.*) Now…for the anatomical and physiological relevance of all of this.

First of all, typically, because of their mirror image incompatibilities, different enantiomers of chiral compounds often taste and smell different. Therefore, enantiomerism is one mechanism by which your body's chemical senses can distinguish among different testants and odorants—that's the good news. The bad news is that, as chemical reagents, different enantiomers can have vastly different (often toxic!) effects on the body. Thus, here's the bottom line:

- The way(s) in which each of the mirror images of a pair of enantiomers act on corresponding substrates is not identical.

- Reaction rates, and/or potential products of biochemical pathways can be drastically different—even toxic. In the extreme, a desired biochemical reaction might not even occur at all!

- Pairing up the *right* enantiomer with the *right* substrate is crucial (as in, for example, proper typing and cross-matching in blood transfusions or organ transplantations and…yes…*pairing up the right client with the right type of music!*).

To summarize: there is definitely a *need* to have asymmetry in biological materials. Thus:

> *The human genome codes uniquely for the L-form of amino acids and the D-form of organic sugars.*

Exactly *why* L- (as opposed to D-) or D- (as opposed to L-) for amino acids and organic sugars, respectively, remains a mystery, with theories that range from purely random natural selection, to extraterrestrial considerations, all of which scientists are still hotly debating with no consensus in sight.

Be that as it may, carbohydrates—designated by the suffix, -ose, such as *hexose*, the six-carbon sugar glucose—are all of the D-form. Amino acids, on the other hand, are all of the L-form, it apparently having a better inherent stability against being broken down, than does the D-form. In any case, histocompatibility schemes rely upon the chiral, "jigsaw puzzle-like" architecture of our anatomical microstructure, and on the requirement that there be *exact* congruence among the "pieces" that make up that very complicated structure. If a "piece"—for example, a foreign protein with the *right* HLA geometric configuration—"fits" into the puzzle matrix, it is presumed by the lymphocyte (the physiologic analog of a "quality control engineer") to "belong there," and thus becomes *biocompatible.* If the piece *does not fit*—i.e., has the *wrong* HLA configuration—the lymphocyte so "tags" it. Granulocytes recognize these tags and proceed to dispose of the "foreigner" by enzymatically digesting it and delivering the remains to the body's garbage-disposal units.

The immune response relies heavily on the participation of *antibodies, activated T-cells* ("killer" lymphocyte cells), *activated macrophages* ("angry" white blood cells), *plasma cells, memory cells* (that store the genetic code of the foreign materials with which they have previously come in contact), *lymphocytes*, and *histamine*. This response also underlies the very essence of the concept of blood grouping and typing, according to the HLA configuration of the cell membrane of erythrocytes; and furthermore, it relates directly to our discussion in Chapter 2 of food allergies, wherein the allergen is (incorrectly) identified as a "foreign" protein.

Some closing remarks

To this point, we have identified "this thing called me" to be an *electrochemical* (not heat!) *engine* (or "instrument," if you prefer), one that is:

- alive (Chapters 1, 2, and 6)
- mobile (Chapter 3)
- digital (Chapter 4)
- sentient (Chapter 5)
- responsive (Chapter 6)
- controlled (Chapter 7)
- fertile (Chapters 1, 2, and 7)
- accommodating.

We have said very little about this last feature, for good reasons! *Physiologic accommodation* goes directly to answering the question, "How does 'Me' work?" which is addressed in Part II of the book. It also provides further insight into answering two other questions raised in Chapter 6, i.e., "*Why* is my body responding to error signals?" and, "*How* is it responding?"—two questions of particular interest to the music therapist. Thus, we begin Part II by taking a look in Chapter 8 at the "*Why?*" and in the remaining Chapters, at the "*How.*"

The music therapist, of course, is interested in *how* the elements of music—rhythm, melody, harmony, timbre, dynamics, and form—can influence (stimulate) the control systems addressed in this chapter, as these respond to the needs and drives (Chapter 8) of the client and his/her *perception* of "threats" to his/her survival. In particular, the therapist seeks to use *music* as a "control signal" to suppress the manufacture and persistence of *stress hormones* when their presence is not desired. Such suppression is intended to *drive the organism*, eventually, to *physiologically adapt*. Let's explore further.

PART II

HOW DOES "ME" WORK?

CHAPTER 8

The *Motivated* Living Engine/Instrument

Why is my body responding to error signals? The short answer is, "To stay alive!" Indeed, the reason we are motivated to heed the warning signs implicit in error signals is that we are *driven*—first and foremost—by the need to *survive*, both as an individual and as a species.

The longer answer is embedded in the very definition of an *error signal*, i.e., the "gap" between where the body *is* at any given time and where it would prefer to *be!* In turn, "where it would prefer to be," is quantified by the "preferred" *operating set-points* that govern the function of all of the body's systems. Such rigorously established set-points (or *physiological reference signals*) are space/time "target values" toward which *anatomical controlled system* configurations aspire to equilibrate, i.e., reach *stationarity*.

The problem, of course, is that the *maintenance* of "preferred configurations" is not *sustainable*, because anatomic systems in real life are constantly being bombarded by *disturbances* that upset their then stationary state—hence, *error signals*. Among the worst of these disturbances, especially from the point of view of the music therapist, is *stress*, most notably, *bad stress!*

Bad stress!

One of my most impressionable experiences in medical school occurred when a professor came into class one day and declared, "Let's get something straight right up front: cancer doesn't kill you; heart disease doesn't kill you; strokes don't kill you; diabetes doesn't kill you," and after going down a long list of debilitating medical afflictions that do not "kill you" he paused, looked us straight in the eye, and concluded with, *"Stress kills you!"* He went on to emphasize that the deadliest lethal diseases with which we humans are afflicted derive not from the *symptoms*—see Table 8.2—for which we are clinically treated, but from the stress, both psychological and physical, to which we subject our bodies on a day-to-day basis—see Table 8.1.

Table 8.1 "Top 20" sources of stress

1. Personal finances and financial concerns
2. Careers and career decisions
3. Excessive responsibilities, including marriage
4. Special events, such as weddings, bar mitzvahs, etc.
5. Health issues, especially failing health
6. Having and raising children
7. Loneliness
8. Sex and sexual issues
9. Relatives and relationships with relatives
10. Neighbors and relationships with neighbors
11. Religious issues/spirituality
12. Fear, perceived or otherwise, including exam anxiety
13. Time constraint issues, especially meeting deadlines
14. Space constraint issues, including claustrophobia
15. Sensory disturbances, such as:
    - Putrid/rotten/decaying smells
    - Bitter/acrid/sharp tastes
    - "Screeching" sounds, such as chalk on a blackboard
    - Emergency vehicle sounds, including sirens
    - "Dissonant" musical sounds
    - Visual glare; flashing lights
    - Pain (nociceptive reflex)
    - Tactile disturbances
    - Cold stress/heat stress
    - Extremes of pressure
16. Unrealistic expectations, especially in competitive situations
17. Moving/relocating
18. Dietary issues and food sensitivities/allergies
19. Political issues/war/unrest
20. Issues triggering strong emotional reactions

Table 8.2 Some stress symptoms			
MUSCULO-SKELETAL	**CARDIO-VASCULAR**	**ENDOCRINE**	**GASTRO-INTESTINAL**
• Muscle ache/ pain • Muscle weakness • Muscle tightness • Twitching/ spasms • Tension headaches • Back pain • Clumsy movements • Wobbly legs/ pacing • Trembling/ shaking • Shaky voice • Nervous tics • Facial pain/ frowning • Grinding/ clenching teeth • Startling reactions • Jaw pain/ache • Rheumatoid Arthritis • Fibromyalgia • Tension myositis	• Chest pain • Faintness • Dizziness • High blood pressure • Migraine Headaches • Tachycardia • Heart palpitations • Cold hands • Increased Perspiration • Cold feet • Sweaty palms • Arhythmia • Visual problems • Fast pulse	• Arthritic joint pain • Infertility • Fatigue • Polydipsia • Skin rash • Hypothermia • Hyperthermia • Bloating • Menstrual Problems • Diabetes • Skin pallor • Hot/cold flashes • Acne • Bone pain • Bulimia • Dysphagia	• Abdominal pain • Belching • Diarrhea • Gas pains/gas • Constipation • Nausea • Vomiting • Urination problems • Acid stomach • Appetite changes • Heartburn • Intestinal pain • Cramping • Gastritis • Ulcerative colitis • Irritable bowel syndrome • Peptic ulcers

BEHAVIORAL	EMOTIONAL	COGNITIVE	IMMUNE

• Sleep problems
• Chronic lateness
• Hyperventilation
• Shallow breathing
• Procrastination
• Bad dreams and nightmares
• Restlessness
• Sexual issues:
  ◦ Difficulty
  ◦ Disinterest
• Accident prone
• Avoidance
• Social issues
• Fidgeting
• Foot/finger tapping
	• Exhaustion
	• Anxiety
	• Depression
	• Agitation/alarm
	• Guilt/anger
	• Anxiousness
	• Fear/fright
	• Frustration
	• Helplessness
	• Hopelessness
	• Impatience
	• Panic attacks
	• Loss of control
	• Tense/jittery
	• Uneasy/shaky
	• Self-consciousness
		• Confusion
		• Daydreaming
		• Distracted
		• Racing thoughts
		• Fearful thoughts
		• Distorted thoughts
		• Negative thoughts
		• Lack/loss of concentration
		• Memory loss
		• Loss of objectivity and perspective
		• Preoccupation
		• Loss of creative thinking
		• In a fog/daze
		• Indecisive
			• Asthma
			• Chronic disease
			• Allergies
			• Herpes
			• Mouth Sores
			• Psoriasis
			• Frequent colds/flu
			• Cancer
			• Mono-nucleosis
			• Strep throat
			• Frequent infections

RESPIRATION	SKIN	GENERAL
• Choking sensation • Feelings of lump in throat • Pressure in chest • Rapid breathing • Shallow breathing • Shortness of breath • Sighing • Chronic cough/phlegm • Raspy throat • Strained voice • Halitosis (bad breath)	• Acne • Flushed face • Generalized sweating • Hives • Hot and cold spells • Itching • Pale face • Psoriasis • Changes in color • Strained face • Worrisome look	• Careless in taking medications • Changes in eating, drinking and smoking habits • Loss of interest in physical appearance • Impulsive behavior • Immobility • Dissociation • Always in a haze • Neuritis/neuralgia • Moodiness/cranky • Generally irritable, nervous, restless

At the top of his list of daily sources of stress were what he called "artificial, self-inflicted 'bad' stresses"—such as those listed in Table 8.1. These are "bad," in the sense that they "attack" our body in ways that our civilization has *created* for itself, through activities of daily living over which we *do have significant control!* That's the operative word here—*control!*

We distinguish, then, the items listed in Table 8.1—"bad" stresses—from what my professor termed "natural, 'good' stresses." The latter include, for example, *environmental extremes* that provoke our senses in ways over which we have *little or no control!* For instance, we talked in Chapter 3 about how our body handles extremes of hot or cold. In Chapter 5, we noted that there are pupillary reflexes that can adjust how much light reaches the retina under extreme conditions of darkness or brightness; how our sense of taste handles extremes of sweet or sour; how we can adjust our sensitivity and reaction to odors that range from pungent to bland, and so on.

Indeed, in all cases, these "natural stresses" are "good," in the sense that they trigger responsive reflexes that are indigenous to our instinct for survival. Thus, being exposed to them—*when our responsive reflexes are working right* (music therapists take note!)—is actually "healthy," in that the body is equipped (see Chapter 7) to handle them "naturally." It is thus able to maintain an effective vigilance against potential or impending annihilation—that vigilance being manifest in autonomic and stress-hormone responses, as described briefly in Chapter 7 (see, also, Tables 7.1, 7.2, and 7.3). However, remember the musculoskeletal issues encountered by Napoleon and Hitler (see Chapter 3). Think, also, about the long-term consequences of a very fast heart beat (tachycardia), and high blood pressure. Look carefully at the impressive list of symptoms and afflictions itemized in Table 8.2. Think about the words of my medical school instructor and it becomes immediately obvious that:

Stress hormones are not intended to hang around!

They are "first responders;" they exist only to handle acute, emergency situations over which we have little or no control; their intent is to deal *immediately, temporarily,* and *effectively* with these emergencies, and then go away.

Indeed, if stress hormones linger for more than brief periods of time, their effects, as shown in Table 8.2, become just the opposite, i.e., they are *toxic* chemicals, in the sense that they instigate unsustainable, long-term, pathological physiological responses that are dangerous to one's health. Acute, emergency situations become, instead, a "stressed-out way of life," and a very hazardous one at that! Again, paraphrasing my professor, it is those very adverse *reactions* (Table 8.2) to prolonged exposure to "bad stress" that eventually "kill you!"

Sources of bad stress

Listed in Table 8.1 are the "top 20" sources of stress. For the sake of the interested music therapist, it's worth saying a few additional words about some of them, to the extent that they contribute to our self-imposed, *unhealthy*, prolonged and enduring state of "fight-or-flight" existence.

Meeting deadlines

For better or for worse we, in an effort to maintain some degree of efficiency and effectiveness in the way our society functions, inflict on ourselves the requirement that things be done in a timely manner, i.e., that we "hit" prescribed target dates and times. For instance, the normal filing deadline each year for U.S. Federal income tax returns is April 15. Colleges and universities adhere to strict deadline dates by which admission applications are due. The same is true for submission of research proposals and/or progress reports to granting agencies. Indeed, for just about any activity that has associated with it an application process, there is always a "must be postmarked by (or received by) such-and-such a time and/or date" tagged on to the application form. We race to get to the bank or post office before it closes; journalists, editors, reporters and writers race to make publication deadlines; we race to pay bills on time to avoid having our accounts assessed for interest and late-penalty charges, and so on; the list is long. We impose on virtually all aspects of our life some time/date deadline that sets off unhealthy "fight-or-flight" alarms and corresponding "bad-stress" responses. Perhaps that's why it is called a *dead*-line!

Taking tests

In every aspect of life, humans are obsessed with judging and evaluating performance. This makes test anxiety a leading cause of "bad stress" responses. From the day we are born—and even before that, *in utero*, when the developing fetus is "tested" for possible congenital abnormalities and signs of anomalous "percentile deviations"—to the day we die, and even after that, post-mortem, when one might undergo an autopsy to determine the cause of death (lest it be other than "natural"), we experience continuous testing to:

- determine intelligence
- determine aptitude and/or "potential"
- determine scholastic achievement
- assess the condition of body fluids such as blood and urine
- establish whether or not the heart, liver and thyroid gland, among others are functioning properly

- get a driver's or pilot's license
- meet the qualifications for a job
- obtain academic or experiential credentials for employment
- determine athletic performance ability.

Here, too, the list is endless. Even worse, testing often combines performance-anxiety with the above-described deadline-distress, because, in the vast majority of cases, examinations are administered with an associated time limit for completion. Thus, with testing, one gets a double whammy of exposure to "bad stress!" All of which one could, perhaps, justify, if one could also prove that the testing is meaningful, objective, unbiased, and relevant—but that's a topic for another book!

Competing

Undoubtedly derived from, and complementary to, our instinctive drive to survive is the drive to *compete* in:

- various sports and athletic activities (including the winter and summer Olympics, together with all of the allied enterprises that go along with them)
- sibling rivalries
- pageants, spelling bees, races, television game shows, board games, and a plethora of contests of all sorts
- the "dating game," courtship and marital relationships
- the inter-personal "games people play"
- the work place and industry
- personal interactions with others, especially relatives and neighbors, including the "keeping up with the Joneses" syndrome and significant *peer pressure*
- capitalistic economies
- religion!

You name it, whatever we do, the element of competition always creeps in to make the activity stressful because, by its very nature:

- To "compete" connotes devoting one's best efforts to win or gain something that others (usually rivals), desperately want and, by implication, to *beat them out* in the process, i.e., be the *first* to succeed.
- For me to win, somebody has to lose! There are no win-win solutions in strict competition. I win at your expense. I succeed *only* if I *make* you fail! We can't *both* win in a true competition.

Unfortunately, competition can escalate to *conflict*—often *armed combat*—and eventually all-out war! But short of this extreme, the *fact* of the human competitive spirit is real, and cannot be denied, even if the *wisdom* of it might be debatable (Schneck 2012). And along with it, we have this "numero uno" fetish—this need to somehow prove (and *continue* to prove) that we are "number one" and nobody does it better.

In and of itself, the desire to excel is a noble objective, but when one pursues this objective in the spirit of competition, success comes at the expense of somebody else's failure, and that's the part that generates enormous "bad" stress, which is to say, being competitive goes hand-in-hand with experiences that produce "bad stress" responses. That's not good! There is such a negative mindset—a stigma—that gets attached to being a "loser." By contrast, there is all too often a conceited air of "superiority" and arrogance that gets attached to a "winner."

As we pointed out in (2) above, our society is obsessed with *judging*—with *ranking* every single aspect of our lives on a scale from best to worst. We are preoccupied with *critiquing everything*, from one's hairstyle, to how we dress, talk, walk, eat and drink! We examine and grade *ad infinitum* academic performance. We evaluate lifestyles, athletic abilities, job performance, marriage relationships, etc.

Ironically, those trying to cope within such competitive environments—and perceiving themselves as not being successful in those efforts—are the ones most likely to turn to drug and alcohol abuse, or worse, as an escape from their frustrations. Without belaboring the point, suffice it to say that from a physiological point of view, *competition—no matter in what amount it exists—is always stressful and destructive.*

Diet

Fact: we concern ourselves more with the fluids and fuels that we put into our *automobile* engines than we do with the fluids and fuels that we put into our *anatomical* engine! There is this prevailing myth that our body, in its infinite wisdom, will extract what it needs from what we feed it, and "fix up" any disparities that might exist between what it *gets*, and what it *wants/needs* to maintain its health. But think about it: your body has nothing more to work with than the raw materials with which you provide it. Provide it with junk, and it can only produce junk; and junk is metabolically toxic, hence "stressful" in a bad way. There is a popular maxim that says it all: *Junk In...* *Junk Out*—the "JIJO principle." Stated another way: if you build a house with inferior materials, your house won't last very long. Indeed, junk:

- generates immune responses
- causes disease and other physiologic afflictions
- leads to premature aging
- upsets the delicate metabolic balance required to maintain stationarity

- can result in attention deficit hyperactivity disorders (ADHD) and serious learning problems
- can be responsible for wild mood swings, restlessness, sleepless nights, and psychic disturbances
- can, as illustrated in Table 8.2, also show up as a whole host of adverse physiologic reactions to "bad stress."

Yet, we foolishly think we know better. We feed our bodies junk, and then wonder why we are always getting sick. Moreover, we often fail to make the connection between diet and various symptoms that (we find out much later) could actually have been attributed to food allergies/sensitivities (see discussion in Chapter 2, and Schneck 2004). In fact, we proceed at first (out of ignorance) to blame these symptoms on everything *but* our dietary habits, even (at least in the past) having professed so in medical schools. A prime example of this oversight involves the causes of certain types of migraine headaches (Schneck 2004, 2012), but there are many others. The same can be said for exercise.

Exercise

Yes, the human body is a mobile engine specifically designed to be *used*—it is a kinematic machine (see Chapter 3). But, the body's engineering design is not intended to be *abused*. In that sense, I categorize exercise the same way that my medical school professor categorized the two types of stress, i.e.:

- On the one hand, there is the "good" exercise to which the body should be subjected quite naturally as it is *used* actively to perform normal activities of daily living. This is healthy exercise that falls within the envelope of human performance capabilities. It keeps us hale and hearty.

- On the other hand, there is "bad" exercise that *abuses* the body by subjecting it to artificial forms of exertion that accomplish nothing more than anatomical wear and tear. These are activities that "create" body movement—for the sake of body movement, alone—with no particular objective in mind other than "just moving!"

Without getting into any more detail at this time, suffice it to say for the purposes of our current discussion, that "bad" nutritional habits, and "bad" exercise regimens both contribute to a type of "bad stress" that is artificially imposed on the human body to produce bad results!

Special events

Not all "bad" stress is necessarily associated with "bad" physical and emotional lifestyles. In fact, quite often, we experience the symptoms and complications of "bad" stress from undertaking activities that we normally think of as being inherently pleasant, happy occasions—although they, too, derive from egocentric drives peculiar to, and created by, our own form of social structure. "Special" events, such as:

- weddings, bridal showers, engagements
- bar mitzvahs, birthday parties, anniversaries
- buying a new car or major appliance
- buying a new house or selling a new or old one
- starting a new job or "moving up in the company"
- moving to a new neighborhood, relocating.

And so on. All contribute to self-inflicted stresses that promote the flow of stress hormones. Engaged in these activities, our bodies pour into the bloodstream a host of biochemical agents that mobilize the organism to endure stress (see Table 7.2). In the short term, such mobilization, as already mentioned, is essential for survival, and so is quite desirable ("good" stress). However, maintained for longer than the short term, and/or, triggered all too often by a lifestyle that includes all of the above on a fairly regular basis, such mobilization—including the persistent exposure of body organs and tissues to the effects of stress hormones—will eventually lead to many of the symptoms listed in Table 8.2, and all of the problems that we *think* kill us.

Other sources of "bad stress"

Briefly, a few other sources of "bad" stress derive from:

- activities associated with estate planning and management of personal **financial affairs**
- **peer pressure**—most especially during one's most vulnerable juvenile/adolescent years, but more generally, all through life
- those times in our life when we make **career decisions**, especially when those decisions are made on the basis of what we "think" others *expect* of us, rather than on considerations related more appropriately to where our heart leads us—and the lifetime consequences we are destined to endure by not heeding those considerations (see also below)
- spreading ourselves too thin, **over-committing** ourselves to the point of having too many responsibilities that cannot be handled effectively, in a timely manner
- trying to do the "right" thing in **raising children**—according to some rather arbitrary standards that really don't make much sense when critically examined
- attempting to be the "perfect" **sex partner**—again, by whose standards?

- being **lonely**; and finally (although the list is virtually endless), but perhaps most important of all:

- our failure to recognize and appreciate that **we are human!** And even more: that to be human is to *not be perfect!* This is where our intellect and our emotions come into direct conflict. Our intellect attempts to deny our human-ness, refusing to accept as being "okay," such human frailties as emotional reactions to stressful situations, fear, crying, failing, and so on. But, our emotions always prove otherwise, even though we won't admit it! That is to say, whether we like it or not, speaking strictly anatomically and physiologically (as we shall see when we discuss anatomic information-processing), *Physiologic optimization principle number 6,* introduced at the end of Chapter 4, reminds us that:

We are human! being human makes us, first and foremost, creatures of emotion, not reason!

Our natural instincts for survival are *emotional.* We are "reasonable" only when we have the time…and *if* we are inclined to be so (Schneck and Berger 2006). In a nutshell, anatomically and physiological speaking:

Emotion trumps reason…that's why music works, when other forms of clinical intervention do not; that's why music elicits such effective and profound physiologic effects. (Schneck and Berger 2006)

Going one step further, disharmony between *intellectual denial* of our human-ness, on the one hand, and *emotional avowal* of our human-ness, on the other, is a leading cause of the "bad stress" that manifests itself in many disease states and physiologic dysfunction. Indeed, in many ways, our basic ignorance (or denial) of "how 'me' works" misleads us into expending enormous and unnecessary volumes of energy functioning in conflict with the very processes we are trying to understand.

Bearing all of this in mind, let's get back to the issue at hand, which is to say, whereas one could argue *ad infinitum* the pros and cons of all of these self-inflicted "bad" stresses, the bottom line is the same: *they ain't healthy!* Moreover, they don't really have to be there! *We* put them there, and they are under *our* control! *We* inflict them upon ourselves, and then *we* try to figure out how to live and deal with them, and survive in the process. It seems that we are not capable of being happy unless we're miserable—arguing, fighting, and in constant conflict with one another—attempting to satisfy certain needs and drives. What are they? In this chapter, we begin to address several prominent human needs and drives from which physiologic operating set-points derive. Some of these are basic, survival-driven ones that are common to virtually all forms of life; others are strictly *anthropocentric*—unique to us humans. As such, they, like many sources of "bad stress," are under our control and can be managed as such. But to be successfully and effectively satisfied, all of them depend on six fundamental *processes* that the music therapist can exploit in managing his or her clients, including:

- cellular/tissue/organ/systemic metabolism

- the anatomic/physiologic handling of data/information

- translation of information into conscious awareness

- the body in time, including biorhythms

- physiological optimization principles, including mechanisms of entrainment and physiological adaptation

- anatomical design criteria, including principles of self-similarity: the body in space.

Note that we addressed several of these briefly in Part I, but mainly in the context of *structure*, not so much *function*. In Part II, we will elaborate somewhat on the latter, adding additional insights, while concentrating on the most notable human needs and drives, beginning, of course, with *the* most important one.

Survival of the self: the *enduring* living engine/instrument

As advertised, by far the single strongest of all human drives is that intended to satisfy the need to *survive as an individual!* This so-called *drive for sustentive fulfillment* relies on *Physiological process number 1: metabolism*, which actually begins in the *zygocyte*, very shortly after initial conception. That is to say, recall from Chapter 1, that *any nucleated cell in the human body is coded to produce one entire human being.* However, early on, the single fertilized cell that was destined to become *you* goes through a series of divisions that eventually produce over 200 types of cell. Each cell type is programmed to perform a very specific, different task. This first of at least eight metabolic *mechanisms* designed to "guarantee" survival of the self goes by the name: **cellular differentiation.** Others include:

1. **Biochemical catalysis/enzyme kinetics,** as it relates specifically to those metabolic mechanisms concerned with the maintenance of:

    - stationarity/homeostasis (discussed in Chapter 6)

    - vital signs (discussed in Chapter 5, see Table 5.5)

    - survival parameters, such as those operating set points listed in Tables 5.5 and 8.3.

Table 8.3 Some important physiological operating set-points		
VARIABLE	**"NORMAL" RANGE OF VALUES**	**EXTREMES**
Body Mass Index BMI = Weight (kg)÷ [Height m²]	19–24.9	<15 = Emaciated 15–18.9 = Underweight 25–29.9 = Overweight 30–39.9 = Obese ≥40 = Morbidly obese
Blood Calcium Concentration (mg/dℓ)	8.4–11.0	>11.0 = Hypercalcemia <8.4 = Hypocalcemia
Hematocrit (%)	38–54 Adult male: 42–54 Adult female: 38– 46	<30 = Anemia >60 = Polycythemia
Blood Glucose Concentration (mg/dℓ Plasma)	80–120 resting <160: two hours after eating	<70 = Hypoglycemia Hyperglycemia Acute >200 Chronic >100–126
Type II (adult onset) diabetes mellitus: >126 Chronic		
Heart Rate (beats/minute)	60 – 100 At Rest	>100 = Tachycardia <60 = Bradycardia
Blood Alkalinity	7.35 ≤ pH ≤ 7.45	>7.45 → Alkalosis <7.35 → Acidosis
Blood Pressure (mm Hg)	120 Systolic 80 Diastolic	>160 = Hypertension <90 = Hypotension
Body Core Temperature (°C)	36.0–37.5	≥39°C = Hyperthermia ≤35°C = Hypothermia
Respiration Rate (breaths/min.)	8–18 at rest	>18 = Hyperventilating <8 = Hypoventilating
ICF/ECF Ratio	2:1–3:1	Low ratio = excess ECF High ratio = dehydration

2. **Paw-to-jaw reflexes,** discussed in Chapters 4 and 5, representing the body's most basic attempts to satisfy its need for:

    - water (thirst)
    - food (hunger)
    - warmth (clothing and shelter)
    - air (breathing)
    - musculoskeletal balance and equilibrium (see Chapter 3).

3. **Fight-or-flight instincts,** more accurately called the *general adaptation syndrome* (GAS), also discussed in Chapter 4 and elsewhere (e.g., Schneck and Berger 2006; Tortora and Grabowski 1993). The GAS occurs in two stages: in stage 1, the *alarm reaction*, the liver, lungs, and spleen are immediately activated by the autonomic nervous system to make available huge amounts of glucose and oxygen—*fuel*—to be delivered by the cardiovascular system to those organs and tissues that need to be mobilized *right away* to ward off danger. These are mainly the central nervous system (for alertness and control), and the musculoskeletal system (to "run away," or "stand your ground"). In stage 2, the *resistance reaction*, the H-P-A axis, kidney, and thyroid gland (see Chapters 6 and 7) are activated as a follow-up to the more immediate alarm reaction. Following the lead of the hypothalamus, the organs involved in the resistance reaction pour into the bloodstream all of the stress hormones that we have been talking about (i.e., see Tables 7.1, 7.2, and 7.3).

   Together, the two stages of the GAS represent the body's most basic metabolic attempts to respond to emergency or stressful situations—*real or imagined* (music therapists take note!)—by fighting against, or fleeing from the perceived threats. Included among the many GAS responses are a:

   - temporary resetting of the body's operating set-points, e.g., heart rate, blood pressure, respiration rate, and blood sugar levels, to (usually higher) values that are more suited for handling the perceived emergency. This is called *reflexive adaptation*, and, again, note the use of the word "temporary." Indeed, these responses are intended to be of short-term duration, not a long-term solution to a perceived problem

   - *temporary* readjustment of feedback/feedforward control mechanisms to ensure an optimized response to the threat

   - mobilization of anatomic/musculoskeletal *first responders*, including biasing the activity of muscle spindles to make them hyper-sensitive to the slightest stretch (which also results in knees and hands shaking, and various other nervous tics and twitches)

   - stabilization of acid-base balance

   - slowing of digestive activity (which also gives one that feeling of stomach queasiness)

   - mitigation of disruptive inflammatory responses

   - dilation of the pupils of the eyes, to increase alertness

   - disruption of rest, relaxation, and sleep habits, also intended to increase levels of alertness and responsiveness.

Plus, an:

- enhancement and optimization of fuel-supply mechanisms, waste-management protocols, and associated biochemical reactions

- increase in sweating and panting, hyperventilating to exhaust the additional heat generated by higher metabolic rates

- inhibition of urinary and reproductive activities

...and/or in general, to do whatever it takes to escape from predators, get out of harm's way, handle an emergency situation, deal with strenuous physical activity, react to a real or imagined threat to survival and...stay alive!

As one would expect, suffice it to say here that, in support of this most important and basic of all human drives, there has evolved a plethora of industries and social establishments—far too numerous to discuss here (and beyond the scope of this text). The interested reader is referred to Schneck (2011b, 2012) for further details. Thus, before we get side tracked, let's move on to another metabolic mechanism that is of importance in meeting the organism's drive for survival of the self.

4. **Nutrient-energy-transduction.** As previously defined, recall that this is a term that refers to the conversion of something (mainly energy) from one form to another. It is derived from the Latin prefix *trāns-*, which means "across," and the verb *dūcere*, which means "to lead." Hence, "to lead across" from:

- solar energy, to the caloric value of food

- the caloric value of food, to the high-energy bonds of ATP

- the high-energy bonds of ATP, to endergonic biochemical reactions, including the contraction of muscles

- the elastic energy of muscles, to the fluid dynamic pressure generated by the heart to drive blood through the vascular system

- hydrostatic pressure, to fluid convection across capillary walls

- osmotic pressure, to trans-cellular transport

- adequate stimuli manifest as light, heat, sound, electrical, chemical and mechanical forms of energy, into corresponding action potentials, the syntax of the human body

- any given form of energy, by all physiologic conversion mechanisms anatomically available, into another form!

Indeed, transduction mechanisms are at the very root of both the:

5. **Transport** and

6. **Utilization** of mass, energy, and linear and angular momentum by the human body. The basic principles by which both mechanisms 6 and 7 operate were addressed briefly in Part I of this book, to the extent that the music therapist needs to know about them, and we shall say some more as the need arises. Again, the interested reader is referred to Giancoli (1989), Schneck (1990, 2011b), Tortora and Grabowski (1993) for much more detail. Suffice it to say here that there are five fundamental *laws of physics* that govern all physiologic processes (Giancoli 1989), to wit, the laws of:

   - *Conservation of Energy*, also known as the *First Law of Thermodynamics*, which asserts that, "Energy can neither be created, nor destroyed, just converted (*transduced*) from one form into another." In other words, "You can't win!"

   - *Conservation of Mass*, which follows directly from the First Law of Thermodynamics because, as Albert Einstein showed, mass and energy are interchangeable, i.e., mass is one form of energy.

   - *Conservation of Linear Momentum*, which establishes the fact that, as Isaac Newton showed, "When the net external force acting on any system is zero, the total linear momentum of the system remains constant" or stated more simply, "Absent any net disturbance, a body at rest tends to stay at rest, and a body in motion tends to *stay* in motion."

   - *Conservation of Angular Momentum*, which follows directly from the previous law, but applies to *torques on rotating bodies*, rather than *forces on translating bodies*, i.e., "The total angular momentum of a rotating body remains constant if the net torque acting on it is zero."

   - *Generation of Entropy*, basically says, "Not only can't you win (i.e., the First Law of Thermodynamics), you can't even break even!" In other words, no process is 100 percent reversible—some useful energy is always lost, or remains unusable (*entropy*). In most situations of interest to us, such as mechanical friction and exergonic (energy-releasing) biochemical reactions, the non-usable form of energy released shows up as heat. This brings us full circle to the idea that we are an *isothermal* engine, unable to process and use heat energy, and thus require sophisticated metabolic mechanisms of thermoregulation.

7. **Thermoregulation.** To this point, we have said a great deal about thermoregulation (see Chapters 2, 3, and 7), so there is no need to belabor the point here.

To summarize, the first of the six major processes by which the seven basic features of our living engine/instrument become manifest is *metabolism*. Its function subscribes to operating set-points that govern mechanisms responsible for:

1. Cellular differentiation

2. Biochemical catalysis/enzyme kinetics

3. Paw-to-jaw reflexes

4. Fight-or-flight instincts

5. *Nutrient*-energy **T***ransduction*

6. Passive and active **T***ransport* of mass, energy, linear and angular momentum

7. Utilization of same; and, the last of the "three 'T's,"

8. **T***hermoregulation.*

That having been said, we move on to human need/drive number 2.

Survival of the species: the *perpetuating* living engine/instrument

Again, it should not be terribly surprising to learn that second only to the human drive for *personal* survival is the drive to perpetuate the species—a drive affectionately referred to as the one seeking *sexual fulfillment*. Recall from Chapter 6 that, complementary to being able to metabolize, this drive to reproduce is also among the major attributes that something must be endowed with in order to be classified as being "alive." However, when talking about perpetuating the species, it is important to distinguish between:

- *simple replication*, as in just "proliferating," which generally refers to *localized* processes that merely involve cell division and/or replacement (mitosis, meiosis, healing, etc.) intended primarily to repair and maintain the *actual* living organism, itself

- *complex reproduction*, as in producing "offspring," which refers specifically to generating an *entirely new, whole and complete organism* separate from the parent.

Furthermore, in the latter case one distinguishes between:

- *asexual reproduction*, such as *binary fission* of an ameba, or *budding* of a plant— wherein the offspring have been essentially *cloned* to be *exact duplicates* of a single ancestor

- *sexual reproduction*, wherein the offspring may be a somewhat revised, perhaps even drastically different version of their predecessors.

Asexual reproduction requires only one parent, and no special reproductive architecture/structures. The offspring are identical to (or at least remarkably similar, within the context of physically imperfect processes) to the parents. *Sexual* reproduction, however, requires the union of a male gamete—a *haploid* germ cell (usually *sperm*, having "half a nucleus" containing only 23 chromosomes)—with that of a female haploid germ cell (usually an "egg," or *ovum*) in a process called *fertilization*. Thus, a brand-new, *unique* cell (*zygote*) is formed—one containing half its chromosomes (23) from the biological father, and the other 23 from the biological mother. If a successful pregnancy ensues, the zygote will develop into an entirely new individual (Schneck 2001a). Sexual reproduction, then, endows species with the added advantage of being able to *change* the characteristics of the progeny, i.e., "adapt," and "evolve," in the Darwinian sense of *natural selection.*

In that respect, it is worth emphasizing *Physiological optimization principle number 7*, namely, that:

> *Human sexual reproductive processes concern themselves not only with perpetuating the species, but with breeding it, as well.*

That is to say, *breeding*—through *sexual* reproduction—connotes not only producing offspring derived from a common ancestor, race, stock, etc., but also by allowing the union of *different* varieties of male and female gametes, *improving* (it is hoped!) each generation of offspring.

But here's the catch—in order for the species to survive, a male has to be *motivated* to have sex with a female! One has to *desire* sexual fulfillment. Thus, although in weight, size, shape, etc., compared with other organs and systems in the body, human *gonads* (sex organs) are *anatomically* inconspicuous (i.e., they do not particularly distinguish themselves), they are certainly not so *physiologically!* No sir! They are, in fact, quite domineering and in control of life! Indeed, so important is the body's drive to reproduce, that we derive from the process of conceiving a child through sexual intercourse one of the most pleasurable of all physiological sensations, i.e., that of sexual climax. That's the primary (though not necessarily the only) *motivating* factor for pursuing sexual fulfillment, and it illustrates yet again, *Physiological optimization principle number 6*, i.e., that *we are creatures of emotion, not reason. Sexual* hormones (see Table 7.1), just like *stress* hormones (see Table 7.2), always trump reason and cognition. (*Aside:* the euphoric feeling that derives from having sexual relations can be taken out of context, i.e., the joy and pleasure of it can become ends in and of themselves, as opposed to its intended purpose, which is to consummate the act of conception…but we won't go there).

Instead, we will close our discussion of this second basic human need by noting first, that reproductive organs in both males and females are also not vital to the life of the individual, or to maintaining homeostasis. Their main function is to produce offspring. As such, therefore, the reproductive system is essential for the *survival of the species* only, rather than contributing also to the survival of the individual, per se. And finally, both *survival of the self,* and *survival of the species* are drives that are common across the board to all forms of life on this planet. What we are about to examine are *anthropocentric* needs and drives that seem to be peculiar to humans, rather than to the animal kingdom at large. We begin with the recognized third most important of all human needs: the drive for *spiritual fulfillment.*

Survival of the "soul": the *spiritual* living engine/instrument

The use here of the term *soul* in conjunction with human *spirituality* seems justified because the two words, *spirit* and *soul*, share common attributes. *Spirit* derives from the Latin *spīrāre*, which means "to breathe" (Sanskrit, *prana*), implying an airy, ethereal quality; and *soul* derives from an Old English word *sāwol*, which refers to the *essence* of the body—its *spirit*—as opposed to its physical manifestation. Thus, the *soma*, the *physical* body (from the Greek *soma*, for same), is believed by many (including, perhaps, some of your music therapy clients) to house, and be *animated* by, the *soul*— the "life force," or *ch'i*, (from the Chinese for "bodily energy"). In other words, the soul is the body in *essence*, rather than in *fact*, and it is considered to be the part of the body that is actually *alive*—that thinks and feels—and from which its actions derive (Prophet and Spadaro 2000; Schneck 2000a; Tsuei 1996).

In turn, then, *spiritual* connotes a corresponding caring for the *essence* of life, rather than the materialism of it—the *soul*, rather than the body. Moreover, the *concept* of spirituality implies a devotion to the immaterial realm of the human experience—a "higher" realm, if you will, rather than the one that is merely "worldly." Finally, the *essence* of life is neither corporeal (of the material body) nor otherwise formed out of palpable (capable of being perceived) matter; and so, the human drive for *spiritual fulfillment* reflects one's basic need to experience those very non-materialistic pleasures of life that derive from, for example:

- the intense desire to love and be loved

- unselfish, altruistic activities intended solely to benefit the welfare of others

- being absolved (forgiven) for our human frailties—and, likewise, forgiving others for theirs

- fulfilling a strong desire to give some meaning and purpose to life other than just survival of the self and of the species, per se

- humanitarian activities that reflect our inherent belief, as stated in the United States *Declaration of Independence*, in the inalienable rights of all individuals to "life, liberty and the pursuit of happiness"

- philanthropic benevolence, generosity and downright human decency, as defined by the "Golden Rule," i.e., treat others as you would expect them to treat you)

...and so on.

It is important to realize further that, while often *equated* with religious faith, "spirituality" and "religion" are *not* synonymous by any stretch of the imagination! That is to say, by definition *religion* connotes a pious reverence by worship, custom, and tradition to some holy set of scriptures and doctrines. It *requires* an obligatory reaffirmation of faith; a creed, devoted loyalty, and unquestioning belief. In fact, the very word, *religion*, derives from the Latin *re-*, a prefix meaning "again;" plus *ligare*, a word meaning "to bind," and the suffix *-onis*, which means "to show respect for what is sacred." Thus, *religion* implies "to bind again," to reaffirm one's faith in what is sacred. How it came to be associated with human spirituality will be explained after we lay some foundation.

There are those who argue that religion probably originated (at least in part) from our ignorance to explain the forces of nature. That ignorance, still prevalent even today, caused us in the early days of our heritage to invent and worship idols and "gods," who were believed to be responsible for such profound forces and experiences, for which we had no "earthly" explanation. In fact, this very reasoning also led to the Greek idea that there were nine heavenly "goddesses"—*muses*, from which the very word *music* derives—who were responsible for our awareness of the fine arts and sciences. The ancient Greeks believed that achievements in the arts and sciences were *divinely* inspired—in that order, i.e., *first* through the arts ("emotion"), and *second* via scientific thought ("reason"). It seems that even way back then, we were recognized to be creatures of emotion *first*, since in ancient Greek culture, the arts were held in much higher esteem than were the sciences—much higher than they are in today's society, but I won't go there, either!

Instead, I will point out that the motivation for thus ascribing divine inspiration *first* to artistic achievements was, for the Greeks, directly connected to the particularly moving emotional experience that could be attributed to those achievements. It was totally inconceivable to the populace of this ancient civilization that anything— especially music—that could elicit such profound physiological effects could derive from a source other than the sacred daughters of the almighty Zeus (the chief god) and Mnemosyne ("Memory," his Titaness lover). In other words, going back thousands of years, long before scientific advances could provide a rigorous basis to explain it, it was already recognized that certain sensory inputs in the audible range of perception could evoke intense physiological responses, manifesting themselves as *emotional* responses. And, since those responses could not be explained in any other way, they *had to be* of divine (godly) origin. This divine association firmly established the importance of music in the human experience. Furthermore, along with it came the additional abstract realization that this form of sensory stimulation, acting through the body's self-regulating mechanisms, had the profound ability to allow the organism to express its healing potential (music therapists take note!).

Getting back, then, to the relation between spirituality and religion, those same individuals who attributed *divine* (based on *faith*) origin to human experiences that were otherwise unexplainable, also extrapolated to equate that very faith with *spiritual fulfillment.* Why? Because most religions profess the very same non-materialistic ideals that were enumerated earlier in this discussion—ideals that seemed to be attributable to *divine* inspiration, akin to the Greek muses. However, it is important to re-emphasize that the ideals so-listed came *first*, and religion second, not the other way around!

Organized religion grew out of both our ignorance to explain the forces of nature, and our need for spiritual fulfillment, as defined above. What has evolved is a cultural attribute that defines particular systems of worship, divine reverence, and reaffirmation of faith, including the beliefs and axiomatic convictions that are the basis of these faithful devotions; and the rituals, activities of daily living, and traditions that are considered to give credence to it. Bottom line: when discussing the *concept* of spiritual fulfillment as a human need, be very careful to distinguish it from *religious* cultural attributes that are presumed to go a long way towards satisfying it. Attributes that include:

- appreciating "higher," immaterial realms of experience
- being aware of manifested, abstract interrelationships between body and mind (Schneck 2000a)
- the search for a *divine purpose*, perhaps accessible only at higher levels of consciousness
- a need for salvation, recognizing that only a "higher power" has the ultimate ability to forgive our less-than-perfect human-ness
- altruistic, unselfish attempts to see to the welfare of others, as a means for "satisfying" this "higher power"
- a humanitarian appreciation and respect for the "inalienable" rights of others
- genuine, and generous philanthropic benevolence.

That having been said, we move on in Chapter 9 to explore some additional, *anthropocentric* human needs, to the extent that they are responsible for:

- establishing physiologic operating set-points
- affecting the second of the six major processes by which the seven basic features of our living engine/instrument become manifest, i.e., *central nervous system handling of data/information.*

Both should be of great interest to the music therapist.

CHAPTER 9

The *Anthropocentric* Living Engine/Instrument

In Chapter 8, we addressed the three primary needs that drive the human body to operate the way it does. These could best be summarized by one S-word—*survival*, i.e., the need to survive as an individual, a species, and an ethereal "spirit." The first two needs result in drives that motivate the behavior of *anything* that can be classified as being technically "alive," i.e., they are *generic* requirements common to all things *animated*, as defined at the beginning of Chapter 6. The third one, survival of the *soul*, seems to be a need that is unique to humans, i.e., it is manifest as an *anthropocentric* drive.

In this chapter, we carry the idea of anthropocentric drives a bit further by exploring three more human "needs" that, this time, can be summarized by another S-word: *searching*: searching for (i) *knowledge*, and through it, *truth*; (ii) *self*, and through it, *identity*; and (iii) *interpersonal relationships*, and through them, some *meaning* and *purpose* to life (Schneck 2005c, 2012).

The desire to satisfy these three human—*anthropocentric*—needs also drives the body to establish operating set-points that cause it to function the way that it does. Thus, we begin our discussion of *searching* by recalling—when we addressed spiritual fulfillment in Chapter 8—the idea that religion evolved, in part, from our insatiable thirst for a way to explain the "unexplainable." Why? Because of yet another human need/drive, i.e., to be empowered to *predict* the future and *control* our own destiny! In other words, to *know!*

The human search for knowledge, and through it, *truth,* and *power*

In our discussion of *sensory integration* (Chapter 6), we talked about the seven basic *elements of knowledge*, namely: frame of reference, scale of perception, resolution, structure, order, relation, and synthesis. We *gain* knowledge via many paths (Schneck 2007c, 2011b), such as, by:

211

- *inheriting* it from our biological parents, via the human *genome* (*nature*), which also includes *intuition*, the body's "sixth sense"

- extero-interoceptive, sensori-motor *experiential* **per***ception* (*nurture*), which may include one or more of the following:

  o *reading* and/or, being exposed to the *media*—radio, television, movies, and other agencies, and especially the world-wide-web—through which information can be communicated indirectly

  o *learning*—formal (institutional), or informal (from one's parents, peers, mentors, and, before writing was formally invented, stories passed on from generation to generation by word of mouth)

  o *extrapolation* from what we *do* know to what we can *infer*, that is, in those cases where we *know* what we *don't* know!

  o *axiomatic* convictions (i.e., *givens*—things accepted to be true *universally*, without formal proof); inspiration; *intuition* (again), and *faith-based revelation*; this is as opposed to:

  o *assumptions*, which are (often wrong or unfounded!) things taken to be *provisionally* true for specific, well-defined situations

  o *serendipity*—"accidental," unanticipated knowledge derived from unforeseen events, "being in the right place at the right time," or fortunate discoveries that are come upon entirely by chance

  o *miracles*—unexplained but experienced marvels that seem to be beyond the known laws of nature (especially in medicine)

- **con***ception*, through *the creative process*, i.e., *self*-stimulated generation of knowledge *de novo*

- *transcendental*, objective realizations, i.e., *metaphysical* things that *do*, or *can*, at least in theory, exist, but are beyond our ability to know about them due to constraints such as those discussed below, which is to say, what we *don't* know we don't know

- rumors and "old wives tales;" including, perhaps, *mythology*

- potential (possibly *extrasensory*) and *paranormal*, basically "unexplainable" *realizations* that are beyond our experience

- the *scientific method*—*verifiable* observations and experiences, followed by formal confirmation and cognition from which *theories* can be formulated by *inductive* reasoning (i.e., going from the specific to the general). Then the stimulation by such theories of the creative process to make predictions based on *deductive* reasoning (i.e., going from the general to the specific), all leading to what we *think* we *do* know (Schneck 2011b).

With respect to the latter, especially, be forewarned that this *method* must be used with care and extreme caution because often standing in the way of pure, absolute, totally objective inquiry are many obstacles and constraints to knowing! (Schneck 2011b). In other words, as opposed to both the *elements of*, and many *paths to* knowledge, the anatomist/physiologist (and music therapist) is more concerned with the many *constraints* to knowing, among them:

- *Technological constraints:* these limit our ability to *measure* everything—totally, objectively, at any scale of perception (especially sub-microscopic and super-cosmic), to the finest degree of resolution, to the most precise accuracy, and human/technologically error-free.

But, even if we *could*…

- **Anatomical/physiological/sensory-input limitations** prevent us from experiencing, altogether, no more than a miniscule fraction of the multifarious manifestations of energy. As noted many times in this book, our body is endowed *only* with those anatomical sense organs that we need to survive… and no more! Thus, we can experience adequate stimuli derived from energy in certain electromagnetic, acoustic, thermodynamic, chemical, etc., forms…*and no other!* The rest is imperceptible, *to us*, even with technological help!

But even if we *could* anatomically *transduce all* forms of energy…

- *Anatomical/physiological/information-processing constraints* further filter out and modulate the sensory adequate stimuli to which we *are* responsive. In addition to factors related to the *type* of adequate stimulus (energy) involved, its *strength* (requiring a *threshold* value), *persistence* (that can result in *sensory adaptation*), etc., (see Chapters 4, 5, and 6) there are additional constraints that we shall address in the next chapter, where we discuss the body's handling of data/information.

But…even if these *processing* constraints did *not* exist…

- *Anatomical/physiological/perceptual limitations* limit even further—and seriously bias—our ability to interpret *objectively* the information that *does* eventually make its way to consciousness. Indeed, as we shall also see in subsequent chapters, satisfying the body's needs, as we are currently defining them, leads to *subjective skewing* of our responses to biased interpretation of information. Perceptual subjectivity might derive, for example, from:
  - strong personal beliefs (including religious)
  - unavoidable, needs-driven human bias (subjective orientation)
  - jumping to (often false) conclusions based on "first impressions" and/or, circumstantial (often not verified) evidence

- circular reasoning (inherently and inadvertently *assuming* a conclusion in the process of arriving at it)

- ulterior motives, again anthropocentrically driven

- the self-fulfilling-prophecy trap—"predicting" something that one then goes about, however innocently, inadvertently and sub-consciously, making *sure* it happens

- subliminal influences that one might not even be aware of (especially prevalent in advertising schemes)

- peer and professional pressure to get positive results

- counterfactual reasoning (i.e., assuming the validity of evidence presumed to *verify* favorably a biased point of view, when that very evidence clearly contradicts known facts, and, indeed, is valid in just the opposite sense, *contrary* to that view point)

- failure to properly account for confounding variables that cloud the issue of objective interpretation of information

- failure to properly "connect the dots"

- the existence of long-standing, prevailing, "state-of-the-art fads"—the "we've always done it that way" syndrome

- human error! (none of us is perfect)

- the *dualism* trap, which is considered further below.

But, even if all of the above could be successfully managed and dealt with, one cannot get around the fact that:

- *The senses can be fooled!* At your leisure, google the Federal Aviation Agency's film, *FAA Pilot Disorientation,* or visit the websites: www.youtube.com/watch?v=-jU7BS-iv6U and www.youtube.com/watch?v=G-lN8vWm3m0 ("The McGurk Effect") to get some first-hand experience in how easy it is to get the senses to misinform the central nervous system. There are many such examples (Ackerman 1990; Coren and Ward 1989), but the bottom line is that *you can't always trust your senses* to be supplying you with a faithful representation of what's really going on. Thankfully, *sensory integration* (see Chapter 6) is available to help mitigate this dilemma, but don't let this give you a false sense of confidence that all is well and reliable when it comes to your senses—*be a skeptic!* Moreover, be also wary of the above-mentioned dualism.

Dualism as a mental constraint to knowing

What often comes up in the "search for knowledge" category of human needs is the question, "Where, as a species, did we come from, and when?" Invariably, this question causes heated debates between those who espouse the *science of evolution*, and those who prefer the *creationist/intelligent-design* theory based on *faith* (Baker and Miller 2006). The evolutionists attempt to satisfy our need to know the answer to this question by seeking a better, *scientific* understanding of the natural world *without regard for meaning or intent*. By contrast, based solely on *faith*, creationism/intelligent-design attempts to satisfy (to a certain extent) our *need for spiritual fulfillment*, by answering this question within the context of purpose and intent *without regard for rigorous proof* (Baker and Miller 2006). The fact is, that each approach—in its *own* way and subscribing to its *own* set of unique axioms/beliefs—satisfies its *own* respective need, i.e., for *rigorous proof* without regard for *intent*, in the case of science, and for a *reaffirmation of faith* in the *ultimate intent* of "higher powers," in the case of religion, quite effectively. In other words, to the extent that each serves a different purpose—to satisfy a different need—science and religion should, in principle, be able to co-exist in peace and harmony. But they don't! Which brings up more basic questions related to the mentality of reasoning:

1. Since neither science, nor religion has (yet!) the, *unequivocal* answer to the original question posed and, since *both* have unresolved issues that seem to be at an impasse, is it not possible that in our quest to "know" how we came about as a species, these two might not necessarily be the *only* possibilities that deserve our attention?

2. Might there be alternative explanations, not yet conceptualized or appreciated, that could satisfactorily resolve this highly controversial Theory of Evolution vs. Creationism/Intelligent Design debate in a way that embraces the positive attributes of both?

3. Is our "either/or" dualistic mentality so deeply embedded in the way we think and reason, that we *force* ourselves to choose *only* between these two prevailing, yet clearly disparate, *polarizing* alternatives for explaining how we got here—neither of which has all of the answers?

I raise the debate in question not to resolve it, but because it illustrates an inherent flaw in the way we tend to reason, i.e., this "either/or" mentality associated with what is known as *dualism* (Shneck 2007b).

Dualism is a theory that divides objective reality in any particular domain into *only* two, mutually irreducible, independent, more-or-less equal, yet diametrically opposite classes of constituents, such as:

- "rational" left brain and "emotional" right brain (Edwards 1989)
- good and evil; love and hate; pure and impure

- manic-depressive alternating mood swings
- mind and body (Schneck 2000a)
- winners and losers; rich and poor; "haves" and "have-nots"
- up and down; north and south; east and west
- in and out; on and off; yes and no
- positive and negative electric charges
- north and south magnetic poles
- right-wing and left-wing political viewpoints
- matter and anti-matter in physics (Giancoli 1989) and, of course, the famous,
- *yin and yang* of Buddhism.

According to *dualism*, although each constituent of the pair *functions* essentially independently of the other, neither can *survive* by itself, in the absence of the existence of its diametric opposite. The two *must* co-exist, doing a precisely choreographed dance of complementary extremes that express themselves in what we experience as *reality*, or *being*.

Plato (429–347 B.C.) introduced the concept of dualism in his *Phaedo*, postulating the existence of eternal "forms" (spiritual *soul* being one of them) that make the world possible and intelligible to humans. According to this Greek philosopher, the human body is a temporary, imperfect incarnation of some of these forms, hence the duality: body and soul (more generally, *ephemeral vs. eternal*). Moreover, the division "by the Gods" of the human race into males and females is a further example of this dualism—one that also makes us social creatures, and gives rise to our search for inter-personal relationships (see below).

In postulating that, "in the beginning," the human species consisted of *androgenous creatures* that embodied both male and female sexuality which the Gods later separated, Plato might not have been as "far out" as one might think. Some neuro-endocrinologists claim that the presence of nipples and other breast tissue in men indicates that the basic body *blueprint* for men and women is identical. However, early developmental (cellular *differentiation*, see Chapter 8), and later hormonal influences (see Chapter 7) prevent feminine features (such as lactation) from maturing in men, and masculine features (such as beard growth) from coming of age in women.

Centuries later, the French philosopher/mathematician René Descartes (1596–1650) championed the cause of *dualism* with his contention that the *mind* (his "spirit") is separate and distinct from the *body* (his "matter"). In three major works—his *Discourse on Method* (1637), *Meditations on First Philosophy* (1641), and *Principles of Philosophy* (1644)—Descartes developed his *Theory of Dualism*. In it, he separated the mind—which is presumed to *reason*, objectively, by means of linear, spatial-temporal cognitive modes of cerebral information processing (Descartes' *Spirit*, which may or may not be *left-brain centered*)—from the body, which is presumed to *react*, subjectively, to holistic, sensory-perceptive, emotional modes of mental function (Descartes' *Matter*, which may or may not be *right-brain centered*, see Chapter 4). Descartes thus ascribed to the former (the mind) a position of authority relative to the latter (the body)—the spirit (mind) being capable of interacting with the body (matter) but being quite separate from it and, in principle, not needing it to exist and/or survive (Schneck 2007b).

By inference, then, *dualism* suggests that the mind is somehow more basic (yes, in Cartesian philosophy, even "godly") than is the body (mere mortals are we); that rational thinking is somehow more reliable and *justifiable* than is emotional reacting; and that, therefore, activities—like the arts—associated with *emotional* attributes are inferior to those—like the sciences—associated with *mental* attributes. Thus, with *dualism* came the denial of our human-ness (see Chapter 8 and *Physiological optimization principle number 6*). Dualism dealt a huge blow to the arts, in general, and music, in particular. We are still dealing with it!

But perhaps more to the point, given the aforementioned constraints to knowing, one *must* admit that virtually all theories, laws, etc., that exist in the domain that we call "knowledge," are just that—theories! They are nothing more than relative, subjective, intrinsic mechanisms that *we* have *invented* to enable us to formulate *descriptions* of "reality," and to explain and quantify various aspects of the human experience. In many (dare I say "most?") cases, these descriptions work not *because of,* but *in spite of* our limited understanding of the fundamental principles involved. And indeed, history has proven to us that most of them are wrong (see Schneck 2011b, 2012)!

All that having been said, there might be more fundamental, anatomical/physiological reasons that dualism and mind/body theories still prevail—reasons that have everything to do with the nature of human decision-making processes. We shall say more about such processes in Chapter 10. Suffice it to say here that there is an as-yet unidentified mechanism by which the brain seems to prefer processing information in "either/or," so-called *inverse couplets*.

Consider that in a study reported in the July 1995 issue of *Prevention Magazine*, when hundreds of doctors were asked to decide among *three* options for treating a hypothetical patient, virtually all of them got so confused that they could not decide on an optimum choice, opting instead to make no choice at all! By contrast, those same physicians, when given only *two* options, had no trouble choosing one of them as being the most desirable method of treatment.

Similarly, when legislators were asked a policy question that involved choosing among *three* options, they, too, froze and couldn't decide; but when only *two* options were offered, they chose easily between them. Perhaps this dualistic means for dealing with decision making derives from our awareness of the biological cycles of life and death, and/or the alternating periods of day and night. Could it be that *these* observations have been "coded" into anatomical paradigms that cause us to think in terms of opposite extremes? However, maybe such either/or thinking can be attributed to our qualitative perception that various forms of energy lie between previously discussed (see Chapter 5) anatomical sensory limits, such as, for light, blindingly bright to barely visible; sound, deafeningly loud to almost inaudible; heat, scaldingly hot to ice cold; and for tactile sensations: firm and solid to delicately soft. (*Aside:* we do, however, appreciate that these extremes represent the outer, "black-and-white" limits of continuous functions that have many shades of "gray" in between.)

Maybe thinking in sets of opposing pairs derives from observing that the human body has a certain bilateral, left-right symmetry about an anatomical midline, including two eyes, ears, nostrils, arms, legs, etc., not to mention left and right kidneys, lungs, sides of the heart, and parts of the brain itself.

Whatever the underlying reason(s)—and it may very well be none of the above (we just don't "know," and are still searching for answers)—one thing is definite:

We humans are preoccupied with the concept of dualism!

However, as we progress into a new millennium, perhaps it is time finally to discard dualism as a concept, most especially as it relates to war and peace! Indeed, there is no definitive anatomical/physiological evidence to support the idea that there is a structural basis for dualism—one that would justify the formulation of a parallel-track set of information-processing pathways, in Descartes' either/or sense. Quite to the contrary, as formalized by Chapter 8's *Physiological optimization principle number 6*, which we shall justify in Chapter 10, speaking strictly in a *human* sense,

Emotion always trumps reason!

That is to say, what the evidence *does* show is that our need to satisfy fundamental drives such as those described here, has evolved into an organism that is first and foremost a creature of emotion, i.e., it is *reactive*. The "reasoning" comes later, *after* the information has been processed *first* perceptually and holistically. Go into a crowded theater and yell, "Fire!" and see how *rationally* the folks respond!

As we shall see in the next chapter, mental function proceeds through neural networks arranged in *series* (in an "and" sense) as opposed to in *parallel* (in an "either/ or" sense). There is no evidence-based separation between mind and body that would make the body subservient to the mind; in fact, if anything, the situation is exactly the opposite! This realization, based on the rapidly accumulating "hard" evidence to support it, helps to explain the effectiveness of the visual and performing arts in affecting adaptive behavioral responses—so much so that the scientific community is being forced to rethink its long-standing attitude toward the arts. No longer must they be considered to be somewhat "less basic" than are cognitive subjects such as English, math, science, and history.

In particular, we (including music therapists!) must now recognize that there are some very fundamental anatomic/physiologic/scientific reasons to explain why music originated in the first place; and how it has evolved to play the major role that it does today in satisfying basic human adaptive functions (Schneck and Berger 2006; Schneck and Schneck 1997). But we digress. Getting back to the pursuit (and power) of knowledge, note that one can satisfy and strengthen one's perpetual search for truth by carefully applying to this process the following trifecta that characterizes sound inquiry:

1. An adherence to fundamental principles of abstract, critical, and logical thinking.

2. Formulation of *relevant* and sound systems of axioms and assumptions that comply with:

   - first principles

   - universal laws (especially of physics, see Chapter 8)—and the corollaries that go along with them

   - initial conditions in time

   - boundary conditions in space

   - compatibility and other identified constraints.

3. A sincere willingness to be skeptical, open-minded, admit when one is wrong, and be prepared to "change course" if the evidence points in that direction (Schneck 2011b).

And again, why this search for knowledge? Because...

Knowledge can empower one to fulfill the need to control one's own destiny

In this regard, there reigns yet another perennial debate between those who subscribe to the doctrine of *determinism*, and those who prefer to believe in *free will*—total control over one's own destiny. The *doctrine of determinism* asserts that all mental processes, including every decision/choice we make, and the actions that derive from them, and/or, our consciousness of all aspects of the human experience, are all the result of a specific sequence of causal events. Stated another way, each successive state of consciousness is born of, and qualified by, all states that preceded it, thus effectively negating the exercise of a 'free will,' or a 'free mind,' or, for that matter, a 'free' *anything!*

At first glance, it seems reasonable to surmise that any current state of affairs can, indeed, depend, in the most general sense, on both past events (an accumulating *integral* effect), and, perhaps, those that have yet to transpire (a rate-dependent *differential* effect). It is this notion of the *relevance of past and future to present* that is the basis for the *doctrine of determinism*. This doctrine states, simply that, first of all, what we are experiencing now *was destined to happen*, given the antecedents as they were; every phenomenon is determined mainly by its history; its attributes are not free, but pre-determined, given the sequence of events that led up to it. This type of reasoning is consistent with the Buddhist/Hindu concept of "karma," a word derived from the Sanskrit word for "deed," i.e., all the acts, words, and thoughts of a present generation invariably determine the outcome—which is to say, that person's fate (*karma*)—in his/her next stage of existence. Cause and effect are inseparable. Not only is an effect preceded by a cause (determinism), but, the cause *invariably* leads to a corresponding effect (Schneck 2011b).

Determinism and causation preclude phenomena from occurring spontaneously, or "at will," in general, and certainly not *free will*, in particular, as a means for controlling one's own destiny. However, as "rational" as it sounds, this is a concept that on the surface is difficult to "digest." For example, isn't it true that I move my arm when I *want* to? And don't I *pick* my friends; *decide* where I want to go on my vacation; *choose* the car I want to drive, where I *want* to live, my career path, etc.? Thus, contrary to the doctrine of determinism, we have the complementary (*dualistic?*) *doctrine of free will* (choice). The latter asserts that all actions derive entirely from the desires, personality and character of those who execute them; they originate entirely from within the individual's consciousness, and he/she accepts full responsibility for the future result(s)/consequences of such actions; little or nothing is pre-determined. The proponents of "free will" are quick to concede that much of their behavior and actions are, indeed, *constrained* by:

- anatomical design criteria and physiological optimization schemes such as those that we have been developing in this book

- physical boundary (spatial), temporal initial, and circumstantial compatibility conditions that might prevail in any given situation

- a wide variety of external influences

- one's need to satisfy fundamental drives for survival

- one's quest to be validated by searching for identity, truth, and purpose…and so on.

However, even given all of that, the bottom line is that, *within those constraints* there prevails the underlying need to rest comfortably with the idea that one is *in control!* One is empowered to satisfy one's needs one's *own way*…and through that freedom of choice, is able to *control* one's own destiny, not have it pre-determined or imposed by some external forces. An individual *wants* that *right*…that *freedom*…to pursue his/her own happiness, and to accept the consequences of failure in that effort. Thus, notwithstanding the possibility that *fate* (determinism) might have *something* to do with the ultimate outcome, i.e., the *end point* might be pre-determined, the *means* to that end, proponents of free will argue, should be *path-independent.* One should be "free" to control *how* one gets to that end!

Some advocates of determinism use the human genome as a paradigm. According to them, all behavior is *programmed* into your genetic code which, in turn, is determined by heredity and evolution. Thus, your 'will' derives by *chance*, not *choice.* On the one hand, in the sense of *nature* (determinism and causality), this is arguably true. But on the other hand, keep in mind that the genome you inherited only provides you with, if you will, the "Leggo blocks" that you have to work with. What you *do* with those blocks, i.e., how, and which one(s) of those embedded 'potential' attributes actually become *realized* during the course of your existence, this—contrary to what the "conventional wisdom" would have you believe—is entirely up to you (*choice*), your environment, and your experiences. Thus, in the sense of *nurture* (free will and control of one's own destiny) one can argue that evolution and heredity determine only a "chancy" *trend*, not a pre-determined *fait accompli*—a thing already done and therefore no longer worth changing.

Thus, we are not necessarily at an impasse here concerning the *dualistic, nature versus nurture* paradigm. It may very well be that the *seemingly* mutually contradictory doctrines of determinism and free will *can* be reconciled by considering a "mediation," a *third choice* that takes the form of a *doctrine of compatibilism*. According to this choice, determinism does *not necessarily* rule out actions that originate (free will) with the one who executes them. Rather, determinism just proposes that there be some *causal* background that is *consistent* with the eventual *outcome*, i.e., some underlying basis for the *results* obtained, irrespective of how they might have been *arrived* at. A convenient way of thinking about this is to recognize that one is "free" to choose the *path*, even though the *destination* might be a foregone conclusion. For example, we might all have wound up in New York, but some of us might have come from California via Chicago, others from Virginia via Richmond, still others from Texas via Atlanta, and so on. The *destination* is the same (determinism)…but the *path* varies considerabliy (free will), depending on the motivating factors that influenced (*cause*) its trajectory (*effect*). Moreover, *along* that path, one can exercise the "freedom" to pursue personal goals, and endeavor to satisfy specific objectives that, indeed, *may be* path-dependent (again, determinism).

Regardless of which of these "doctrines" you subscribe to (if any!), here are some things to consider:

- Have we become *obsessed* with the concept of "free will?"

- If so, can "free will" exist in the wake of such an obsession?

In other words, if the mind is preoccupied with the drive for free will (or any other idea or inclination), is it, in fact, free at all? To be truly "free" precludes functioning in an obsessed state of compulsion, for *any* form of obsession (free will included) burdens one down, anchoring one to that obsession. Thus anchored is not "free" at all, but *chained* to a fixation, a "free-will fetish!"

Moreover, if one subscribes to the premise that, "All humans are created equal," then there can be *no* "free will," because freedom and equality, by their very definition, are mutually exclusive concepts and so cannot co-exist. That is to say, that which is "free," by definition *cannot* be restricted by arbitrary standards of "equality." True equality imposes the constraint that nothing can deviate from some arbitrarily designated set of *criteria* for parity, and hence, negates the very *concept* of freedom if that "freedom" requires compliance to a set of standards. It's like saying, "We have free speech in this country, as long as you say what's *expected* of you, and don't make waves!" Which brings up more questions:

- Do *freedom of choice*, the right to *pursue happiness*, and *liberty* give one license to do what one *wants* to do, or what one *ought* to do?

- Who decides what is meant by "ought?" In other words, how much leeway does one have in exercising the *privilege* of controlling one's own destiny? How much *responsibility* goes along with that privilege; and at whose expense is it exercised?

Finally, we are constantly being subjected to subtle influences of a subliminal nature from various sources and things, the existence of which one might not even suspect, much less be consciously aware of. These produce *evoked responses* that we are not always in control of, hence are lacking in "free will." Instead, we are the subjects of almost hypnotic temptations that lead us to do things that we *think* are of our own volition ("free will"), but, in point of fact, are not!

So…what's it to be: (a) determinism; (b) free will; (c) compatibilism; (d) all of the above; or (e) none of the above? Lots of questions—few answers—so it's best to move on.

The human search for *self,* and through it, *identity:* will the *real* you please stand up?

Do you suffer from *dissociative identity disorder,* formerly known as "multiple personality disorder?" Technically, this refers to a medical affliction wherein, within the same body, there exist two or more distinct identities—"split-personality states"—that affect the person's behavioral patterns. These are often bizarre and contradictory, as in, the famous 1886 Robert Louis Stevenson novella entitled, *The Strange Case of Dr. Jekyll and Mr. Hyde,* which gave birth to a psychiatric syndrome known as a "Jekyll and Hyde personality." On that basis, it would not surprise me if most of you answered, "No," to the original question, since the syndrome is not one commonly experienced.

But speaking more generically, I would suggest that *all of us* should answer, "Yes!" because, if truth be told, we *all* have, living in the same body, multiple personalities that manifest themselves in various ways under different circumstances. They, too, affect our behavior as it derives from: what we think of ourselves, what others think of us, what turns us "on," what turns us "off," how we react to each other, to music, to challenges in life, and so on. For example, consider the following attributes of one's identity, and see how they might apply to *your* "multiple personalities." The various "yous," if you will, are categorized according to whether you are examining yourself from inside-out (i.e., what *you* perceive) or whether you are viewing yourself from outside-in (i.e., what you think *others* perceive).

1. First, there's the *emulated* personality, the "whom" that we (perhaps secretly) would like (or pretend) to be. In the 1947 movie, *The Secret Life of Walter Mitty*, Danny Kaye daydreams about all of the marvelous things he could accomplish if only he could be the heroes about whom he fantasizes—the crowds roaring and cheering, the accolades flowing incessantly. Most of us have a secret hero in our lives—an athlete we worship, a political icon, a member of the clergy, a relative we admire, a spouse we adore, a dear friend, a teacher who has influenced us the most, a Hollywood star, a famous astronaut, an accomplished musician or artist possessing talents we *wish* we had, etc.—someone we look up to as a role model and strive to emulate. Indeed, we *need one*...speaking of human needs! A person (including music therapists!) can learn a great deal about an individual by knowing who his/her role models are. Make that a routine part of your diagnostic protocol.

2. Getting back to reality, there is the *perceived* personality, the "who" that we really think we are (as opposed to the individual we would like to be, i.e., the *emulated* personality). This is the person who, for whatever reason, we envision ourselves to be—genuinely believing that this is who we really are. Unfortunately, because of a variety of external pressures—social, peer, family, professional, etc. (see *Sources of "bad" stress* in Chapter 8), we guard the perceived personality very carefully, lest it enter the world to become vulnerable to attack, prejudice, hurt, judgment, and/or humiliation and embarrassment. The perceived personality, therefore, remains our own personal secret, just between you and you. It's much safer that way.

    However, should we be fortunate enough to meet someone we really trust—that *very special person* (music therapist?) who will accept us for who we are: human, frail, sensitive, far from perfect, but well-meaning folks who just want to love and be loved in return—then we very cautiously let that perceived self come reluctantly out of hiding, just a little bit at a time, and hope for the best. This mutual, unconditional acceptance of one another's perceived personality is the key to a healthy, honest, and open relationship between any two people, be it a parent and child, student and teacher, or husband and wife. As the expression goes, "A true friend is somebody who knows all about you, and likes you anyway!" Moreover, to know you are not being judged has a tendency to bring out the very best in you. But, alas, in our society, the above is rare, and so, the perceived personality, more often than not, gives way in a functional (social) sense to the *persona*.

3. The *persona* is the "who" that we want others to think we are. It is our protection, the public impression we want to project; our *outward* appearance as we attempt to express it; our façade, the image behind which we can safely hide. This personality comes in two forms:

- One is derived from *external* pressures, which give rise to the person that we *think* others, such as our peers, parents, professional colleagues, professors, or prevailing public, *want or expect* us to be—whether or not we can live up to those expectations (see *image* personality below).

- The other is derived from an *internal motivation* driven primarily by the reward system that gives rise to the person we *want others to think we are*—a "role-playing" self, if you will, that we attempt to convey to the general public, our friends, and family (see *projected* personality below). Indeed, the *persona* is the identity to which William Shakespeare refers in Act II, Scene VII, of *As You Like It*, when Jaques declares, "All the world's a stage, and all the men and women merely players."

To the extent that we are able to play the role that we *think* is *expected* of us…and if we are successful actors…life is good, but not necessarily satisfying or fulfilling, because deep down, hidden well below all of the above personalities, is the one that few if any of us ever find, i.e., one's *real* identity.

4. The *real* identity is the "who" that we really are, the "concealed" personality that—like DNA tucked safely away in the nucleus of a cell, or the valuables that we keep securely locked away in safety deposit boxes, or the queen ant that never leaves the nest—*never* emerges from hiding, ever!. This is the personality that is so well camouflaged, guarded, and ill-defined, that *we* might not even be conscious of it *ourselves!* And yet, we seem to spend our entire lives in search of this "self," this *true identity*. Perhaps our *real* personality is that aspect of "us" that people refer to when they speak about a *soul*; or maybe the pursuit of this identity is embedded in concepts such as *altered states of consciousness*.

    Could it be that the personality we really are exists only momentarily at the instant of birth, to be subsequently buried by experiences that derive from exposure to the outside world? Does this "self" give way to the person that eventually emerges, having gone through a process whereby a youngster first internalizes the activities of caregivers, and later, the *expectations* of the society in which he/she will live out the rest of his/her life? Did a "real" you (*nature*) once exist, briefly, in the womb, yielding to the "now" you, who is just a victim of circumstance and experience (*nurture*)? Do we, therefore, have a sub-conscious memory of that brief moment in time—a "strange attractor" (in the language of Chaos Theory)—that drives us to spend the rest of our lives trying to recreate that original, innocent experience in some asymptotic sense? Is that yet another, subliminal, sub-conscious need that manifests itself as an abstract, ill-defined drive? Once again, there are more questions than answers. Turning, then, away from *you*, per se, how about the person that *others*—looking through their eyes—would *like* you to be, i.e., an *image self*.

5. The *image self* is the individual that *others* create for you, a personality that exists in their minds as they see you, together with their own expectations of you. That is to say, it is the person *they* think you should endeavor to become, irrespective of whether or not *you* can live up to their preconceived expectations of you. This is the person that fails your admirers if, for example, you are an athlete who does not live up to your "potential"—potential by whose standards and/or criteria: yours or theirs? More often than not, in the case of their perceived *image* of you, it is *their* criteria, although, in developing your own *persona*, you strive to *emulate* what *you think* their expectations of you are. The imaged "self" is destroyed when we do not live up to others' expectations of, or fantasies about us, as was the case for people such as athletes O.J. Simpson and Pete Rose, disgraced bicyclist Lance Armstrong, televangelist Jim Baker, and, yes, even former U.S. president Bill Clinton. Once they ceased to fit the image the *public* had created for them, these "heroes" fell from grace; their image was shattered in the eyes of their loyal followers; the role models were no longer *models to be emulated.* The image self is very close to, yet different in subtle ways from, another type of identity—the *projected personality.*

6. The *image* and *projected* personalities are alike in that both have to do with how others perceive you. They differ however, in that, whereas the *imaged* ("imagined") personality is created in the minds of others on the basis of *their* pre-conceived expectations of you, the *projected "self"* is created in the minds of others on the basis of the *cues they get from you,* i.e., on how *you* actually come across to them, based on what *you think* they are looking for, will accept, and reward.

    Furthermore, the image you are *trying* to project (see the *persona* above),— i.e., the signals you are sending, may or may not be the same as the image they are getting, i.e., how they see you and the signals they are receiving, whether those signals are what you *intended* them to be, or not. In other words, something may be "lost in the translation," so that there may be a significant disconnect between a) what they are *actually getting,* and what they are *expecting;* and b) what they are *actually* getting and what you *intended* for them to get, what you *think* you are *projecting.* Therein lies a significant source for the lack of communication that often exists among individuals and, in a more global sense, among governments and nations, especially if that communication is coded into several different foreign languages. Again, something invariably, and *literally* gets lost in the translation!

As a music therapist, you must keep this in mind when using music as the means for communication with your clients, i.e., you and they might not always be "on the same wavelength." What you think you are transmitting, might not be what they are receiving and/or transducing/translating one to one!

In describing these various personalities, we have barely touched on but a few of the many complex aspects of human behavior (see, for example, Liebert and Spiegler 1994). Indeed, our society makes living quite complicated, and stressful because we conjure up a myriad of behavioral games, with associated anthropocentric rules that are established to govern how we will navigate the path through the maze that takes us from birth to death. Though not necessarily *all* bad, regrettably, a good number of these games, and the rules that go along with them, are among the major causes of human stress, conflict, lack of communication, prejudice, deceit, corruption, self-interests, and lots of other bad things (see Chapter 8 discussion of bad stress). Suffice it to say for now, that the pursuit of self and through it, identity, includes an introspective, critical examination of one's deepest thoughts and emotions, to the extent that one is even *aware* of them. It also follows from a drive to "be all that you can be," to strive for excellence in a *self-actualized* effort to fulfill one's maximum "potential;" and a *self-sufficiency* that goes along with *self-determination*. Those drives, perhaps coupled with the need for spiritual and sexual fulfillment, also make us *social creatures* as discussed below.

The human search for relationships: the need to be *validated*

Indeed, we *are* social creatures (perhaps à la Plato's androgynous formulation that causes us to seek a complementary *soul mate?*). We *need* to:

- be *loved* (*unconditionally!*) and to love in return
- be *secure* (and provide security for others)
- have a support system (a "net underneath us")
- feel *validated*, i.e., to *matter*
- contribute something meaningful to our society
- feel that life has some *purpose* and meaning other than just to survive as an individual self and a collective species.

That being the case, we all search for some effective ways to interact with others in a meaningful, satisfying, and self-preserving way. Presented in Schneck (2012) are several "social skills" embedded in basic principles that are proven means for successfully getting positive results—*most of the time*—in dealing effectively with people, and bringing out the best in them. That is to say, constantly and routinely applying the principles listed below will achieve highly satisfying relationships with others. Why? Because (as we shall see in Chapter 10), information encoded into these *positive* principles will invariably be processed through the brain's "rational/ reasonable" hippocampus. This is as opposed to a syntax encoded into *negative* language and/or attitudes that are *perceived, rightly or wrongly,* to be "threatening," and hence, diverted to be processed by cerebral pathways that invariably trigger hostile, amygdala-driven fight-or-flight, "fear spiral" responses (Schneck and Berger 2006). The reader is referred to Schneck (2012) for specific details. Here, we simply summarize these principles.

Thus, to deal effectively with your fellow human beings, consider living a life-style governed by the following principles:

- *Empathy and concern*—reflects sincere compassion for another's plight. It sends the message that you hear, care, understand, and want to help in any way that you can.

- *Forgive and forget*—says, "I recognize that you are human. To be human is to be less than perfect. To be less than perfect is to make mistakes. Don't fret about your mistakes; in most cases, they can be fixed. If they can't, together, we can work around them and make the best of difficult situations."

- Perhaps *the most basic* principle in dealing effectively with people is embedded in this version of The *Golden Rule*: *Ask not of others what you would not do yourself.* Treat them as you would want to be treated.

- The *principle of effective communication* implores you to *"Say what you mean, and mean what you say!"*

- A maxim guaranteed to make you an agreeable person, one with whom others will gladly enjoy working and interacting is embedded in the *principle of good leadership*. A person who abides by this principle knows and appreciates the subtle differences between ruling and leading!

- Embedded in an optimistic, encouraging *principle of certainty* is the well-known fact that: *A positive attitude makes most, if not all, things possible.*

- The *principle of acclamation* encourages one to use *praise* as a means to show confidence in others. Learn to recognize, encourage, and nourish talent! And react to self-directed achievements and greet accomplishments with, *"You did a really great job!"*

- The *principle of honesty and humility* recognizes that, *"I admit it... I was wrong!"* are six words that have perhaps done more to promote peace and good will among humans (not to mention save marriages!) than have any others.

- Going one step further, few short sentences are so powerful in making folks feel important and a "part of the action" than those that actively seek their input. Thus, *"What do you think?"* illustrates the *principle of engagement*. We all have a need to be validated and made to feel like we matter, *really* matter!

- Three sets of three words each definitely lead to success, involvement, and commitment. They illustrate the:

- ○ *Principle of politeness:* "*Would you please?*"

- ○ *Principle of persistence:* "*Practice makes perfect!*"

- ○ *Principle of dependence:* "*I need you!*"

- The *principle of gratitude:* "*Thank you!*" is a winner!

- Last, and perhaps as important as the Golden Rule, those folks who operate according to the *principle of selflessness* routinely use the words "*we,*" and "*us.*" There's no "I" in "we" or "us."

Again we, *all of us*, are social creatures in search of identity, purpose, and relationships with others, and through them, discover a satisfying, self-fulfilling *meaning* to life. We all share a need to communicate, experience social interactions, be validated, and be *nurtured*, deriving from these, love, support, security, and self-empowerment. Two mechanisms that have evolved to help us reach these goals are various modes of *self-expression*, and *recreational activities*.

One's search for identity can be greatly enhanced by exploiting the human need for *self-expression*

In talking about self-expression, we distinguish between those "practical" aspects of the human experience that can be classified as strictly scientific, ethical/moral, social, etc., and those that relate to an "abstract" appreciation for what is *beautiful* and *pleasurable*…in, of, and strictly for *itself*. The latter represents a societal attribute called *aesthetics*, from the Greek *aisthánesthai*, meaning "perceive;" and the related *aisthētikós*, meaning "sensitive." Thus, *aesthetics* is generally associated with the "sensitive perception" that is embedded in the *arts:* creative arts and crafts, fine, and literary arts. Within that context, it further derives from, and complements both our search for personal identity, and inter-personal relationships, since self-expression is but one realization of that search. That is to say, as an *outward* display of one's unique perceptions, self-expression provides a way for a person to establish and project his/ her own identity and individuality into the world outside the "self." It thus further establishes a means for self-empowerment and validation by involving an individual in activities classified as the:

- *visual arts*, which include painting, drawing, sculpture, architecture, landscape design, photography, ceramics, jewelry, textile design, clothing, movies, fashions, and anything else that titillates one's special sense of vision

- *performing arts*, including vocal and instrumental music, dance (ballet, modern, ballroom, tap, etc.), drama, acting, live theater, pantomime, radio, television, movies, and anything else that is associated with one's physical rendering of an active accomplishment

- *skilled crafts*, which include carpentry, plumbing, weaving, crocheting, electrical design, woodworking, knitting, construction work, furniture design and manufacture, sewing, glass-blowing, and similar work involving artistic design and creative "use of the hands"

- *literary and oral skills*, including *writing* for stage (e.g., plays) and screen (e.g., movies, television); literature (e.g., novels, short stories, poetry, biographies, creative writing, etc.); and writing for commercial publications such as newspapers and magazines; *language* skills (e.g., debating, oratorical forensics, etc.); and any other form of vocal or written expression

- other *artistic* activities, such as producing and directing shows; creating original musical compositions; arranging scores and charts; choreographing dance numbers; producing documentaries; conducting; and many, many more.

One's search for identity and relationships can be greatly enhanced by exploiting the human need for *recreation*

On December 10, 1948, the United Nations General Assembly unanimously adopted a *Universal Declaration of Human Rights*, which included the stipulation that *leisure* is considered to be one of those "unalienable" rights that can neither be given nor taken away. Derived from the Latin *licēre*, which means "be allowed," the word *leisure* connotes time away from required work...in other words, *free time* during which one may:

- pause and reflect, become introspective (search for self)

- rest and relax ("re-charge one's batteries")

- amuse oneself (discover what "turns you on? ...off?")

- pursue hobbies

- do the things one *likes*, rather than *has* to or is *committed* to do.

Among those "things" are activities that can be generally categorized as being *recreational*, a term that dates back to the late 14th century. From the Latin, *re-*, meaning "again," and *creare*, meaning "to create, bring forth, beget," *recreation* suggests that one is involving oneself in activities that "refresh" and "revitalize" the body, "creating it anew." Activities that can be classified as recreational are many, and are highly dependent on one's individual interests. They include, for example:

- playing and/or listening to music

- participating in or watching a wide variety of sports activities

- working in the garden, planting, harvesting

- hunting and/or fishing
- pursuing hobbies such as woodworking and others
- traveling (and going on vacations)
- going to the movies or enjoying them on TV
- reading
- taking classes of interest at local schools
- playing cards, Bingo, the Lottery…even gambling
- playing pool, billiards and other table games
- bowling
- painting and sculpting

…and so on…all intended to be pleasurable and self-fulfilling. Needless to say, as is true for all human needs and drives, whole industries have evolved to satisfy the human need for recreation. Moreover, the leisure life of a nation is highly reflective of its values and character, not to mention providing millions of jobs and pumping billions of dollars annually into its economy. Perhaps Aristotle said it best when he declared, "If we are the play things of the gods, then let us live life as play." Or, as the English writer Gilbert Keith Chesterton (1874–1936) put it, "The true object of all human life is play. Earth is a task garden; heaven is a playground." So… maybe this human need, though listed here last, is certainly not least! In fact, we could have added many items to this list, noting that the parameters that define and quantify human needs and drives establish *physiologic operating set-points* to which we, collectively, as *controlled systems*, aspire. One can then say that physiologic operating set points are established by the organism's drive to satisfy *at least* its need to:

- survive (sustain itself), as an individual
- survive (endure, perpetuate itself), as a species
- be spiritually fulfilled (a great source of musical inspiration on both the creative (composing) and receiving (listening, responding) ends)
- control its own destiny (be "in charge")
- know (become enlightened, empowered)
- have some identity (be validated; mean something!)
- socialize (relate to others)
- express itself (emote, another outlet served so effectively through the medium of music)
- compete (gain mastery, prevail)
- recreate (play, revitalize itself; music "to the rescue" yet again!)
- rest and relax (it is hoped, to relieve stress!).

Note, in particular, how many of these needs are serviced so effectively through the physiologic effects of music.

A bit of perspective

Think about all of the operating set-points that derive from one's desire to satisfy fundamental human needs. Then think about the various systems that have evolved to satisfy those needs: political, anthropological, religious, economical, intellectual, aesthetical, social/societal, etc. Consider these to be "degrees of freedom"—which is to say, all of the unrestricted and independent ways that the human experience becomes manifest—and furthermore, think of these as representations (*projections*) of all of *humanity*, i.e., human beings taken as a *group*. Finally, thinking of the "group" in some multi-dimensional, holistic sense, note that we *experience* those *projections* in our own, *very limited* space/time domain, highly restricted as it is.

All of this reasoning makes me think of the great Austrian mathematician, J. Radon. In 1917, Radon proved that any two-or-three-dimensional object can be uniquely *reconstructed* from the infinite set of all of its *projections* into the *next lower dimension*, i.e., two-dimensional objects mapped into one-dimensional lines, three-dimensional objects projected into all possible two-dimensional planar views, and so on. Essentially, what Radon proved is that if you piece together enough two-dimensional views, you can uniquely reconstruct a three-dimensional object. Indeed, this theory forms the basis for many of the modern non-invasive medical imaging modalities, such as computed X-ray tomography (CT scanning), magnetic resonance imaging (MRI), and clinical ultrasound.

But as I think about Radon's formulation, and relate it to the above paradigm describing the whole, multi-dimensional human experience and its various "projections," I can't help but wonder if, in a very generic sense, there may be more to his discoveries than he himself might have realized at the time. That is to say, by inference, Radon introduced the more generalized concept that in order to define and understand, to the point of being able to uniquely reconstruct, *all* of the features of any multi-dimensional process, that process must be studied in *all* of its realized manifestations, giving none of them a higher priority than any other. Thus, applying Radon's theory to the human experience as formulated above:

- *if* we replace "two-or three-dimensional object" in Radon's theory with "multi-dimensional humanity (as a group)" in our formulation, a humanity (*object*) that is realized through an infinite number of manifestations ("systems, projections")

- *if* we replace "infinite set of all of its projections" in Radon's theory with "multifarious (having great variety) degrees of freedom (for humanity)," as defined above

- *if* we recognize that, given our anatomical/physiological/technological limitations, and the constrained, four-dimensional space/time domain within which we live, we can *only* experience/perceive, and examine these degrees of freedom as a *finite* set of "projections" into (in "Radon language") the "next lower dimension," i.e., that within which *we* experience ("see") humanity functioning

- *if* we therefore admit that *we* experience humanity (the "object") in a domain that limits *our* perception of its overall, multifarious degrees of freedom (equivalent to Radon's three-dimensional object viewed only in its next-lower, two-dimensional projections)

- *if* we *ever* expect to derive a *comprehensive* understanding of the *whole* of the human phenomenon, to *reconstruct humanity* enough to uniquely define and understand it

- *then* we must take into consideration *all* of the manifestations ("projections, points of view") of that experience in the domain in which *we* are examining it (i.e., the next lower dimension, in Radon's terms)… *ascribing to no one of those projections any more or less importance than is given to any other.* No weighting factors; no judging; no bias!

Stated more succinctly, we must "take into consideration each and every manifestation of humanity—all *anthropocentric projections*—treating them equally." Indeed, to derive a self-consistent theory that accurately explains *all* forms of behavior that is uniquely human—*everything* that is "us"—we must assign equal importance to *every* "projection" that reflects *every* form of human endeavor, lest we create a disproportionate picture by arbitrarily enhancing one point of view, such as the "scientific" one, at the expense of another, such as the "religious," or "aesthetic" one. But alas, recent history has shown that we don't do that—our tendency to *judge* what is "basic" and what is "not" has resulted in our taking a disproportionate point of view in appreciating the role that the arts, in general, and music, in particular, play in the overall human experience. Regrettably, the arts are one "projection" of humanity that has hitherto been disparagingly minimized in prioritizing the importance of the things we do— most especially in our public education system, and thanks, in part, to the nearly 360-year-old Cartesian philosophy that we addressed in our earlier discussion of dualism. But that's another topic for discussion. For now, we note that the body's efforts to function in accordance with its designated operating set-points is reflected in what today's world of *computer* networking calls *information technology* (IT). In the anatomical world of *neural* networking, it goes by the name of *Physiological process number 2*: the handling of data/information, which we address in Chapter 10.

CHAPTER 10

The Human *Information Technology* System for Handling/Processing and Managing Data and Information

In Chapter 4, we noted that your body has its own GPS (global positioning system) for *locating* the anatomical source of sensory action potentials. We now observe further, that it also has its own information technology (IT) system for *dealing* with these sensory signals. That's not so easy, because, potentially, the organism can be literally bombarded—from both internal (*interoception*) and external (*exteroception*) sources (see Chapter 5)—with as many as 400 *billion* bits of adequate stimuli per second! Thus, hypothetically, your body can be asked to handle just under 35 *quadrillion* (that's 35 thousand-trillion!) sensory inputs per day, across the entire energy spectrum. Talk about information overload and sensory gridlock!

Well, fortunately, we don't have to respond to that much sensory stimulation. First of all, the data that is even eligible to be processed is but a miniscule fraction of the pool "out there" from which it can potentially derive. That is to say, at the risk of belaboring the point, it is worth repeating yet again, that we are not anatomically endowed with the hardware that would be required to transduce into action potentials all the multifarious forms of energy—across the entire frequency spectrum—to which we are routinely exposed on a daily basis (see for example, *constraints to knowing* in Chapter 9). It's just not possible; we have specific *adequate stimuli constraints*.

Second, recall also, from Chapters 4–6, that the sense organs we *do have* will not respond to stimulation unless the incident energy is of sufficient (threshold) strength, duration, persistence, and, on occasion, *urgency*. So, we also have additional anatomic constraints embedded into: (i) neurological *potentials*, i.e., resting, receptor, threshold, depolarization, action, etc.; (ii) *refractory* periods, absolute and relative; (iii) *biasing* mechanisms, e.g., hyper-polarization, hypo-polarization, etc.; and (iv) *sensory adaptation*, to "ignore" persistent, benign inputs (Jacob *et al.* 1982; Schneck 1990; Schneck and Berger 2006; Tortora and Grabowski 1993).

Result: adequate stimuli-specific sensori-motor responses are also "highly selective," such that, an incredible 99.975 percent of the energy to which we are

233

exposed never even gains access to our body. We are not even aware of it (a sobering thought!). But that *still* leaves a hypothetical excitation rate of 100 million adequate stimuli per second, nearly nine *trillion* pieces of information per day and way too much for our central nervous system to handle in a manner that is effective, practical, manageable and not overwhelming. Enter the *reticular activating system* as a first step in resolving this dilemma.

Information-processing paradigm in the central nervous system

The CNS IT paradigm is basically a three-step process that involves three T-words, i.e.:

- adequate stimulus-specific, selective sensory *transduction*

- neural-network *transmission* of digitized raw data

- sensory integration and *translation*/interpretation of information.

We have already discussed sensory transduction (as above), transmission (see Chapter 4), and sensory integration (see Chapter 6). Before we talk about translation and interpretation of information, we need to "fill in" some more "IT blanks." First, to recapitulate briefly, adequate stimuli that do gain access to the body are transmitted as raw *data* through nearly 50 miles of "wiring," i.e., neurons—the *anatomical* units of information processing. The signals "buzz" through nerve networks that form the architecture of a sophisticated communications system—the *nervous system*. En route to (*afferent*) and from (*efferent*) the *central nervous system* (brain plus spinal cord), this communications network handles, collectively, *trillions* of "bits" of data, digitally encoded into *binary*, compound, electrochemical, *action potential pulse trains*—the *physiological* units of information processing. These are relayed by intervening biochemical *neurotransmitters* that are "squirted" into *synaptic junctions*. Thus, digitized pulse trains make their way to and from the CNS, in accordance with *Physiological optimization principle number 5*, which one might call the *principle of economization of limited resources* (see discussion in Chapter 6), There, further processing takes place to reconstitute digitized raw *data* into integrated, meaningful *information*. The sensory-to-motor nerve ratio is about 3 to 1. So, how does the body deal with all of this data? The short answer is, "It doesn't!" Before we even *get* to the level of sensory integration, data must manage first, to get through the reticular formation!

The reticular activating system

We were first introduced to the reticular formation in Chapter 4, and mentioned that we would get back to it in Part II. Well...here we are. Recall that this "netlike" (hence its name) formation is a tangled, densely packed cluster of nerve cells, about the length of the little finger of one's hand, that extends from the uppermost portion of the spinal cord, up through the brainstem (*medulla*), and, via the *pons varoli* ("cerebral bridge"), into the *mesencephalon* (midbrain) and portions of the *diencephalon* ("through brain").

Because the *interneurons* within the reticular formation are very short, messages can be relayed quickly from one nerve cell to the next, allowing them to process data at incredible speeds (on the order of *micro*seconds). Thus, this formation acts as a *reticular activating system* (RAS). That is to say, it functions as a type of "data-sieve," continuously sifting through and filtering hundreds of millions of bits and pieces of afferent data that converge upon it and deciding which ones it will allow to "activate higher cerebral centers," and which ones can be discarded without consequence.

Also known as the **e**xtended **r**eticular **t**halamic **a**ctivating **s**ystem (ERTAS) because of its intimate connection with the *thalamus*, the RAS (or ERTAS) decides whether or not a *response* to the sensory inputs is even necessary, and, hence, also makes judgments as to what (if *any*) data will get through to "higher" regions of the CNS…as opposed to what can simply be discarded as being "useless." The decision-making process is based, too, on *which* neurons (or neural networks) are firing, at what *frequency*, how *persistently*, from *where* in the body, and so on.

Only the data that the *reticular nuclei* deem appropriate for further processing, because it is essential, unusual, threatening (imminently dangerous), action-provoking, novel, interesting, stimulating, arousing or whatever other criteria the RAS uses to evaluate it, is allowed to "pass through the gate" to be forwarded on to "higher" levels of the brain for further processing. The RAS also *controls* various life-support systems that ensure a *paw-to-jaw* existence, i.e., pure, instinctive survival! If the RAS decides that no response to the corresponding inputs is necessary, and, further, that the data need not be saved for further processing, they are simply discarded—gone!— without ever reaching consciousness. Incredible as it may sound, that is the ultimate fate of as much as another 99.9995 percent of the afferent signals that do gain access to the CNS via sensory nerve networks, leaving but 500 bits of data per second, or just over 43 million per day for the brain to handle. Now we are getting a bit more reasonable…but we are not done yet!

The data that makes it through the reticular activating system works its way up the *spinothalamic tract* to be "greeted" by the thalamus, the brain's "reception center." *All* data coming in to the brain—except that derived from our special sense of smell, *olfaction* (remember, this data goes directly to the "smell" brain, the *rhinencephalon*)— undergoes a preliminary *classification screening* in this oblong mass of gray matter located towards the back of the forebrain. Here, specific regions are specialized to receive particular kinds of digitized inputs. Once classified, data is now starting to become *information*. As such, it is immediately dispatched to the "almond-shaped" amygdala (fear center), where it undergoes *sub-conscious evaluation* to effect, if necessary, instantaneous responses to *perceived* imminent threats to the safety of the organism, or to any of its basic drives (see Chapters 8 and 9).

The amygdala—the emotional living engine/instrument

It is at this stage of information processing that we part company with *dualism*. If there is any doubt about our being, first and foremost, creatures of *emotion*, one has just to trace the path of information as it courses through the brain. Leaving the thalamus *it goes first to the amygdala*, the body's "fear center" and the place where *emotional* life-and-death decisions are made. If the amygdala senses "danger"—real or imagined—it issues forth distress messages, "SOS" *error signals* that mobilize into action corresponding "911" controlling systems (see Chapter 7). It also truncates any further *cognitive* information processing. In fact, it goes even further than that: an active amygdala draws increased blood flow to that area of the brain, while triggering an inhibitory reflex that shuts down the hippocampus. As always: *emotion trumps reason!* Moreover, under conditions of *prolonged* stress, *Physiological optimization principle number 8* kicks in:

Use it, or lose it!

That is to say, in its effort to optimize physiologic function, the body does not endeavor to keep and support anatomical regions that have fallen into disuse. Thus, *sustained* neurological inhibition of the hippocampus, combined with compromised blood flow to that cognitive region of the brain, cause it to start *atrophying*—it begins to waste away, degenerating to dangerously low levels. So much for reason!

"Distress"/error signals generated by the amygdala are in the form of outgoing, *motor*, compound action potentials that travel via A-H-P (amygdala to hypothalamus to pituitary gland) tracts, *hypothalamo-hypophysial* pathways, and *hypothalamo-autonomic* routes to trigger the release from target organs and tissues of neurotransmitters and/or hormones that elicit "fight-or-flight" responses (Chapter 8). *Only if the amygdala sounds an "all clear"* does information track *next* to the "sea-horse-shaped" hippocampus (cognitive center) and sensory regions of the cerebral cortex, where *momentarily delayed, conscious perception* allows it to be processed further, and, perhaps, eventually stored elsewhere. For storage and recall purposes, in both the amygdala and the hippocampus, information is fine tuned by *stimulus coding* it.

Stimulus coding in the limbic system

The purpose of *stimulus coding* in the limbic system—by the amygdala in the case of emotional responses, or the hippocampus in the case of cognitive responses—is to give processed information *temporal* sequential significance as it proceeds further up the line to still "higher" cerebral centers, where it may eventually be filed away in, and recalled from, *memory*. Indeed, as we shall discuss later, such physiologic sequencing of afferent information gives birth to the concept of *time*, a primary dimension of human *consciousness*. The tagging may be accomplished in one or more of the following ways:

- The region comprising the front part of the frontal lobe of the brain (i.e., the *prefrontal cortex*) has temporary, "working," or *primary memory slots*—"mailboxes," if you will—that are filled in a particular sequence so that, for example, "box A" is filled first, followed by "box B," then "box C," and so on. In recalling the information stored momentarily as "post-it notes" in primary memory—based on its anatomical location—the brain then knows that the material retrieved from location A came in before the material stored in location B, which preceded the material that can now be found in location C, and so on.

- In addition, the tagging centers of the brain actually *code* the incoming information *stereochemically* by endowing the neurotransmitters associated with it with a biochemical "label,"—in much the same way that clothing-check persons tag items for subsequent retrieval at night clubs or restaurants. Thus, for example, an item coming through first might receive a triangular biochemical tag; the next one, a circular biochemical tag; and the next one, a square biochemical tag. In recalling the stored information, the brain then knows that the material carrying the triangular tag came in before (i.e., preceded in time) the material carrying the circular tag, which took place in time prior to that material carrying the square tag, and so on.

There might very well be other, yet-to-be identified ways in which information is tagged by the brain to give it temporal significance, but the point is that such tagging and storing in working memory for later identification and possible resorting is what gives us a sense of sequencing and, as a result, a sense of time. Those individuals in whom temporal tagging/storing of sensory information has gone awry—such as, some on the autism spectrum, or others who suffer from Alzheimer's disease, or have experienced a stroke, brain damage, a serious accident, etc.—might have an impaired sense of time, poor short-term memory recall ability, and/or experience difficulty in making sense out of the adequate stimuli that they perceive. To them, the world is confusing, which may explain much of their bizzare behavior. For example, read this: *My name is Dan Schneck.* If your brain is sequencing material properly, with the words perceived in their intended sequential order, then this sentence should have made "sense" to you. But suppose you read read: *Is Schneck name my Dan,* with the words all jumbled up. Get the point? *Correct sequencing of information is a prerequisite to correct interpretation of information.* Thus:

> *Music therapists take note: Your client might not be hearing, seeing, or otherwise sensing things in the same order or perceptual configuration in which you are presenting them! That might result in confusion, defensive tactics, withdrawal symptoms, stress responses, and other seemingly unexplainable reactions to words, music, and other forms of communication.*

> *Don't assume that what you are transmitting is what the client is receiving!*

Again we note that the thalamus, amygdala, hippocampus, and hypothalamus, together with the parolfactory area, mammillary body, and fornix (Latin for "arch") constitute a group of interconnected cerebral structures called, collectively, the *limbic system*—the "emotional," or *sub-conscious* brain. *Bottom line:* the *emotional, sub-conscious* brain, after *integrating* and *evaluating* afferent inputs from all sensory modalities (see *Sensory integration* in Chapter 6), only "heeds" about 10 percent of the signals coursing through it, i.e., some 50 bits per second (about four-and-one-third-million per day), thus preventing 90 percent of what made it through the reticular activating system from "percolating up" the CNS to the level of conscious awareness. *Talk about constraints to knowing!* Moreover, for most types of sensori-motor tasks of daily living, processing rates of under *half* that amount—i.e., 20–25 bits per second, equivalent to an information-processing rate of 50–40 msec per bit—usually suffice to produce acceptable results. Even slower processing speeds, up to several hundred msec per impulse, are required for more complex tasks, such as recognizing and interpreting printed words. However, music therapists again take note:

> If you are stimulating your clients at incident rates greater than they can process, they might experience "drop outs," losing vital pieces of information that might cause it not to make sense.

> On the other hand, if the stimulation rate is too slow, they might perceive it to be "jerky," thus losing any sense of "temporal continuity" in the information being processed, and again, it won't make sense.

> Bottom line: to optimize your management of any given client, learn the cerebral information-processing rate of that client, and structure your clinical intervention within that constraint.

But we're still not done with the IT paradigm, so, what's next?

The momentary stop in primary memory

Information that makes it through the limbic system and into *primary memory* gets processed further. This is only a momentary stop, lasting but a few seconds (to no more than a minute) and involving some 7–10 pieces of information at a time. But the stop is significant in several ways.

First, remember in Chapter 7 when we talked about the body's *immune system*, mentioning that there were "memory cells" that could store the *genetic information* uniquely identifying *foreign materials* which the system had come in with contact previously? Such stored information allows the body to *recognize immediatley* previously encountered "invaders," thus optimizing its all-important speed and effectiveness in responding to such potentially threatening invasion. Well, guess what? The pre-frontal cortex *also* has "memory cells" that store *sensory information*, uniquely identifying the attributes of a previously encountered experience. This allows the body to *immediately recall* having had that experience in the past, and further explains why, each time the nervous system encounters the *same* type of stimulus, it *processes* that stimulation that much faster and easier. In other words, *Physiological optimization principle number 9* asserts that:

> *The human body learns most effectively through constant repetition and reinforcement, embodied in the famous expression that "practice makes perfect!"*

We'll get back to this concept, since it is actually the first step in the process of entrainment, as a means for physiologic adaptation. For now, we note that the enhanced ease and increased processing speed of previously encountered experiences is called *facilitation*, and the mechanism that allows for facilitation is called *memory of sensation*. Memory of sensation is also another way that the body experiences time, in this case by becoming aware through memory of the cyclic periodicities that are inherent to the nature of our universe.

Perhaps equally important, though, is the fact that *primary memory* allows the body to discard yet more information that, based on memory of sensation, is identified as having "come through this way before," and been previously discarded because it was deemed to be "useless." Thus say "good-bye" to at least half of the information that got this far! But we are *still* not done yet…so where do we go from here?

The extended stop in secondary memory

Continuing "up the ladder," and recruiting the services of the parietal and occipital lobes, and parts of the basal ganglia, the brain now *recodes* the information derived from primary memory. It does so:

- *semantically*, i.e., the information's *syntax* may be re-defined
- *temporally*, i.e., its *sequence* may be re-ordered
- *spatially*, i.e., its *structure* may be geometrically re-configured

as the signals move into *secondary* or *auxiliary memory*. Such sorting out, reorganizing, filing, cataloging, and transferring usually takes place in 24-hour cycles surrounding sleep/wake states, as the body continues to prioritize and further identify what it might ultimately want to do with the information, if anything! That is to say, believe it or not, at this stage in the processing of information, the body *still* reserves the right to discard any information it decides—for whatever reason(s)—not to retain permanently. That often results in as little as half a million total bits of information per day being retained—an *average, equivalent, net, compound action potential information-storage-rate* of nearly six stimuli per second, which amounts to some 1.5×10^{10} bits of information in an 80-year lifetime. Compare this *permanent* storage situation with the estimated 8.0×10^{10} *tertiary* memory cells in a "typical" cerebral cortex, and one can see why scientists claim that we only utilize on the order of 10–20 percent of the total capacity of the brain in the course of an average lifetime.

Be that as it may, information can wander around in the neocortex for minutes, hours, days, weeks, months, even years, before, if not discarded in the meantime, it lands in a "final resting place"—"cold storage" or tertiary memory.

The permanent stop in tertiary memory

The ultimate fate of information that our body *does* finally choose to store on a long-term basis is *tertiary memory*—the *permanent* storage sites that retain this information *for a lifetime*, barring:

- brain damage that results from injury, disease, aging, and/or degeneration
- a systematic, long-term *adaptive* reprogramming that neutralizes the information stored by:
  - overlaying and replacing it
  - reciprocally inhibiting it from becoming realized
  - by-passing it with newer, more dominant neural networks, a process called *plasticity*—the ability to be molded
  - all of the above.

There is no specific, localized, identifiable cerebral *center* for tertiary memory, it is simply a generic term designating the *locus* (collection of points that satisfy a given condition, in this case, the storage of information) of all anatomic regions where are contained information intended to stay there *for life!* The information in tertiary memory is derived, cumulatively, from the total of all of our life experiences. This is as opposed to information that comes to us *pre-programmed* and permanently inscribed in our genetic heritage. Somewhere in between *inherited*—genetic, *nature*, "read-only memory" ("ROM")—and *acquired*—experiential, *nurtured*, tertiary, "programmable memory" ("PROM")—is *"random access memory"* ("RAM"). This is a term coined to identify systemic operating set-points that can be continuously altered in response to persistent anatomic stimulation, and it begins with *memory of sensation*, which results in *facilitation*. The process of *entrainment* then goes on to exploit the attribute of *plasticity* to generate neural networks *de novo* ("from scratch") as a means for satisfying the *adaptive* needs of the organism. In other words, as we shall see, one may think of *physiologic adaptation* as the RAM component of our body's information-processing networks—becoming PROM in the "short term" i.e., single lifespan of experiences, perhaps persisting through many generations of progeny, and ROM in the "long term," i.e., undergoing continuous updating through generations of persistent exposure to stimulants and experiences that result in "permanent," evolutionary changes to the body's operating set-points.

It is worth emphasizing again, that when information finally embeds itself in the tertiary memory slots of the cerebral cortex it stays there forever, permanently implanted in our brain as if by a branding iron! True, we may have to "dig deep" to retrieve stored memories that we might, for whatever reason(s), be *consciously or sub-consciously suppressing*, but nevertheless they are there! One way of extracting them is through the suggestive techniques of deep hypnosis, wherein one is encouraged to extract and "relive" the events hidden away in the "attic" of tertiary memory, events so buried, that they would not be retrievable by any other means. But once so-realized, they may help to explain behavioral patterns that can then be effectively managed, especially through music therapy. More details about this paradigm for cerebral information processing may be found in Ackerman (1990), Berger and Schneck (2003), Coren and Ward (1989), Ornstein and Thompson (1984), Schneck (1990, 2011b, 2012), Schneck and Berger (1999, 2006), Schneck and Schneck (1997), and Woody (1982), among many others. So we now say a few words about the final step in the body's IT paradigm: *translation of information.*

Translation of information: the Gestalt Laws governing the conscious perception and organization of sensory information

The best way to discuss what our brain does with the information stored in tertiary memory is to summarize what are known as the *Gestalt Laws* (Coren and Ward 1989). We were first introduced to these somewhat informally in Chapter 6, when we talked about the sixth element of knowledge, *relation*, in the section on *sensory integration*. Here, we now formalize them into five laws:

- *Law of proximity*, which addresses the body's ability to discriminate among individual elements of adequate stimuli that are received very close together in space and/or in time. This is a function of the *resolution* limitations of sensory transducers, wherein if ambient-somatic monitoring mechanisms are unable to distinguish as being "different from one another," incident sensory inputs that arrive closer together than the sense organs can handle, the respective inputs are perceived to "blend together," i.e., to coalesce into a single unit, or figure. In fact, even if sensory transducers *can* resolve a set of adequate stimuli into their individual elements, all of those that share attributes in common and are "close enough to one another" in space and/or in time are assumed to constitute a self-contained, homogeneous unit.

- *Law of directionality*, which addresses the body's ability to "connect the dots." This is a function of the *tracking* characteristics of the CNS's information processing networks. Thus, in the absence of any obvious discontinuities in incoming information, consecutive individual elements of adequate stimuli that are perceived to follow one another in the same direction, tend to be grouped as defining a continuous path in that direction. That is to say, the sequential pattern of incident sensory inputs is perceived to be tracing a smooth, unbroken, continuous trajectory in the given direction, such that the next incoming stimulus is *expected* to follow suit, in that direction. If it doesn't, it is *discarded* as being an "odd data point," one that doesn't belong in the group.

- *Law of similarity*, which recognizes that the body's information-processing networks are uniquely endowed with the inherent ability to extract essential *common denominators* that may be embedded in adequate stimuli. Thus, those stimuli that share identical/greatly similar generic features, or are otherwise comparable in the attributes that define them, tend to be perceptually grouped together into the same object category, *even if they are not in close proximity to one another* (that's how this Gestalt Law differs from the first one).

- *Law of closure*, which derives from the body's basic desire to avoid "loose ends." Thus, for example, if a physical space or region is bounded by a continuous curve that may or may not be closed, the brain, nevertheless, tends to *perceive it* as a self-contained, closed figure. That is to say, the body "closes" any existing breaks in information—"filling in the gaps," so to speak. This is actually the case for *any* type of sensory input, not just visual, i.e., the body will automatically fill in the details that it *thinks* should be there in order to, again, "connect the dots," i.e., create a continuous flow of information with a logical ending.

- *Law of pragnanz*, which, from the German term for a "good figure," stipulates that in an effort to evoke the most effective *response* to specific adequate stimuli (if, indeed, the body decides that a response is even necessary), *sensory differentiation* and *integration* mechanisms embedded in all of the preceding laws attempt to create the most stable, consistent, and meaningful *interpretation* of those stimuli (see Chapter 6). That is to say, the body, being *purposeful*, seeks to glean the *essence* of the information contained in the stimuli (the "spirit of the law," so to speak), as opposed to its *absolute* content (the "letter of the law"). But this is easier said than done, given all of the anatomical/ physiological limitations and constraints that we have been talking about thus far. Nevertheless, to illustrate the concept of *pragnanz*… I challenge you to read the following (there are no typographical errors!):

    > *If you cn raed tihs… yuo've porevn my pinot. The hmaun mnid deosn't need the lterets in a wrod to be in the rgiht oredr. As lnog as the frist and lsat lteetr are in the rghit palce, yuor bairn deos the rset… rerarnagnig the gebibirsh to mkae snese of the mses!*

I rset my csae! Except to note that the last stage in the IT paradigm translation, followed by meaningful interpretation, results in *awareness*, from which derives *Physiological process number 3: Consiousness* (Dennett 1991).

Human consciousness

To summarize, the second of the six major processes by which the seven basic features of our living engine/instrument become manifest is *information technology*— how the body processes the syntax encoded into sensory action potentials. This includes mechanisms responsible for:

1. adequate stimulus-specific, selective *sensory* energy **T**ransduction

2. neural-network **T**ransmission of *digitized* raw data

3. filtering of data by the *reticular activating system*

4. stimulus coding by the *limbic system*

5. recognition/identification by a momentary stop in *primary memory*

6. recoding/evaluation by an extended stop in *secondary memory*

7. permanent storage in *tertiary memory*, and the last of these "3-Ts"

8. **T**ranslation of *information* following *sensory differentiation/integration*, leading to *consciousness*.

The World Book Dictionary defines *consciousness* as, "an awareness of what is going on about one; the power of the mind—whether rational or not—to be aware of acts, sensations, or emotions; the mental activity of which the individual is aware." The dictionary then goes on to give the etymology of this word, i.e., it derives from the Latin prefix *com-*, which means "with," to which is attached the word *scīre*, which means, "know" (the same root from which comes the word *science*). Hence:

Consciousness is the human instrument of knowing.

Schneck (1990) distinguishes complex *awareness*—consciousness—from simple *awakeness*. The former is an *active* physiological state of possessing knowledge, *and realizing (i.e., being "conscious" of the fact) that such is the case*. The latter is simply a *passive* state of being subject to *sub-conscious* arousal and sensory stimulation, *without necessarily attributing any particular significance or meaning to such stimulation*. So, of what are we aware?

The most basic form of awareness is our ability to retrieve from memory, *stimulus-coded, sequential sensory information*, and to attach to it a significance embedded in the fundamental dimension of perception that we call *time*, yet another T-word! Thus, one might say that:

Time is the primary dimension of physiologic consciousness.

Going one step further, what are the attributes of "time?" i.e., what does stimulus-coded information make us "aware of," that results in our conceptualizing *time* as a primary dimension of consciousness? Basically, three things:

1. Cause and effect do not (indeed, *cannot*) occur simultaneously because of a fundamental principle of physics, which is to say:

    The default configuration of any physical system is the status quo (see the laws of physics in Chapter 8).

This is illustrated in physiology by the *principle of stationarity* (see Chapter 6) and in nature, in general, by the facts that:

a) systems of any kind have an inherent *inertia* against any form of change. In politics, we call it *conservatism;* in the classroom (and perhaps even in the practice of music therapy), we face a *resistance to being taught;* in social systems, we constantly encounter the "we've always done it this way" mentality, and so on. But even if we could overcome that inertial resistance…

b) energy conversions of any kind cannot occur instantaneously—they are inevitably *delayed.* Why? Because the system must first pass through a *metastable* state of equilibrium, i.e., it must first "accelerate" from a *potential* state to a *kinetic* one, and that requires a brief *pause* (see Chapters 3 and 5). Your car, for example, does not start to move the instant you depress the accelerator pedal. It takes a moment to react.

c) our perception of that delay, and the inertia that preceded it, is embedded in the brain's ability to tag, sequence, store, and retrieve sequential information.

2. As we have already noted, there is an inherent *periodicity* that characterizes events in our universe. Our perception of that periodicity, too, is embedded not only in the brain's ability to tag and sequence information, but also in its ability to recognize certain incoming cues as ones that it has previously encountered, i.e., it *remembers having seen them before.*

3. Any given event has associated with it some *duration,* embedded in the velocity and displacement that result from the previously induced acceleration. The latter can be *tracked* by our IT mechanisms to document how long it took for the event to occur. "How long" translates into the perceived "time it took" for a system to transition from one equilibrated state to another. Thus, again, by retrieving from memory, information stored in some logical sequence, one can identify events as:

a) having already taken place—a consciousness derived from medium-term secondary and permanent tertiary memory that give us a sense of *past*

b) taking place even as we are experiencing them—a consciousness derived from short-term primary or working memory that gives us a sense of *present*

c) not yet having taken place at all, i.e., no memory, which gives us a sense of *future.*

Finally, given that:

- *time, is a fundamental dimension of perception derived from the physiological attribute of memory*
- *consciousness, is a physiological process derived from time*
- *knowledge is derived from consciousness…*

…we close this brief discussion of human consciousness by observing that our body's *knowledge* (obtained via sub-conscious, even un-conscious, semi-conscious or conscious mechanisms from which derive our *awareness* of the inherent periodicities in our universe) has evolved into adaptive *biorhythms, Physiological process number 4* in our developing paradigm, which we will address in Chapter 11.

Information-processing rates

The *rate* at which the brain can receive, tag, store, and retrieve sensory information from within the body (*interoception*) or from the surrounding environment (*exteroception*) is called its *cerebral information-processing rate* (IPR). This rate constrains, among other things, our CNS's ability to *resolve* sensory input (Gestalt Law number 1), and it is unique to any given individual. As an illustration, recall from Chapter 5 that the human sense of vision—because of the ways in which optic neurons fire when stimulated, and the resolution characteristics of the visual system—is capable of processing images at the maximum rate of about 50–60 per second. That is to say, digitizing real-life continuous motion into a series of "still frames" that are cast on the retina of the eye at rates on the order of 50–60/sec will make the motion *appear*, to the observer, to be continuous, even though in reality it (i.e., the motion) is being projected onto the retina in discrete, sequential time steps.

It may just be a coincidence, but it is interesting to note that the lower limit of this digitizing process—the 24 frames/second "flicker speed" for the eye—is the same as the 24 cycles/second "beat frequency" that is the threshold for perceived dissonance when two sounds differing in frequency by that amount are presented *simultaneously* to our hearing apparatus (Schneck and Berger 2006). Recall further, that the human auditory system also requires at least 50–100 milliseconds to lock onto and identify any given sound, so if *consecutive* sounds impinge on the ear drum at rates in excess of about 10–20 per second, they will exceed the brain's auditory *resolution capability* and it will not be able to tell one sound from the other. The bottom line, as mentioned earlier, (*again, music therapists take note*) is that:

Each of us is endowed with an individual-specific, unique, characteristic, nature-and-nurture-derived capability to process information at specific rates which will vary from individual to individual.

However, as we shall see below, there are times when this *inherent IPR* can be *biased*—up or down—by mechanisms not unlike those that can also lead to *sensory adaptation* (see Chapters 4 and 5). One can call this biasing "IPR adaptation." For now, we note that one can postulate that:

- *if* the brain is *processing* information (*cerebral IPR*) at the same rate at which this information is coming into the central nervous system (*incident information rate (IIR)*)

- *then* the individual is *perceiving* events in "real time" in a one-to-one correspondence with the *actual* rate at which they are occurring. "Real time" and "perceived time" are equal.

Any deviation from this one-to-one correspondence is more the rule, than the exception. We already noted in *Physiological optimization principle number 6* (Chapter 9), that *emotion always trumps reason*, which is another way of saying that the body *reacts*, a split second before *consciousness* sets in. Things "happen"—in *real* time—before we are aware of them, in *perceived* time (Schneck and Berger 2006). We also noted this in our discussion in Chapter 5 of *Physiological optimization principle number 4* on delayed consciousness, and shall have more to say about biasing and *IPR adaptation* in the section below on *physiologic relativity.*

But before we get there, we must mention that all stimulus-coded time cues received through sensory extero- and interoception converge eventually on the *suprachiasmatic nuclei* (SCN) of the hypothalamus (see Chapter 5), which, as we shall see in the next chapter, establishes the *biorhythm* that we associate with most (probably all) physiologic processes. Thus, just as the *sinoatrial node* (Chapter 2) acts as a natural *cardiac* pacemaker for the heart, the SCN, located near the preoptic area of the anterior ventral hypothalamus, acts as a natural *cerebral* pacemaker. The SCN, responding to time cues, synchronizes the body's internal processes with the daily (circadian), monthly (menstrual), and yearly (circannian) cycles of our environment. Of significance here is the further concept embedded in *Physiological optimization principle number 10:* phase regulation.

> *Phase regulation is an optimization scheme whereby the activity of one set of anatomical structures is coordinated and synchronized with that of another, leading to a phenomenon known as co-acting, in order to minimize the energetic demands of physiologic function and thus optimize performance.*

In phase regulation, one finds that the operating *frequency ranges (bandwidths)* of individual organs or tissues are not *independent* of one another. Rather, they are *co-dependent*, meaning that the operating frequencies of said organs and tissues are related to one another by, in some cases, simple whole number ratios. (This is not unlike those frequency ratios that characterize musical intervals, suggesting that there may be a type of *harmonic order* to physiologic function. We shall get back to this point in Chapter 13.) As examples of phase regulation, consider that:

1. Up to 30 percent of the heart's energy is conserved because:

    a) the ejection of blood from this organ is timed to be in phase with the rhythmic oscillations of the elastic arterial system

    b) the beginning of the respiratory cycle is timed to coincide with the end of one of the ejection phases of the cardiac cycle

    c) the *ratio* of the cardiac period to the arterial pulsation period is maintained at approximately 2:1 (a perfect octave in the musical realm! Is there a message here?). Consider further that:

2. The musculature of the stomach "cranks out" a new peristaltic wave every 20 seconds, but the wave *lasts* about a minute, so that three waves at a time travel down this organ, and the ratio of peristaltic duration to muscular period is about 3:1 (a musical twelfth; see, also, Chapter 2).

3. For the cardiovascular and respiratory systems, the whole-number ratio for several system parameters is optimized at 4:1 (a "double octave").

4. Although during the day, the ratio of pulse rate to respiration rate can vary from 2.5 to 7.0, it equilibrates to a value of 4.0 between midnight and 3 a.m., when physiologic function is optimized according to a so-called *nightly normalization of the rhythmic functional order* principle that prevails during restful sleep. In fact,

5. Harmonic co-acting (synchronization) of *all* physiologic processes is especially prevalent during sleep, thus reducing and optimizing the energetic demands of the organism. This results in a state of *physiologic consonance*, which optimizes healing, as well. On the other hand, *stress*, during one's wakeful hours, upsets this balance/equilibrium, leading to *physiologic dissonance*, with all of its adverse consequences on health and well-being (see Chapter 8).

As we shall see in the next chapter, our expanded awareness (perception of time) is also intimately linked to our consciousness of the *biorhythms* that characterize all physiologic processes, to wit:

- the cyclic beating of the heart
- periodicity of the firing rates in neurons
- rhythmic breathing patterns
- oscillating peristaltic movements in the gastrointestinal system
- diurnal variations in body temperature
- timed release of urine (bladder function) and fecal wastes (rectal function)
- timed release of endocrine hormones to correspond with their role in metabolic processes

- sleep/wake cycles
- periodic 90-min sleep-stage cycles
- female menstrual cycles
- patterns of gait
- the 4–6-hour cravings for food (hunger cycles)

…to mention just a few. All of that having been said, as promised, let's get back to how all of this relates to "real" time vs. "perceived" time.

The physiology of relativity

"Has it been only ten minutes? I feel like I've been here for hours!" "Doesn't time fly when you're having fun?" "A watched pot never boils." These are but a few of the expressions we use to describe the subjective nature by which we experience time. Indeed, in 1905, Albert Einstein showed that time cannot be perceived objectively. He noted that two events that *appear* to be simultaneous to one observer, relative to his or her specific *frame of reference* (remember the very first element of knowledge? see Chapter 6), might not appear to be so to another observer moving in a different frame of reference. Thus, the *physics* concept known as the *theory of relativity* was formulated. Einstein and those who followed after him went on to prove—*from the point of view of pure physics*—that there is no such thing as an absolute, purely objective observation. Rather, any measurement will ultimately depend not only on:

- the extent to which the *process* of measuring actually *disturbs* the event being measured (a point health-care practitioners must always keep in mind, especially as it relates to non-invasive and invasive techniques of diagnostic imaging, and other clinical procedures)
- the *scale of perception* (second element of knowledge) at which the measurement is being taken
- both the *resolution capabilities* (third element of knowledge), and *sources of error* in the measuring system itself,

but also on:

- the *frame of reference* of the observer making the measurement, hence the term "relativity."

But one very important aspect of the entire concept of relativity involves a question that was never raised by the authors of the *physical* "theory of relativity," and that is

- To what extent is the observation being *processed*—anatomically/ *physiologically*—at the same time rate at which the event is *actually occurring* in "real" time? How does the body handle visual, auditory, etc. *cues* that it receives through adequate stimuli that are incident on its various sensory systems? How does it translate these into meaningful *temporal* information—which is what we have been talking about thus far in this chapter? In other words, *objective, inanimate, purely physical* reference frames aside, what about *subjective, living, anatomic ones*...and the "relativity" that *they* introduce into an observation because of individual-specific differences in the ways that incoming sensory information is eventually processed by the unique IPRs of the IT systems of various *anatomic* observers? *This should be a question most often asked by clinicians of all kinds (Schneck and Tempkin 1992)...but certainly, music therapists in particular!*

Establishing a "standard" unit of time

In order to answer the above questions, one must first establish a *standard*, a point of reference against which "time" can be measured. Since, according to *relativity*, it is apparently impossible to formulate a purely *objective* measure of time, suppose we do the next best thing and define what can be called an *intersubjective* timescale based on what we will call the *standard second;* and let's define this "standard second" in a way that all of us can agree on, which is what is meant by *intersubjective*. That is to say:

- when there are certain realities experienced by a critical, statistically significant mass of sensing subjects, e.g., human observers and...

- when they all agree that these realities have certain similar (or identical) attributes, i.e., common denominators uniquely recognized by this critical mass of "observers," in the sense that they all describe those realities in essentially the same, virtually exact way, then...

- we have what is called *intersubjective consensus*, based on which we can then go on to establish certain *standard criteria* that can be applied to "define" that particular reality. For example, our "definition" at the beginning of Chapter 6, of what it means to be "alive," is derived from a set of criteria established through intersubjective consensus; enough folks *agree* that if "something" satisfies those criteria, "it" is "alive."

By virtue of intersubjective *consensus*, one can then proceed to *arbitrarily* quantify the attributes agreed on to define the corresponding reality. In the case of *time*, for example, the *standard second* has been scientifically defined in terms of the frequency of radiation emitted by cesium atoms when they pass from one equilibrated state into another (see Schneck 2011b for details, which are beyond the scope of this book). This quantified variable thus becomes the *standard*, "objective" unit of time that we all agree to use in describing and calibrating how long it takes for events to occur. Let's call it *externalized time* to the extent that it is:

- as observer-independent as technology will allow

- arbitrarily calibrated against an intersubjective, mutually agreed-on, universal standard

- not necessarily related on a one-to-one basis to individual-specific, subjective *perceived time*, as we shall define it below.

Externalized time, based on the standard second, is the quantified dimension that shall be used to describe the "real" rate at which events in our experience are occurring, independent of "us." This rate, then, is also presumed to be the rate at which data (in the form of adequate stimuli) derived from "outside" (i.e., the events under observation) arrive at our sense organs. Call it the *incident information rate* (IIR)—the rate at which our sense organs are sequentially stimulated—and the rate at which we can, *at least hypothetically*, perceive the corresponding events to be taking place in "real" time (as objectively as it gets, based on intersubjective consensus).

But…hold everything! What about the fact that each of us perceives the passage of time in accordance with our own, unique, personalized *cerebral information-processing rate* (IPR), determined at least in part by our own, individual, genetically inherited ability to handle data at a particular speed? How does this affect how we perceive in time the data/information to be processed, data derived from the above-mentioned sensory stimulation? Is this perception yielding or *not* yielding results that are *in phase with* (and hence, giving us a "true" representation of) events as they are "really" occurring? Are these events occurring at the same rate as that associated with our own biological clock ("internalized" sense of time)? To answer *these* questions, we must go one step further and *calibrate* our "internal" clock with the "external, standard" one.

Establishing a "physiological" unit of time

First of all, I cannot give you a specific, "intersubjective" number for this unit of time, as I did for the "standard" second, because, by definition, it is *not* standard; it is unique for each of us, individual specific. All we can say about it is that, at least:

- *anatomically* we inherit a pre-programmed ability to process information at a certain rate. This ability is embedded in the anatomical design criteria of neural and vascular networks, and in physiological optimization principles, both of which we have been developing herein.

- *physiologically* we can bias that rate to a certain extent, depending on our mood, state of health, interest in the subject matter being perceived, and a variety of other factors (see below).

- the previously identified *suprachiasmatic nuclei* located in the anterior hypothalamus have much to do with setting the pace for information processing. Specifically, they synchronize and coordinate it with the daily (circadian) rhythms of our environment (see Chapter 11).

- the *limbic system's* IT responsibility to *stimulus code* and sequence data is constrained to function at a specific rate.

- the *transduction* and *transmission* of data, its conversion into "information," followed by storage and retrieval from primary, secondary, and tertiary memory, and its final *translation* into consciousness are all constrained by rates that depend on the *synaptic transmission characteristics* and *neurotransmitter properties* of specific nerves and neural networks.

Bottom line: our internalized "clock" is ticking away at its own IPR, providing us with a *subjective*, relative sense of time. This may, or may not be in phase with sensory inputs, IIR, derived from the "real" physics of our universe. The latter is arbitrarily "timed" according to an *objective*, external, "standard" clock, ticking away on your wall or desk. However, that doesn't mean that one can't *calibrate* one's *natural*, internal clock by *nurture*. Let's see how this works by considering the following hypothetical example.

As I observe an event (a "jigsaw puzzle?"), suppose my body receives information about that event, coded into, say, 36,000 bits of "real" data (the "pieces" of the jigsaw puzzle). Recalling the fourth element of knowledge, we can say that the *structure* of the event is coded into 36,000 *adequate stimuli* delivered to my sensory systems at a certain rate, which is the *incident information rate* (IIR). Suppose further that the "real" event transpired over a "standard" (wall clock) time interval of ten minutes—600 "standard" seconds—so that IIR = 36,000/600 = 60 adequate stimuli per second.

Now…suppose my *natural* IPR is such that I can *normally*, i.e., when awake, sober, well rested, thinking clearly, etc., process these data (*without drop-outs*) at the rate of, to make the math easier, 60 bits at a time. That natural rate sets my *personal* clock, which is to say my own, internalized, biological clock *normally* ticks off (36,000/60) = 600 of my *personal* units of time to process this data.

So, finally, *after* I have processed these data by my *own*, internal clock, I look at the external clock on the wall and, lo and behold, note that these data represented events in "real" time that *actually* transpired in an elapsed time of ten minutes. I can thus *calibrate* my internalized sense of time—time as I perceive it—with the external, standard units of time as defined by intersubjective consensus. In other words, to tell myself that what I was experiencing (IPR) bore a one-to-one correspondence with what was *actually* happening (IIR), I now *equate* the 600 units of *my* perceived (personal) time to the 600 *standard* seconds of intersubjective time, so that my personal unit of time is now equivalent to the intersubjective unit of time. A "second" of "standard," *external* clock time is now the same as a "second" of "my" *internal* clock time—*normally*, as long as I maintain my IPR (we'll get back to this).

Internalizing the sense of time

That being the case, after enough such experiences (*nurture*), my body commits to permanent, tertiary memory, the fact that, cognitively, it is to *assume* that 36,000 bits of incident data is always associated with events having taken place in 600 seconds of *both* perceived *and* "real" time. In other words, I have now committed to permanent memory, a *reference unit of time*, e.g., a ten-minute interval required to process 36,000 adequate stimuli (keep in mind that the numbers used here are only to illustrate basic principles). I am now in a position to compare my *internal* clock against an *external* clock for all subsequent experienced events, which is what makes "time" *relative*. I have *trained* my body by *nurture*, i.e., stimulus coding, conditioning, **en***trainment*, and permanent, tertiary memory, to calibrate its *natural* tendencies so that they will correspond, one to one, with *experienced* reality as it is actually happening. Now my body will always *perceive* events coded into 36,000 adequate stimuli, as having occurred in ten standard minutes of "real" time…*provided* again I am experiencing these events in a wakeful, sober state, and processing information *normally*. Once calibrated, my body permanently *remembers* this one-to-one correspondence as a *conditioned reflex, whether or not it actually holds in other situations*. What do we mean by that?

Biasing information-processing rates

SCENE 1: TEMPUS FUGIT…"TIME FLIES!"

Suppose I am asleep. My eyes are closed, cutting off visual input; the room is quiet, such that auditory cues are minimized; sensory adaptation has dulled significant tactile input; I am neither eating nor sniffing much of anything; I am not in significant pain, and I am a sound sleeper, not easily awakened or terribly reactive to external stimulation. Under these circumstances, it may actually take as many as eight "real" hours—"wall-clock time"—just to *accumulate* 36,000 bits of data (if indeed I accumulate it at all!). Furthermore, in this peaceful state of slumber, my body metabolism has also slowed down considerably, such that my information-processing networks have been *biased* down to, say, a reduced IPR of 20 bits at a time. It thus *should* take my sleeping body $(36,000/20) = 1800$ seconds $= 30$ "wall-clock" minutes to process this data.

But, according to the clock at my bedside, *eight hours have gone by since I fell asleep!* Where did the time go? Where did the other 7 hours and 30 minutes come from? According to my IPR, *only 30 minutes should have gone by* to process 36,000 bits of data at an IPR of 20, but according to my external clock, that 30 minutes of *expected* time *turned into eight hours of actual time! Boy has time flown!*

In fact, even if I *was* awake, the slower IPR would conflict with my calibrated *internal* clock, which says that, based on the *amount* of information processed, only ten minutes of external clock time should have elapsed to process 36,000 bits of data. But in fact, that ten minutes of *anticipated* time turned into 30 minutes of "real" time.

Again, with my internal clock running slow, external time seems to "fly" compared with calibrated time. That's why "time flies when you are having fun"—your IPR slows down to "savor the moment," just as it does when you are deeply engrossed in a major project, and look at the wall clock in amazement at how much time has *really* gone by, compared to how much time you *think* had gone by.

SCENE 2: TEMPUS REPIT; TEMPUS SERPIT…
"TIME CRAWLS; TIME CREEPS"

You are now in a physician's waiting room, running a fever of 103°F, impatiently anticipating your impending physical exam. Through your discomfort, you happen to notice that *clock time seems to be dragging!* "I *feel* like I've been here for ten minutes, but the wall clock tells me it's been only five. What's going on here?" Then you remember: heat speeds up biochemical reactions, hence metabolic rates. Since your biological clock ticks according to its own physiologic information-processing rate (IPR), and since that rate depends on biochemical reactions, it follows that IPR can, again, be biased by altering biochemical velocities. An increase in the latter, e.g., due to higher temperatures, speeds up IPR, which makes your biological clock run fast. Suppose your "heated" IPR jumps from its *normal* rate of 60 to, say, twice that amount, 120. Now, in *real time*, the clock on the wall tells you that the time that elapsed while you were processing that same 36,000 bits of data was only (36,000/120) = 300 seconds = five minutes. But your *sub-conscious, calibrated* clock "remembers" that 36,000 bits of data is *supposed* to correspond to an event that took place in *ten* minutes, not five. In other words, you *think*, because of the amount of information processed, that ten minutes *should* have gone by, but your *heated consciousness* informs you that, in fact, it has been only five. Real time (five minutes) seems to lag behind perceived time (ten minutes)—*time is dragging!*

Indeed, external clock time does seem to drag when you are ill and running a fever, as it does also when you are suffering from boredom, where disinterest tries your patience and thus speeds up your IPR, or at any time that your internal clock is running fast. *That's why a watched pot never boils*—in your impatience, your IPR soars, and what seems like hours on your biological clock turns out to be only minutes of external clock time.

AND FURTHERMORE…

While we are on the subject, conversely, lowering body temperature decreases the speed of biochemical reactions, hence making your biological clock run slow compared to calibrated external clock time. Hours of external *clock* time now seem like mere minutes of internal *biological* time. The above considerations have several implications. For example:

- As we mentioned in Chapter 3, in *hyperthyroidism* (overactive thyroid gland) there is increased metabolic activity, known as the *calorigenic effect*. The latter leads to higher body temperatures, more heat, faster biochemical reactions, increased IPR, and consequently, seemingly slower passage of external clock time, so the person suffering from hyperthyroidism is always *early* to appointments!

• On the other hand, in *hypothyroidism*, one's biological clock is running slow, so to this person, external clock time is always racing, causing him/her to be perpetually *late* to appointments!

• Moreover, with age, cellular metabolism slows, due in part to hypoxia, i.e., a decreased oxygen supply resulting mainly from cardiovascular issues. This, and other aging effects on IPR, make external clock time appear to pass more rapidly as we get older. *Time flies with age, too!*

• Then there are the time-perception effects of various *drugs*, such as the fever-producing ("pyrogenic") *mescaline* and *psilocybin*, and others, such as methamphetamine and cocaine, that can increase or decrease physiologic metabolic rates, with possible fever-producing side-effects.

• *Music therapists, especially, take note:* IPRs can be significantly affected by different types of music, forms of meditation, clinical intervention procedures, and other techniques that are used to "drive" the physiologic system in an effort to cause it to *adapt*. All have temporal implications as well. That's one reason, for example, that folks who close their eyes while listening to their favorite music often report drifting into a meditative state and losing all track of time. Hobbies can serve the same purpose.

• IPRs (and hence, *subjective* perception of time) can also be influenced by many pathological conditions, stressful situations (see Chapter 8), fear (Schneck and Berger 2006), anxiety, pain, waiting for some important news, excitement about an upcoming event, experiencing a surge of the hormones acetylcholine (inhibitory) or adrenaline (excitatory), or by any other situation where we are not receiving incident information in "real" time at a rate consistent with that at which we are actively, physiologically processing it. The list is long, but the moral of these various scenarios is always the same:

Your (subjective) clock and the wall (objective) clock are inversely related—when your clock is running slow, the wall clock seems to be racing; when your clock is running fast, the wall clock seems to be dragging. Time, indeed, is relative!

But not only that… by using as examples, the spindles embedded in striated skeletal muscles (see Chapter 3, and Schneck 1992), sensory adaptation (see Chapters 4, 5, and Schneck 1990), and physiological information-processing-rates, we have established *Physiological optimization principle number 11:*

The body uses the fundamental mechanism of biasing to optimize and control the function of anatomical organs and tissues.

Some closing remarks, and a reprise on the fundamental elements of knowledge

Physiological optimization principle number 9 advises us that the human body learns most effectively through constant repetition and reinforcement, i.e., *practice makes perfect!* In Chapter 6, when we talked about sensory integration and developed *Physiological optimization principle number 5*, we noted that before the brain "integrates" anything it first processes *separately* the digitized data encoded into each sensory modality as it "reports in" to the CNS. That is to say, the senses break adequate stimuli down into their essential components (i.e., *differentiate*) and the brain then reassembles them (*integrates*) to generate meaningful information.

It is interesting to note that, if we couple these mechanisms of "learning" with the physiological information-processing paradigm formulated in this chapter there emerges a remarkable correspondence between how the body *naturally* goes about *learning,* and the *cognitive* paradigm that was outlined in Chapter 6. In that chapter, we listed—again, based on intersubjective reasoning—seven criteria that we all "agree" establish the essential elements of "knowledge. Now, observe how closely the elements of *consciousness*—the third of the six major processes by which the seven basic features of our living engine/instrument become manifest—fit into the earlier-developed "knowledge paradigm:"

- First, we have *frame of reference.* Indeed, the human body *is* our frame of reference, constrained by:) (i) anatomical design criteria; (ii) physiological optimization principles; (iii) nature; (iv) nurture; (v) physiologic relativity; and (vi) limitations that we have been documenting throughout the book, thus far.

- Next, we have *scale of perception.* As detailed in Chapter 1, the human body is organized into six levels, ranging in scale from: (i) atomic; to (ii) molecular; (iii) cellular; (iv) tissues; and (v) organs to (vi) systems and eventually, the entire organism.

- Third in the knowledge paradigm, we have *resolution,* which, in the human body, involves spatial and temporal issues related to: (i) the *type* of adequate stimulus to which the organism is subjected; (ii) its frequency; (iii) intensity; (iv) persistence; (v) repetition rate; (vi) anatomical location; and (vii) various biasing mechanisms.

- The fourth element, *structure,* is handled by the body through: (i) *differential* (as opposed to *integral*) mechanisms; (ii) *catabolism* (as opposed to *anabolism*); (iii) transduction; (iv) digitization; and (v) transmission of data/information.

- Fifth, *order* manifests itself as *stimulus coding* and *memory.*

- Sixth, *relationships* becomes: (i) *sensory integration;* (ii) *translation;* and (iii) *interpretation of information*, all of which result in the final element of knowledge:

- *Synthesis,* which we know as *awareness; consciousness!*

These are interesting parallels between our *conception* of what "knowledge" is all about and how the body actually works in achieving it. Keeping that in mind, we now continue talking about "how we work," by moving on to the fourth of the six significant physiological processes. This one addressed the body in time, and more specifically, its *biorhythms* (music anyone?).

CHAPTER 11

The Body in Time

In Chapter 10 we talked about *the* most fundamental dimension of human perception—*time*—and how this measure of the human experience derives from *stimulus coding* of adequate stimuli, which, coupled with *sensory integration*, and primary, secondary, and tertiary *memory*, eventually results in human *consciousness*. We learned about subjective, individual-specific, inherited, internal clocks, and objective, "standard," *intersubjective*, external clocks. We then compared the two by observing that: when your internal clock is running fast, the external clock on the wall can't seem to keep up with it, and hence, external time "drags" behind. By contrast, when your internal clock is running slow, *it* can't seem to keep up with external time, and so, the latter leaps ahead—time seems to be "flying." Finally, we noted that *internal* time has evolved to be calibrated, biased, and synchronized with (i.e., correspond to) the cyclic events that go on in the *external* environment within which we live, so that we can function "in phase" with those periodicities. Carrying this reasoning one step further, in this chapter we elaborate a bit more on this notion of calibrating and synchronizing anatomical/ physiological function with the body's surroundings, i.e., we will address *the body in time*, and the *biorhythms* that derive from it.

Talking about the periodicity of time, reminds one of the words of Mark Twain, who said,

> *Everything which has happened once must happen again and again—and not capriciously, but at regular periods, and each thing in its own period, not another's, and each obeying its own law. (1996)*

I would like to add to Twain's words:

> *And when the 'things' are human, each one subject to its own sense of temporal physiologic relativity.*

Biorhythms

J.J. Virey (1775–1846) is considered by many to be the father of *chronobiology—the study of periodic phenomena in living organisms*. In his 1814 doctoral thesis in medicine, Virey described the human body as a *horloge vivante*, a "living clock." The reasoning behind this is based, in the most general sense, on yet another principle of physics that we addressed in Chapter 5, i.e.,

> *Energy manifests itself as being cyclic… vibrating in all of its realized forms. Indeed, "All God's creations got rhythm!"*

…and the human body is no exception. Any wonder, then, why *rhythm* is the most fundamental element of music, and why it is so basic to the clinical applications of music therapy (Schneck and Berger 2006; Berger 2015)? Indeed, *chronobiologists* have identified over 100 recurring internal physiologic events, and there are undoubtedly more waiting to be discovered. Thus, it is worth emphasizing again that, notwithstanding the concept of *homeostasis*, the processes of physiologic function are *not* expected to maintain a *constant* internal environment. Rather, most of the variables that define these processes exhibit *periodic* behavior that can be broadly classified as:

- *infradian*—repetitious, but recurring *less than once per day*
- *circadian*—cycling *exactly once daily*
- *ultradian*—periodic, but with periods short enough to allow relatively fast cycling rates, i.e., recurring *more than once per day*.

Recall that the *period* of a regularly repeating process is defined to be how long it takes for the process to complete one full cycle. In the human body, it is *process specific*, meaning that it depends on the complexity of the particular physiologic function involved—the more complex the function, the longer its period, and vice versa. But recall, also (see Chapter 10), that all physiologic processes are coordinated and synchronized with one another through *phase regulation*.

The various events that recur in the human body do so within a logarithmic timescale that ranges from *nano(10^{-9})*-seconds to *giga(10^{+9})*-seconds. For example, at one extreme, the neurotransmitter, *acetylcholine*, binds momentarily to a receptor site on the skeletal muscle's motor-end-plate for a *very* brief *billionth* of a second. At the other extreme, a "typical" 75-year lifespan amounts to just under 2.5 *billion* seconds. In general, in addition to being *process specific*, timescales for most physiologic processes also tend to be *spatially specific*. That is to say, their periods increase from 10^{-9} to 10^{+9} seconds in almost one-to-one logarithmic proportion to the corresponding anatomic (and societal!) *level of organization* at which the associated activity takes place (see Chapter 1). Thus, *ultradian* timescales are correlated mainly with biochemical catalysis, physiological information processing, cellular tissue organ metabolism, and the transport/utilization of mass, energy, and momentum. We shall examine some of these later, as well as various *infradian* timescales, but we begin our discussion of biorhythms with those that recur daily, i.e., *circadian* ones.

Circadian biorhythms: physiologic events recurring daily

From the Latin *circā*, meaning "around," and *diēs*, meaning "day," *circadian* biorhythms are physiologic events that, as the name implies, recur in daily cycles. Many of these timed activities have evolved into genetically coded *adaptations* to the inherent cycles of our universe, a major source of our perception of time. For example, we receive visual cues that stem from the inherent cycles of our universe, such as the diurnal (day)/nocturnal (night) alternating light/dark cycles associated with the Earth's rotation about its own axis relative to the position of the sun at any given time. We call each such cycle a day (*diēs*) in our life. We are also aware that each day, the *amount* of day*light*, as well as the amount of *heat* in the environment, both vary in circannian (yearly) cycles that correspond to how long it takes for the Earth to complete one full trajectory around the sun. We call each such cycle a year (*annus*) of our life.

We observe further that the Earth has a heavenly body (the moon) that revolves around it in regular *menstrual* (monthly) cycles, from which derives the corresponding concept of a month (the etymology of the word paralleling *moon)*, and so on. Thus, timed biological responses (biorhythms) have become *conditioned reflexes* that represent genetically coded *adaptations* to these inherent cycles of our universe. That is to say, our environment influenced the evolution of our individual genetic make-up, which now determines our pre-set biological clocks, as discussed in the previous chapter. Specialized genes, programmed to respond to specific adequate stimuli, for example, *light* or *heat*, code for the synthesis of proteins that are expressed in *unique* response to *that* adequate stimulus. In turn, these proteins evoke specific, periodic physiologic events, such as those *circadian* ones described below:

1. For a person on a "conventional" schedule, the endocrine secretion rate of the hormone *cortisol* rises during the night, to a maximum "surge" that begins around 4 a.m.—eventually supplying the body (by the time it awakens) with 25 percent of its daily allotment of this adrenal secretion. Apparently, this ensures that blood levels of cortisol will be at their highest just before a person arises, thereby preparing the body for the anticipated daytime stresses to follow. The hormone levels then fall throughout the day, to a minimum at bedtime.

2. Blood levels of the hormone *adrenalin* also increase in the morning.

3. What will eventually amount to 50 percent (for men) to 80 percent (for women) of one's daily supply of *growth hormone* (secreted by the pituitary gland) starts entering the blood during stage 2 of the sleep cycle (see below), and continues on into stages 3, 4, and rapid eye movement (REM sleep). Much of this blood is delivered to skeletal muscles, where it helps to restore muscle mass and repair "wear and tear" micro-traumas sustained during the previous period of active wakefulness. Thus, the tissue is effectively healed back to full strength.

4. More generally, *hormones* are released into the blood on set daily schedules that range from every two to every four hours, depending on how the endocrine system is "locked on" (*entrained*) to external cues and *diurnal* activities. However, note that many hormones are released in regular 90-minute cycles (i.e., they are *ultradian* biorhythms). The latter also seems to be the "magic number" for cyclic rest and activity, including *sleep*. Indeed, studies (e.g., see Rose 1989) show that during each night's sleep, one goes through four or five 90-minute cycles, the first including four distinct stages, plus an REM phase, and the remaining ones cycling only through varying amounts of stages 2, 3 and 4 REM.

5. Appetite, attention span, cerebral function, tolerance for pain, and several other physiologic processes also seem to operate in regular 90-minute cycles over a 24-hour period—or is it 16–"90-minute hours?"

6. "Normal" *body temperature*, 98.6°F, actually rises during the hours that one is active, reaching a maximum 99°F (±) by around 5 or 6 p.m., local time. Conversely, body temperature gradually falls to its lowest value during the time one is resting/sleeping, reaching a minimum 97°F (±) around 3 or 4 a.m., local time. That's a 2°F swing during the course of an "average" day, which correlates one to one with corresponding metabolic rates, and, interestingly, with those times of the day when muscle contractions are strongest (around 6 p.m., although "grip strength" peaks at 2 p.m.) and weakest (around 3 a.m.).

7. "Resting" *heart rate* can vary by as much as 20–30 beats/min. over a 24-hour period. The average resting heart rate is usually between 80 and 100 beats/min, but it can *triple* under "fight-or-flight" conditions.

8. *Bone marrow* makes more blood cells from 6 to 10 *p.m.* than it does from 6 to 10 *a.m.*

9. Cells lining the *skin and digestive tract* speed up their metabolic activity around 12 midnight to 1 a.m., while slowing down during the height of the day.

10. *White blood cells* are more active during the evening than they are during the day (although the activity of "natural killer" cells peaks in the morning).

11. *Platelets* are "stickiest" around 9 a.m. daily.

12. "Resting" *blood pressure* can fluctuate by as much as 30 percent daily, rising in late afternoon and within a half-hour after ingesting a meal. It also tends to be higher during the winter months.

13. One's *special senses* show circadian peaks and valleys in acuity.

14. Even our *moods, sexual drives, and levels of alertness* undergo cycles, largely under the control of the pineal gland (*epiphysis cerebri*), the brain's "third eye" (partly because of its anatomical location behind the eyeballs), which was introduced

in Chapter 7. Recall that this gland functions only in the dark, and is the source of the sleep-inducing (and gonad-inhibiting) hormone *melatonin*. The activity of the pineal gland peaks around 2 a.m. It is suppressed during the day by a factor of 4–6 under the inhibitory influence of the sympathetic *pineal nerves* that emanate from the bilateral *superchiasmatic nuclei* (SCN) of the brain (remember the SCN?). That is, visual and other time cues perceived through extero-interoception converge on the SCN, located on either side of the third ventricle of the brain.

To refresh your memory, the SCN *is* the body's biological "alarm" clock, or "pacemaker," if you will. It receives cues from what are called *zeitgebers* (German, *zeit* = "time," + *geber* = "giver"), which include various adequate stimuli, mostly, light, via the *retino-hypothalamic tract*. Then, interacting with many other regions of the brain, the SCN generates light-induced, gene-mediated, neuronal/hormonal activities that synchronize the body's endogenous, internal processes with corresponding cycles in its surroundings. Thus, during the day, when the photosensitive SCN is active, the pineal gland is not, and vice versa at night. Some theories suggest that the pineal gland, unlike the SCN, is also involved in more long-term biological rhythms, which leads us to consider *rhythms to the rhythms—infradian biological rhythms!*

TO EVERYTHING THERE IS A SEASON: INFRADIAN TIMESCALES INVOLVING EVENTS THAT RECUR LESS THAN ONCE DAILY

Solomon (*ca.* 970–930 B.C.) declared in the opening verse of Chapter 3 of the Old Testament's *Book of Ecclesiastes* (from the Greek for "preacher") that, "To every thing there is a season, and a time to every purpose under the heaven." So it is that going beyond the *daily* rhythms of physiologic function, one encounters still more recurring events, with timescales that range from days to an entire lifespan (*infra-* is Latin for "below," as in *recurring less times than daily*, or, "beyond" as in *recurring on timescales in excess of 24 hours*).

Now, granted, one could argue that an entire lifespan has only one, *degenerative* half-cycle—from birth to death. But the notion of *reincarnation*—the rebirth (*regenerative* half-cycle) of one's "soul" in a new body—has many sectarian believers. For example, consider that Brahmanism proposes that the *essence* of one's being—the *spirit*, as opposed to the physical body—is continuously *reborn* (see related discussion of the survival of the soul, in Chapter 8). Such reanimation(s) allow it to complete several *spiral-staircase-like* life-death-life cycle(s). Presumably, as one's soul climbs up these progressive levels of embodiment, it advances through an ascending path that eventually converges on enlightenment and absolute purity. Details are beyond the scope of this text, so we revert, instead, to considering well-established timescales associated with the body's *less-than-a-lifetime-but-more-than-a-day* biorhythms, which are classified as being:

1. *Circaseptan*—weekly—from the Latin *septem*, meaning "seven," as in, originally, the annual month of September. Indeed, the body persists in showing patterns that recur in a range from four to ten days, averaging weekly turnovers (Orlock 1993). There is evidence to suggest that as early as 3000 B.C., the development of the seven-day week as an early measure of time was rooted not only in the Bible's version of *creation*, but also in qualitative observations of corresponding psychobiological rhythms of the human organism.

    It is well known, for example, that the "common cold," if medically treated, can be cured in about seven days; otherwise, it goes away on its own in about a week! This tongue-in-cheek observation suggests that *weekly cycles are characteristic of the body's immune system*. Indeed, the most and best investigated circaseptan rhythms *have* involved the immune system—due, perhaps, to the facts that critical post-operative inflammatory reactions tend to peak and then subside in seven-day cycles, and many common disease incubation periods tend to require about a week following exposure before first symptoms appear.

    But that's not all. The observations that:

    a) *blood platelets* live about ten days, as do *taste bud cells*;

    b) the numbers of *T-cells and B-cells* (of the white blood cell category)— immune cells vital for the body's resistance to infections and cancer— fluctuate on seven-day schedules; and,

    c) the accumulation of additional, similar types of evidence…

    all point to the fact that *many cellular regeneration cycles and turnover rates also have weekly periods*. So do some of the body's *adaptive mechanisms*. For instance, *blood pressure* and *heart rate* both take about a week to readjust after being upset by major schedule changes. Add to that, the facts that the *acidity (pH) and salt content of urine* also seem to vary in seven-day cycles, and it becomes clear that the list of circaseptan rhythms in the human body is long and varied, but not all-inclusive.

    Some cellular turnover, immune system, physiologic adaptive, and other cycles spill into two-(*circadiseptan*) and three-(*circavigintan*)-week periods (*Note: vīgintī* is Latin for, "twenty," as in, three weeks = 21 days ≈ 20). For instance, symptoms of chicken pox usually appear about two weeks after exposure. The risk of *organ rejection in transplant operations* (especially kidney) peaks about a week post-op, but continues to exhibit "danger zones" on the 14th and 21st days following the procedure; and *gums* are renewed about every two weeks. Still other cycles recur monthly (*circatrigintan*), and annually (*circannual*).

2. *Circatrigintan*—monthly—from the Latin *triginta*, meaning "thirty." Other than interesting anecdotal endocrinology reports that identify apparent 30-day cycles in the *hormone levels of men's urine*, most notable among circatrigintan cycles are the "almost monthly" *female ovulatory cycles*. These are also called

menstrual, from the Latin, *mēnsis*, for "month"—in this case, closer to the 29.5-day *lunar-*(synodical) month than the average 30.5-day *calendar* month.

At birth, girls have in both ovaries the full complement of some 400,000 immature egg cells. Of these, only about 481 will mature and be released from the ovaries, in a process called *ovulation.* They are discharged from the ovaries at the rate of about 13 per year, for the 37-year "average" reproductive life of the "typical" female—"typical" meaning that she has "regular" menstrual periods. The number 481 is a hypothetical *upper limit* that assumes no pregnancies, because ovulation and menstruation cease during a pregnancy. Realistically, the odds are that only 24 or so of the mature eggs will ever be fertilized by a male sperm cell; and, of course, if a pregnancy *does* ensue, we enter the *human reproductive timescale range* that includes the average period between fertilization and birth. This is generally calculated to be 266 days, or about 8.75 (rounded up to "about" *nine*) calendar months—the human *gestation period* (from the Latin, *gestatio*, meaning "to bear").

Some other periods that go beyond months include:

- peripheral nerve generation, which takes, on average, four to six weeks

- the manufacture of fully mature sperm cells, which takes about two months, although 1000 such cells *reach* maturity each second

- the life of a red blood cell, on average, 120 days

- the life of most liver cells, which averages about five months.

The human gestation period, broken down into three, three-month *trimesters*, also brings to mind the three-month, *quarterly cycles* associated with *seasonal* changes. Most notable among the cyclical events associated with a change in season are *emotional mood swings*. In particular, there is a rather common clinical syndrome known as *seasonal affective disorder* (appropriately abbreviated to "SAD"), first recognized by Hippocrates a long time ago! SAD is a mild form of depression and "moodiness" that usually arrives in late autumn, peaks in winter, and clears up by early spring. It is characterized by undulating mood swings—from happy to sad and back again in four- to six-week cycles—loss of energy, and diminished sexual drive (all symptoms that are not uncommon even among "mentally healthy" individuals!). In fact, anecdotal evidence (Thommen 1987), not yet "scientifically" verified, nevertheless *suggests* that we all experience *biorhythms* with:

- 23-day *physical cycles* that affect musculoskeletal strength, endurance, coordination, energy, and well-being

- 28-day *emotional cycles* associated with the nervous system, creative processes, acute sensitivity, awareness, perception…and moods

- 33-day, cerebral *intellectual cycles* within which alertness, analytical-functioning, logical analysis ability, memory/recall, and communications skills all undergo periodic peaks and valleys.

3. *Circannual*—yearly (from the Latin *annus*, meaning, "year") cycles, and beyond. We are now into periods of time that involve *growth and development*, and *aging:* from (numbers are approximate):

   - a neonate (birth to ten months-old)…to…

   - a toddler (ten months to two years)

   - early childhood (age two to five)

   - middle childhood (age six to ten)

   - late childhood (age 10 to 13, including puberty)

   - juvenile/adolescent teenage years (age 13 to 19)

   - young adulthood (age 20 to 30)

   - middle age (age 30 to 50)

   - senior citizenry (age 50 to 70)

   - senescence (>70 years of age).

   In an even longer-term sense, we can look not only at *total organism* cycles, but, also, at *total societal* cycles and *evolutionary* periods, all of which are beyond the scope of this book. Thus, continuing with our discussion of the body in time, let's now examine some periodic events that recur *more than once daily.*

ULTRADIAN TIMESCALES INVOLVING ANATOMICAL/ PHYSIOLOGICAL EVENTS THAT RECUR CONTINUOUSLY ON A DAY-TO-DAY BASIS

The most convenient way to examine ultradian events is to break them down into timescale ranges as follows:

1. From micro- to milliseconds, taking us from atomic to molecular scales of perception. These are typical of, for example, *enzyme kinetics* and biochemical catalysis. That is to say:

   - Consider the activity of the red blood cell enzyme *carbonic anhydrase,* which, by combining it with water, converts some 60 percent or more of the carbon dioxide generated through aerobic metabolism into carbonic acid. Every second, a single molecule of this enzyme can "turn over" 600,000 molecules each of carbon dioxide and water into as many molecules of carbonic acid. That equates to a catalysis time of $(1/600,000) = 0.0000017$ seconds per conversion, or on the order of two *microseconds!* Such rapid processing times are critical for eliminating metabolic wastes, preventing them from accumulating quickly to toxic, life-threatening levels.

- Similarly, every second, a single molecule of the synapticenzyme *acetylcholinesterase* can "deactivate" 25,000 molecules of the neurotransmitter acetylcholine. It does so by breaking it down into its components: acetic acid and the Vitamin B-complex constituent, choline. This is accomplished in a catalyzed reaction time of (1/25,000) = 40 microseconds. In addition to making the substrates available for *immediate* recycling, such a fast processing rate is vital to ensure that nerve impulses can follow one another in rapid succession, without the synaptic region experiencing a neurotransmitter "traffic jam" that would seriously impede the transmission of life-sustaining action potential signals. It also prevents muscle fibers from being continuously stimulated to a fatigued state following just one firing of an alpha-motor-neuron (see Schneck 1992).

- Indeed, many enzyme-catalyzed reactions *must* proceed at microsecond speeds in order for them to be effective in sustaining life. Some, however—such as several reactions involved in digestive processes—can proceed more slowly without significant consequence. For instance, each molecule of the proteolytic ("protein-splitting") digestive enzyme *chymotrypsin* takes a full ten *milli*seconds to sever a peptide linkage and thereby snip a protein molecule from a food particle. This gives it a "turnover number" of only 100 substrates per second, which takes us to the next level of timed events.

2. From milliseconds to seconds, taking us from molecular to cellular/tissue scales of perception. These are typical of, for example, *neuromuscular kinetics* and the previously discussed physiologic information processing networks. We are now in a timeframe associated with cellular transport processes, neural action potentials, and synaptic transmission rates, many of which are *endogenous*, meaning that they are independent of external cues, and *autonomic*, meaning that they are "self-governed," i.e., not driven by ambient rhythms. That is to say:

    - consider that, because of the approximately 0.0005 sec (range 0.4–1.0 milliseconds) that it takes for a nerve to "reload" enough to "fire" again once it has completely discharged (recall that this is the *absolute refractory period*), nerves are generally constrained to fire, at most, 1000–2500 times per second. (*Note:* although these *milli*second times are *one thousand times slower* than the *micro*seconds that it takes to deactivate the neurotransmitter once the nerve has fired, milliseconds are still pretty fast compared to our typical daily temporal experiences.) However, recall further that in "real life," maximum transmission rates beyond 700–800 action potential "spikes" per second are rarely encountered, and *most* neurons fire at rates closer to 300 temporally sequenced impulses per second. Furthermore, when one takes into account attenuation and consolidation through nerve networks—and sorting and filtering by the reticular formation—it is more likely that responses derived from any given input modality result from "higher centers" having actually attended to and processed only 50, to as few as five *integrated* pieces of information per second, per modality, with corresponding timescales on the order of 20–200 msec. These numbers are consistent with the facts that (see Schneck 1992):

- ° fast-twitch skeletal muscle fibers achieve maximum contracted lengths in 15–50 msec (time to peak) following a single stimulation
- ° slow-twitch muscle fibers require 60–120 msec to reach peak contraction
- ° it takes about 100 msec to establish a good image on the retina
- ° 50–100 msec are required for the hearing apparatus to "lock onto" and identify an incident sound frequency
- ° a typical blink is completed in about 200 msec
- ° at rest, the human heart actively completes a single "beat" in about 250 msec, passively "resting" for some 500 msec between beats
- ° it takes about 5 sec to inhale (2 sec) and exhale (3 sec) once, at rest
- ° arterioles contract and relax in 2–8 sec cycles.

These larger numbers take us to the next timescale level.

3. From seconds to minutes, typical of, for example, tissue/organ *compartmental kinetics* (i.e., fluid transfer from extracellular fluid compartments into intracellular ones, and vice versa), and the systemic *transport* of mass, energy, and momentum. Many aspects of physiologic transport mechanisms are addressed in Schneck (1990). As further examples of this range of timescales, consider that *vital signs* (see Chapter 5 and Table 8.3 in Chapter 8), which include:

- body core temperature
- alkalinity and acidity (measured by pH)
- blood pressure
- respiration rate (8–18 breaths per minute at rest).
- heart rate (60–100 beats per minute at rest).

As mentioned earlier, all recur with periods that fall within this range, the last two having activity levels lying between 0.6– and 7.5-sec cycle times. Moreover, recall from Chapter 2, that the complete journey of blood—out the left ventricle, through the *systemic circulation*, into the right atrium, and then out the right ventricle, through the *pulmonary circulation*, back into the left atrium, i.e., the *circulation time*—takes from as little as 18–24 sec to as much as a minute under "normal" circumstances. Among the many things that blood carries are hormones, which, too, have effects on target organs that last from just a few seconds to several minutes. Thus, one notes that *hormonal function* is orders of magnitude slower than neurotransmitter function (see also, related discussion in Chapter 7 of proportional and differential control).

Going one step further, *macroscopic* transport involving the entire human body also falls within this time range, for example, *gait cycles* average 80–120 steps per minute (on the order of resting heart rate). So, too, do various types of conduction convection radiation transport mechanisms for mass, energy, and momentum (Schneck 1990). Included are those thermoregulatory mechanisms by which body temperature is maintained, and the autonomous smooth-muscle function that generates peristaltic undulations of the gastrointestinal system. Speaking of the gastrointestinal system takes us to the next timescale level.

4. From minutes to hours, typical of, for example, the activity of organs/systems that include *metabolic kinetics*, involving the *utilization* of mass, energy, and momentum. For example:

    - *sleep cycles* recur in regular 90-min patterns

    - the *amniotic fluid* that surrounds an embryo is completely replaced every three hours.

And what could be a more appropriate example of this timescale than *digestion*? Consider that;

    - it takes some 45 minutes to produce digestive enzymes in the pancreas and deliver them to the small intestine

    - food can spend three to five hours (average four-and-a-half) churning around in the stomach

    - it can spend two to four hours (average two-and-a-half) traveling through the small intestine

    - it takes up to eight hours negotiating the large intestine:

        ○ two hours in the ascending colon

        ○ three hours in the transverse colon

        ○ three hours in the descending colon

all the while being *processed*. Then:

- the sigmoid colon can hold the resulting stool for up to between nine and nine-and-a-half hours until it is eventually eliminated via voluntary defecation through the anus.

Thus, a complete trip through the alimentary canal, from lips to anus, can take from as little as 12 to as much as 24 hours, which brings us back around to where we started...*circadian* cycles.

A "tsunami" of information to deal with?

All this talk about the body in time, incident rates of sensory stimulation, stimulus coding, cerebral information-processing rates, sensory integration, Gestalt Laws of Perception, and so on reminds me of an article that I came across in the January, 1999 issue of *Inc. Magazine*. That article is particularly germane to the material discussed in this and the previous chapter, because in it, the author David Shenk bemoaned the, "tsunami of information that is pounding away at us, making all of us more anxious, less effective, and sometimes even sick."

His concern was that the incessant information explosion that is invariably coupled to the human drive to "know," and the enormous proliferation of new knowledge both pose significant challenges to our educational system. Shenk's major concern, among several, was how to incorporate effectively such a rapid output of new material into our classrooms and curriculums. Furthermore, how do we deal with a situation that will undoubtedly threaten our physiologic well-being; and how do we manage to cope when the information is streaming in faster than we can handle it? First of all, in the nearly 17 years that have elapsed since that article appeared, let me point out that none of Mr. Shenk's dire predictions have materialized to nearly the serious degree that he foresaw.

But in a more fundamental sense, he completely missed the point by failing to carry the subject through to its logical conclusion, hence his misgivings about the eventual outcome. You see, by now it should be clear that ours is a history of *cyclical events*, both large scale and small. These events—in the sense of *societal* (analogous to *sensory*) *integration*—cause us to spiral *up* (we call it "progress") to a new plateau, or down (we call it a "mid-course correction") to a more stable state, or neither (a conservative surrendering to the default configuration—the status quo—as discussed in Chapter 10).

Viewed in terms of the issue at hand, which is to say, the information explosion to which we are constantly subjected, one must recognize that our heritage is, in fact, replete with cyclic, *disequilibrating*, unstable periods of information *explosions* that are invariably followed by *equilibrating*, stabilizing periods of information *implosions*. These two states (the stock market being a good example) undulate back and forth like the tides of the sea. If we don't realize and appreciate this fundamental nature of periodicity, we, as did Mr. Shenk, have totally missed the point!

That is to say, history has shown that every time we begin to suffer the consequences of information overload (explosion, the state Mr. Shenk was concerned with), there invariably follows a natural progression of events that leads us to seek *common denominators*—order, relationships—among the plethora of information (structure). Extraction of such common denominators further allows us to distinguish the signal from the noise in the information. Eventually, from such *inductive reasoning*, new fundamental principles emerge (synthesis!). In turn, these fresh new ideas bring insights by which the enormous volume of fragmented information can be effectively condensed into much smaller groups (implosion, the direction in which we inevitably head). These smaller groups have been recognized—by the likes of Newton, Maxwell, Einstein, and others—to be *special cases* that derive by *deductive reasoning* from more *general laws and principles*, and the entire cyclic process starts all over again. This cycling through the basic elements of knowledge is not unlike how the brain processes data to derive meaningful information from them, in order to affect an appropriate response. It also illustrates *Physiological optimization principle number 12*:

> *Information overload is a self-limiting, cyclic process, whereby explosions are invariably followed by implosions, which lead to explosions, and so on... In a never-ending "do loop!"*

Recognizing the periodicity of the human experience is the essence of understanding everything, and we have been emphasizing this throughout this book, to wit:

- we sleep daily
- we eat meals several times a day
- we have a pulse
- we use the bathroom on a regular basis
- we drink a glass of water, and ingest food by alternating swallowing with imbibing/chewing
- we blink our eyes
- we clap our hands
- we walk with a periodic gait pattern
- we rhythmically inhale and exhale
- energy vibrates between potential and kinetic states
- pendulums swing
- the Earth rotates about its axis
- the planets revolve around the sun

- birds flap their wings
- dogs wag their tails
- tides come in and out

...get the point, Mr. Shenk? Rhythm—it's everywhere! So much so, that one can accept as an axiom the fact that *all forms of reality—all human experiences—are cyclic in their regular manifestations*, such cycles being of large and small scale. Thus, *the biological handling of information is no exception.*

So what is all of this concern about the information explosion? It is but one more cycle in the open-ended quest for knowledge. It is an impending opportunity to formulate still another basic principle in math, physics, or some other of the natural, social, and applied sciences in the human experience. It is a means for moving one step closer toward, for example, world peace and prosperity, a "unified field theory" in physics, or an understanding of physiologic processes as they relate to disease, malfunction, and disability in medicine and the allied health sciences (including music therapy!). No, the information explosion does not bode impending "data smog" (Mr. Shenk's words). It is not a cause for alarm; and it is not to be taken as a sign that "we may be on the verge of an attention deficit disorder epidemic" (Shenk 1999). Nor should a mass of accumulating *structure* be seen as a dilemma that foretells doom, but, rather, as exactly the opposite—an *opportunity*; something to look forward to, because around the next corner may be lurking the next great advancement in human history. That's the way it's always been and that's the way it will always be because:

All God's creations got rhythm!

So, with that as a "given," let's close this chapter with some additional observations.

Some concluding observations

By now, it should be apparent that:

- the human body has an optimized, sophisticated, delicately balanced, coordinated, and synchronized hierarchy of operating timescales, each intended to satisfy specific physiologic needs of the organism

- our perception of time is not only derived from stimulus coding of *external* adequate stimuli but, also, from our awareness of these *internal* biorhythms that are associated with physiologic processes. Moreover:

- while the actual ambient cues, with which these biorhythms were *originally* made to coincide, are no longer absolutely necessary in order to elicit a response, it is important to note that:

- if the cues are *not* there, the timed sequencing of important physiologic processes with which they are correlated, such as sleep/wake patterns, eating habits, and menstrual cycles, are still significantly affected. That is to say, if these regular cues are absent, the body gets thrown off schedule (for further insights into these points see also Trivers 1985).

Furthermore, it is important to realize that time, as a fundamental dimension of perception, is a *qualitative* concept that expresses our awareness of such things as past, present, future, and periodicity. To *quantify* time requires that we develop a system of *units* that can be used to scale this perception according to a mutually agreed-on (*intersubjective*) set of standards. Such quantification—briefly discussed in Chapter 10, in the Section entitled, *Establishing a "standard" unit of time*—forms a branch of the science of *horology*, from the Greek *hora*, meaning "time" (the same root from which the word "hour" is derived), and *logos*, which means "telling." Thus, any device that "tells time" is called an *horologe*.

Finally, as we have been professing throughout, depending on genetic make-up (*nature*) and environmental exposure (*nurture*), what are "normal" biorhythms for one individual might not be for another. All numbers and values quoted in this book are *typical* averages most likely representative of any given *general* population. In fact, biological rhythms, timescales, etc., are not only *level-of-organization-specific*, *complexity-specific*, and *process-specific*, they are also *individual-specific*, and should be appreciated as such when discussing them in general terms: *music therapists…be aware!*

All of that having been said, we note that in formulating *Physiological optimization principle number 12* above, we were actually adding to a growing *set* of *principles* that, collectively, illustrate the fifth of the six basic *processes* by which the general features of our living engine/instrument become manifest, i.e., the *group* of processes that can be lumped together as *optimization schemes*…which takes us to Chapter 12.

CHAPTER 12

Physiologic Optimization Schemes, Among Them Adaptation Mechanisms

To this point, we have formulated a dozen physiological optimization principles that govern the *effectiveness* of human body function. Let's briefly review them:

1. *Reaction coupling* (Chapter 3) joins *exergonic* (energy-releasing) biochemical reactions with *endergonic* (energy-absorbing) ones in order to minimize the liberation of non-usable *heat* energy, while optimizing the kinetics of these reactions.

2. *Cascading reactions* (Chapter 3) also ensures that *heat* production is *minimized*, while *maximizing* opportunities for *control* of biochemical reactions, by requiring them to go from substrates to products via a complex sequence of many intermediate, small steps, rather than one huge leap.

3. *Minimum energy* (Chapter 3) forces *reaction coupling* and *cascading reactions* to proceed along paths of *least resistance*, thus ensuring that the metabolic needs of the organism are satisfied both *effectively*, and at *least energetic cost*.

4. *Time-delayed consciousness* (Chapter 5) ensures timely, appropriate, effective responses (if necessary) to sensory stimulation, by having the central nervous system process such stimulation, and respond to it *instinctively*—fractions of a second ahead of their reaching conscious levels of perception.

5. *Reductionism* (Chapter 6) optimizes the storage, retrieval, and utilization of limited resources by first breaking:

   • *mass* (such as nutrients) down into its basic *ingredients (structure)* in a process called *catabolism*

   • *energy* (such as sound) down into its basic *spectral components (structure)* by *frequency-specific excitation*

   • scaling adequate stimuli into *digitized* action potentials

...storing all of these individually...and reassembling/reconstituting them (in a process called *anabolism*) as necessary to meet the body's needs...thus economizing on both, the use of *space and energy*.

6.   ***Emotion trumps reason*** (Chapter 6) complements number 4 above by ensuring that information tracks through the central nervous system in *series* (i.e., sequentially, in an "and" format) rather than in *parallel* (i.e., simultaneously, in an "either/or" format). Information thus travels *first* through emotional, instinctive regions and *second* ("next, then") through cognitive regions associated with *reason*.

7.   ***Natural selection through breeding*** (Chapter 6) allows for the attributes/ characteristics of offspring to be updated, mutated, modulated, or otherwise varied in an *evolutionary* sense, through *sexual*, rather than *asexual* reproduction.

8.   ***Use it, or lose it*** (Chapter 10), the anatomical equivalent of "down-sizing" complements number 7 above in a *generational* (rather than *evolutionary*) sense, by allowing unused organs and tissues in the *individual* (rather than his/her *offspring*) to deteriorate, atrophy, and eventually cease to exist, thus optimizing physiologic function by eliminating "clutter."

9.   ***Practice makes perfect*** (Chapter 10) optimizes the learning process by recognizing that pathways to knowledge work best, and achieve the most effective results, through constant and persistent repetition and reinforcement.

10. ***Phase Regulation*** (Chapter 10) as a complement to numbers 1, 2, and 3 above, optimizes physiological performance by exploiting *co-acting mechanisms* to coordinate and synchronize the activity of one set of anatomical structures with that of another.

11. ***Biasing*** (Chapter 10) optimizes *control* of physiologic function by *skewing* the *sensitivity* of anatomical ceptors to being stimulated. Their responsiveness to deviations from the status quo can thus be directed either *toward* or *away from* designated operating set-points.

12. ***Self-limiting processes*** (Chapter 11) complements number 11 above by imposing natural, *intrinsic*, self-regulating constraints that prevent deviations/ fluctuations from the status quo from reaching unbounded extremes, thus optimizing system *stability* and avoiding "run-away," catastrophic failure.

In this Chapter, we will now add to our growing set of *optimization principles* by considering one that might be called:

13. ***Train it...to gain it*** via *adaptive mechanisms*. As we shall see, this principle has particular relevance for the music therapist.

The general principle of physiologic adaptation

The word *adapt* derives from the Latin prefix *ad-*, meaning "to," and *aptāre* meaning "join," as in *fit together*. Thus, as opposed to *biasing*, which goes to the issue of adjusting a system's *sensitivity* without messing with its *operating set-points, physiologic adaptation* goes directly to the latter. That is to say, it systematically adjusts an organism's *operating set-points*, usually over a period of time, in order to "fit in" with changing circumstances; to *accommodate* whatever conditions prevail at the time. Indeed, faced with varying challenges to its very existence, the body's *survival* depends on its ability to *adjust*, to make the *right* choices out of many possible alternatives, and to *adapt* or cease to exist!

Case in point—bone remodeling

Suppose I weigh 180 pounds. When I stand up, that weight is supported by, and evenly *distributed* among, my load-bearing joints (hips, knees, ankles). Articulating at these joints are bones that have a specific anatomical design—one that includes operating set-points that optimize the skeletal system's ability to accommodate my weight most *effectively*. "Most effectively" means in a way that is metabolically and mechanically conducive to the health of the load-bearing bones/joints involved. Now, among the key operating set-points that ensure such health is the cross-sectional area of the bony substance across which my weight is distributed. This is because: the *larger* this area, the *smaller* the mechanical load-bearing *stress* (force *per unit area*) that the tissue is asked to support...and vice-versa! In other words, distributed over a larger area, my weight poses minimal threat to the health of the tissue being asked to bear it, because each portion of that tissue has less of my weight to support. Thus, for my 180 pounds, my bones have, over time, gradually *adapted* to exactly the right cross-sectional area needed to optimize their weight-bearing function. All well and good...

But, suppose I now choose to become a furniture mover (or gain another 100 pounds!). On a day-to-day basis, no longer are my load-bearing joints asked to carry *just* 180 pounds. Quite to the contrary, they are routinely being asked to support loads far in excess of my previous weight. Unless something changes, my bones can be seriously impaired, even broken! What to do? Answer: *piezoelectrically activated osteoblasts* to the rescue! Recall (Chapter 3) that these are cells that manufacture bone tissue. They do so in response to *piezoelectric* stimulation—literally, electrical signals that are generated in bone tissue when forces are applied to it ("*piézein*" is Greek for "to squeeze, or press," as in "pressure," hence, *piezoelectric*, "pressure electric"). Thus, a *feedback* adaptive pathway is enabled whereby:

- *increased* forces that persist over a period of time, such as regularly moving furniture or gaining weight, *raise* the mechanical stress (pressure) levels in my bone tissue

- which leads to increased *piezoelectric excitation of osteoblasts*

- which proceed to manufacture *more* bone tissue, in a process called *osteogenesis*

- which increases the cross-sectional area of the load-bearing bones, i.e., moves it toward a new operating set-point

- which *lowers* the mechanical stress level in my bones

- which makes them metabolically and mechanically "happy."

- As the stress level drops the piezoelectric intensity falls off, the activity of osteoblasts wanes, and the cross-sectional area of the bone tissue equilibrates at its new load-bearing value, i.e., a new operating set-point has been established.

The above is an example of *functional adaptation*, i.e., adjusting systemic operating set-points in response to functional requirements. In this case, it goes by the name of *bone remodeling*. But wait! Recall (Chapters 3 and 7) that there are also *osteoclasts* that *resorb* (dissolve) bone tissue. What is *their* role in all of this?

Well, *osteoclasts* are after the calcium deposits in bone, and they are under the influence of the parathyroid glands (see Chapters 4, 5, and 7). Thus, what we have here are *osteoblasts* and *osteoclasts* both constantly competing with one another to see who will prevail in controlling *osteogenesis*. In fact, the "winner" depends on which set of circumstances requires the more immediate type of adaptation, i.e., which one is most critical and/or life-threatening:

- lowered blood calcium levels, which allow the parathyroids to prevail, hence, *osteoclasts* and *bone resorption*...or...

- increased load-bearing demands, which allow piezoelectricity to prevail, hence, *osteoblasts* and *osteogenesis.*

There is always a very delicate balance between the two. Moreover, both processes are *reversible*, i.e., *functional adaptation works both ways*, as exemplified by the *use it, or lose it* optimization principle. Finally, while we are on the subject of bones, it seems appropriate to mention another of the many examples of functional adaptation, and that is control by the kidney of *erythropoiesis*.

Another case in point—renal control of erythropoiesis

The activity of osteoblasts, and the bone remodeling that results from this, is an example of adaptation triggered by persistent *mechanoreception*, in this case, *piezoelectric excitation*. By contrast, the activity of osteoclasts, and the bone resorption that results therefrom, is an example of adaptation triggered by persistent *chemoreception*, in this case, *hypocalcemia*. Control of *erythropoiesis* by the kidney illustrates another adaptive mechanism triggered by chemoreception—this time, a lack of oxygen, i.e., *hypo-(or an-)oxia*. To understand how this works, consider the following scenario.

Suppose I am a long-time resident of New York City, having grown up at sea level. Suppose further that, to satisfy its metabolic needs, my body requires 20 milliliters of oxygen per deciliter of blood. This amount of the element is derived from the sea-level air that I breathe, interacting with the capillaries of the pulmonary circulation at the alveolar level of the respiratory system (see Table 2.2 of Chapter 2). Since oxygen does not readily dissolve in blood, it is actively transported in the fluid by the carrier molecule, *hemoglobin*, contained in *erythrocytes* (red blood corpuscles). The quantity and partial pressure of oxygen, O_2, being what it is in moist alveolar air at this altitude, my body's need for O_2 is being satisfactorily met by the following operating set-points (see Chapters 1, 2 and 5, and Schneck 1990):

1. Total blood volume (TBV) = 5.2 liters

2. Hematocrit = 45 percent (percentage of TBV that is red blood corpuscles (RBC))

3. Mean corpuscular (cell) volume (MCV) = 90 cubic microns

4. Mean corpuscular hemoglobin (MCH) = 30 x 10-12 grams per cell

5. Cardiac stroke volume (SV) = (End diastolic volume (EDV)), minus (End systolic volume (ESV)) = 70 milliliters per beat

6. Heart (pulse) rate (HR) = 75 beats per minute

7. Cardiac output = SV x HR = 5.2 liters per minute

8. Respiration rate (RR) = 13 breaths per minute

9. Total number of alveoli (pulmonary air sacs) = about 300 million

10. Total number of pulmonary capillaries = about 3 billion.

The above operating set-points, at sea level, will ensure that the 45 percent erythrocytes in my blood will be almost (97.5%) completely saturated with oxygen as they pass through the lungs, and that I will, indeed, get the 20 ml-O_2/dl-blood that I need to survive at sea level! But…what happens if I decide to travel to Denver, Colorado, to Mile High Stadium, 5280 feet *above* sea level, to catch a New York Giants vs. Denver Broncos football game? The air at this altitude is rarified—not much oxygen available. My sea-level operating set-points are not now sufficient to satisfy my body's metabolic needs. What to do? *Adapt!*

REFLEXIVE, SHORT-TERM, TEMPORARY ADAPTATION

Fortunately, *for the short term*, I don't need to adapt by changing *all* of the above operating set-points. In anticipation of my *returning* to New York City (sea level) soon after the game is over, my body need merely shift into *reflexive adaptation* mode. This involves *temporarily* changing *only* operating set-points 5–8 above. Thus, the endocrine (H-P-A axis) and autonomic (sympathetic) nervous systems go to work to:

1. *Increase end-diastolic volume* by as much as 50 percent—by:

    a) *enhancing* atrial systole

    b) allowing the heart to *fill* longer.

    The latter is accomplished by slowing down the transmission of electrical impulses through the atrio-ventricular (AV) node and musculature of the ventricles, thus *delaying* the onset of ventricular systole.

2. *Decrease end-systolic volume* by a comparable amount (the so-called *cardiac reserve volume*), by allowing the heart to empty faster and more completely, i.e., *enhancing* ventricular systole, an *inotropic effect.* The *ejection phase* of the cardiac cycle is thus a much shorter fraction of the total cycle, which further contributes to a longer filling phase.

3. *Increase the heart rate* to nearly triple its sea-level value—a *chronotropic effect* acting on the cardiac pacemaker…the *sino-atrial node.* Events 1 and 2 above increase stroke volume. Together with the chronotropic effect, all three can lead to a more than *sevenfold* increase in cardiac output, to some 37 liters/minute!

Moreover, at this altitude:

4. *Hyperventilation* sets in. Recall from Table 5.5 that one's normal respiration rate is 8–18 breaths per minute, consuming 5–6 liters of air in the process. Recall further from Chapter 2 and Table 2.2 that one has significant total lung capacity, with, also, *pulmonary reserve volumes* that can be accessed when necessary by breathing more deeply and panting rapidly.

So, faster, deeper breathing, combined with increased blood pressure, and cardiovascular performance all allow me to *reflexively adapt* to the oxygen-poor atmosphere at Mile High Stadium, and live to talk about it!

But, suppose I *don't* return to New York City after the game. What if, while I am in Denver, I meet somebody who makes me a job offer I simply cannot refuse? The job, however, is in Denver, so I must relocate. What now? My body cannot continue to survive on a long-term basis with blood pressures of 190/110, cardiac outputs of 37 liters per minute, heart rates of 240 beats/min, and respiration rates three to four times what they were at sea level; I cannot go on hyperventilating continuously! That simply won't do, *reflexive adaptation* is intended to be a "temporary fix" (see related discussion of stress hormones in Chapter 7 and bad stress in Chapter 8). It thus fails miserably as an adequate means for *acclimating* one's-self to high altitudes. The good news is that there is an alternative, a long-term "plan B" in the form of *functional adaptation,* that kicks in to address items 1–4 and 9–10 of the earlier list of operating set-points.

FUNCTIONAL, LONG-TERM ADAPTATION

To address items 1–4 of this list requires that we take a closer look at renal control of erythropoiesis. Recall that red blood cells are produced in bone marrow. They live about 120 days, with a turnover rate of about one percent daily—2–10 million cells per second being purged from blood by the spleen and excreted in the stool (see Chapters 1 and 2). Recall further (Chapter 7) that under conditions of hypo-anoxia, the *rate* of production of erythrocytes is controlled by an *activated* plasma protein called *erythropoietin*. This circulating alpha-globulin hormone is activated by an *erythropoietic factor* that is secreted from the kidney when blood oxygen concentration is too low. *Activated erythropoietin's* target tissue is bone marrow, specifically receptor sites on the membranes of *hemocytoblast stem cells* that are destined to mature into erythrocytes.

So, I am now a permanent resident of Denver, Colorado, living at an altitude of over 5000 feet above sea level. The *chemoreceptors* in my kidneys are sensing *prolonged hypoxia* (low oxygen levels) and my cardiovascular/respiratory systems are screaming for help! Responding to these pleas, and the sustained lack of oxygen, the kidneys:

- start pouring *erythropoietic factor* into the blood, which

- *activates* circulating levels of *plasma erythropoietin,* which

- finds its way into the *receptor sites* on the membranes of the bone marrow's *erythroblast germ cells,* causing them to actively

- *bias* (skew) the *general* process of *hematopoiesis,* the manufacture of *all* blood cells, toward the *specific* process of *erythropoiesis, the* manufacture of *red* blood cells, which

- causes bone marrow to increase its production of *erythrocytes* (at the expense of *leukocytes* and *thrombocytes*), which

- over a period of several weeks, drives the *hematocrit operating set-point* (item 2 on our attributes list) up to a new, higher value, as high as 60 percent. This will provide *more red blood cells* to carry oxygen to all of the cells and tissues of the organism.

But that's not all, the hypothalamus, acting through the pituitary gland (*anti-diuretic hormone* (ADH)) and, ultimately, the kidney (*vasopressin hormone*), drives the operating set-point for *total blood volume* (item 1 on our attributes list) up about 20 percent, as well, to some 6.25 liters. Even more erythrocytes are now available to soak up oxygen from the lungs. Furthermore, although MCV (item 3) remains relatively constant at about 90 cubic microns, the *hemoglobin content* of each red blood cell (item 4) does increase slightly…to about $30.5 \times 10_{-12}$ grams, making more carrier molecules available to transport oxygen. But we are *still* not done!

In order to further avail ourselves of what little oxygen there is in the atmosphere at this high altitude, we now turn our attention to items 9 and 10 of our operating set-points list. Specifically, we endeavor to provide increased blood flow through the pulmonary circulation—through more blood vessels—to a more abundant supply of alveoli. Thus, after a period of months, we find that the increase in total blood *volume* is accommodated by a concomitant increase in the *total number of capillaries* through which that additional volume is *distributed* in the lung tissue. What *was* about 3 billion capillaries at sea level might increase to 3.5–4.0 billion or more at altitude! This, again, is the result of *piezoelectric, mechanoreceptor stimulation* of the process of *neovascularization*, generating new capillary beds in response to endocrine and autonomic nervous system induced increases in blood *pressure*. Finally, we find, over time, that several million more alveoli join those 300 million that existed at sea level.

Cumulatively, then, higher hematocrit values, increased blood volume, more mean corpuscular hematocrit, a larger pulmonary capillary bed, and a greater number of lung alveoli all allow inotropic, chronotropic and hyperventilation effects gradually to subside, while still providing the cells of the body with the oxygen they need to survive at this high altitude. Blood pressure drops back down to "normal" (which also halts neovasculatization); pulse rate slows down (the sino-atrial node is no longer being over-worked); the heart stops pumping so violently, and respiration rate becomes "tolerable." Except for TBV, hematocrit, MCH, and the number of pulmonary capillaries and alveoli, all of which maintain their *adaptive* values, all other operating set-points seem to revert back to their sea-level values, including circulating blood plasma levels of erythropoietin!

Yup! Over a prolonged period of time *circulating plasma levels of erythropoietin also drop back down to their sea-level values, even though the other variables remain elevated!* That's a type of "Pavlov's dog" situation wherein the *original* stimulus, i.e. *higher* concentration of plasma *erythropoietin*, that triggered these desirable responses (e.g., raising hematocrit levels to 60%) is no longer required for the response (60% hemacocrit) to prevail. *The reflex has become conditioned, or, acquired!*

In order to understand what's going on here, we need to carry functional adaptation to its logical conclusion.

MEMBRANE RECEPTOR SITES AND PERMANENT ADAPTATION

If one examines the number of *erythropoietin receptor sites* per unit area of cell membrane on the *erythroblasts* of residents *native* to Denver, Colorado, one is likely to find a much greater number of such erythropoietin "loading docks" in the bone marrow tissue of *these* individuals, than would normally be found in individuals residing at sea level. That being the case, the tissue of Denver natives is *much more responsive to erythropoietin* than is the tissue of sea-level residents, and so it takes less of this hormone to produce a correspondingly greater effect. That's precisely what happens to the tissue of sea-level residents when they relocate to higher altitudes. The adaptation process eventually produces bone marrow stem cells with a greater number of membrane receptive sites for specific types of hormones, such as erythropoietin. Thus, after functional adaptation is complete, the *sea-level* values of these hormones will now produce the *acclimatized* effect, because the hormone has more ways to gain access to its target cells. Adaptive control of the number of receptor sites on a cell membrane is yet another way of *biasing* the *sensitivity* of target cells toward the desired hormonal effect, illustrating again, *Physiological optimization principle number 11*. Stated more formally, it is also an example of an *Anatomical design principle number 8: architectural design that ensures adaptive criterua that facilitate selective stimulation:*

> *If a persistent stimulus is applied to protein-specific, target-tissue receptors, the anatomy of that tissue's cell membranes functionally adapts, eventually coding for the growth of more available receptor sites for that stimulus. The target tissue thus becomes more sensitive to such stimulation, so that less of it is required to elicit a correspondingly greater stimulus-specific response/effect.*

Anatomical design principle number 8 also provides a basis for the concept of *conditioned reflexes*, i.e., those not inborn or inherited, but, rather, acquired as a result of training (*Physiological optimization principle number 13*). The cerebral cortex plays an important role in regulating the neural mechanisms involved in the establishment of conditioned reflexes, which often requires (*music therapists take note*):

- redirecting CNS information-processing pathways
- reconfiguring *existing* neural networks
- the *neogenesis* of new ones (Schneck and Berger 2006).

The above are elements of the *entrainment* phase of the *functional adaptation paradigm* which also includes the earlier-defined mechanisms of *biasing, facilitation* and *memory of sensation* (see Chapter 10). The latter case involves the activity of a family of mitogen-activated enzymes called *protein-kinase Cs* (Sherrin, Blank and Todorovic 2011; Sweatt 2004). These are important molecular "switches" responsible for, among other things, gene expression (see Chapters 1 and 2), such as that which codes for the manufacture of stimulus-specific, cell-membrane, protein receptor sites, and/or specific neurotransmitters. The switches can be "turned on" by synaptic transmission of certain action potentials (hence, *facilitation*), or by persistent exposure to certain adequate stimuli (hence, *receptor-site neogenesis*). When so-activated, they signal the expression of RNA "memory molecules" that facilitate subsequent transmission through the synaptic junction (thus, *memory of sensation*), a process called *synaptic plasticity* (Sherrin *et al.* 2011). The activated molecules can also signal the expression of proteins that become membrane receptor sites (hence, *permanent adaptation*). But, *caution…*

FUNCTIONAL ADAPTATION IS SELF-LIMITING

Here, too, we still have *Physiological optimization principle number 12* to contend with. That is to say, most physiologic processes, including functional adaptation, are *self-limiting*, to wit:

- There is an upper limit to how many receptor sites any given cell membrane can accommodate; there is only so much room for them on the membrane surface!

- There is also an upper limit to how much erythropoietin the body can manufacture; it does not have an infinite supply of ingredients to work with, nor does the cell have the space in which to store them. Thus, enzyme-catalyzed synthesis of the hormone can only proceed at a limited speed.

When either (or both) of these constraints reaches the saturation point, no amount of additional stimulation, *regardless of how persistent or intense*, can elicit a further response. Indeed, as saturation levels are approached it takes progressively stronger and stronger stimuli to generate a functional adaptation response. Moreover:

- At one extreme, if persistent stimuli are quite deliberate, occur infrequently, slowly, and are spaced relatively far apart, the body treats each one of them as if it is an isolated, acute, temporary event and so might not feel the need to change any of its operating set-points to adapt to them.

- At the other extreme, continuous, persistent stimulation delivered at exceedingly high rates might encounter refractory effects and "dropouts" that can seriously interfere with and impede the adaptation process. (See related discussion of the "flicker speed" for vision in Chapter 5.)

Taking all of the above into consideration, one might say that:

> *Functional adaptation acts both: to reduce the organism's* **need to respond** *to a stimulus—by adjusting its operating set-points—and to reduce the organism's* **ability to respond** *to that stimulus, as a result of self-limiting constraints and saturation effects.*

A few more examples of biasing and adaptive responses

To the above two salient examples of functional adaptation, we can add others that we have already encountered in this book. These actually complement *Pysiological optimization principles numbers 7 (evolution), 8 (arrested development), 11 (biasing), and 12 (self-regulation)*, i.e.:

- In Chapters 3 and 4, we noted that the brain can *bias* striated skeletal muscle spindles (Schneck 1992). This allows them (and hence, the muscle) to become more *responsive to being stretched*. It is an evolutionary *adaptive mechanism* by which the body mobilizes its musculoskeletal system to "fight or flee."

- In Chapters 4 and 5, we introduced the concept of *sensory adaptation* (Schneck 1990). Here, the "firing" thresholds of sensory nerves can be *biased*, so that they become less easily stimulated. This, again, is an evolutionary *adaptive mechanism* by which the body is endowed with the ability to "ignore" ("tune out") persistent, yet benign, adequate stimuli.

- In Chapter 5, we noted further that:
  - the eyes can *adapt* to indulge variations in light intensity
  - the ears can *adapt* to tolerate variations in sound intensity
  - tonic and phasic tactile receptors can *adapt* to accommodate variations in the rate at which they are stimulated
  - nasal chemoreceptors can *adapt* to attenuate lasting odors
  - oral chemoreceptors can *adapt* to nullify persistent testants.
- In Chapter 10 we talked about the *relativity of time*, and how cerebral information-processing rates could be *biased* to affect temporal responses to adequate stimuli. This is an evolutionary *adaptive* mechanism that leads to *Physiological optimization principle number 4: time-delayed consciousness.*

Then, of course, there is also:

- *Behavioral adaptation.* This refers to the various mechanisms by which patterns of action or living are changed in order to better suit the environment in which one finds oneself. Any conduct that helps ensure survival of the self and species can be considered a behavioral adaptation. Thus, examples of this are numerous, including:
  - huge population migrations due to climate or terrain
  - nocturnal (night)/diurnal (day) activities of daily living
  - carnivorous/herbivorous/omnivorous eating habits
  - patterns of male/female courtship, and so on.

All of the various mechanisms and examples of physiological adaptation have particular relevance for the music therapist, because they can all be exploited when using music as an effective clinical intervention for the management of diagnosed populations (Schneck and Berger 2006). Indeed, *music can drive the body to adapt* via the following paradigm.

The physiological adaptation paradigm

Physiological adaptation begins with repetitive, persistent stimulation (such as through the elements of music) of the body's intero-extero-ceptive senses (see Chapter 5, and *Physiological optimization principles numbers 9, 11* and *13*). It ends when, following prolonged exposure to such stimulation, the body's operating set-points are eventually readjusted. They are *retuned,* so to speak, to *harmonize* functionally with the adequate stimuli that instigated the adaptation process in the first place. In essence, the persistent stimuli *drive* the engine ("play the instrument," if you will), allowing it to transition from its then current state of affairs, to a more optimal one.

In progressing from start to finish, the adaptive process navigates through several alternative pathways that can be grouped under the general heading of *entrainment*. It includes one or more of the following:

1. *Stimulated gene expression of first messengers:* We just addressed this when we spoke about the genetic expression of *molecular switches*, and it plays a critical role in both *facilitation* and *memory of sensation*. Nucleic acids that function as *control genes* activate the synthesis of so-called *first messengers*, which include:

    - neurotransmitters

    - hormones

    - enzymes

    - neurochemical opioids

    - immunoglobulins.

    Relating gene expression to music, recall from Table 5.2 in Chapter 5, that when the infrared vibrational frequencies with which the four DNA bases (adenine, cytosine, guanine, and thymine) resonate are transcribed into the audible spectrum, an identifiable acoustic pattern emerges (Alexjander and Deamer 1999). This suggests that our biology may be *harmonically ordered*, exhibiting a symbiotic courtship between the genome and acoustic stimulation. Such stimulation might systematically activate control genes on the DNA molecule, as these *resonate* with corresponding musical-pitch frequencies.

    Indeed, it is likely that further research will reveal that one's body recognizes in *entrained* musical sequences, an *acoustic* pattern that is *unique* to that individual. This is not as inconceivable as it might appear at first, given that the immune system recognizes a unique *biochemical* pattern encoded into the histocompatibility complex (see Chapters 1 and discussion of chirality in Chapter 7), and *enneagrams* can uniquely define personality types on the basis of *instinctual* drives and *behavioral* patterns. Thus, why can't our body react to *acoustic* patterns to endow us with a unique "musical DNA print" to go along with its unique fingerprints and HLA codes? In fact, it may follow that a specific and unique *DNA base pair sequence* is also encoded one to one into a corresponding *individual-specific note or harmonic sequence*, unique to that individual. One may have one's very own, personal melody or chord pattern, which might also help to explain individual musical preferences and why different folks react differently to the same musical style, key signatures, timbres, etc. (Schneck and Berger 2006). *That thought should especially interest the music therapist!*

2. *Activation of second messenger systems:* Second messengers are those organelles, molecules (mostly proteins), and other cellular elements in target organs and tissues that respond to stimulation by first messengers. For example, hormones

(first messengers) travelling down the hypothalamic hypophyseal tract to the pituitary gland cause it to release *endorphins* (*endogenous morphines*). These are second messengers that are very effective pain relievers—the body writes its own prescriptions for pain! Endorphins also induce euphoric feelings of pleasure, thus helping to mitigate many of the adverse consequences of stress. The latter is often called the "thrill effect," commonly experienced by the feeling of "chills running up and down the spine" when one listens to one's favorite music. Since pain and pleasure are among the most compelling forces that drive human behavior, one's ability to control these clinically—*such as through music*—offers a very effective means for non-pharmaceutical medical management of a patient.

Acting mainly through the H-P-A axis (see Chapter 7), the autonomic nervous, and endocrine systems, second messengers can influence the activity of virtually every organ and tissue in the body, their effects being generically classified as:

- *excitatory*, i.e., *instigating/enhancing* function
- *inhibitory*, i.e., *blocking/suppressing* function
- *biasing*, i.e., skewing the response *sensitivity* of targets
- *sedative*, i.e., having a *calming/quieting* effect
- *arousing*, i.e. *activating*, stirring to an active state
- *aesthetic*, i.e., providing an *entertaining emotional diversion*
- *therapeutic*, i.e., *remedial*, helping to heal, ministering
- *ameliorating*, i.e., making at least *tolerable*, if not "better"
- *inciting*, i.e., stimulating *adaptive* processes, in a positive sense
- *abrasive*, i.e., actually *producing* stress, in a negative sense!

3. *Rhythm entrainment:* That the human body can actively entrain, and hence be driven by ambient rhythmic patterns—to the point of functioning in accordance with them—is amply illustrated by the infradian, circadian, and ultradian examples discussed in Chapter 11: "The Body in Time." Think, also, about what happens when you listen to a lively polka, or a rousing march, or your favorite jazz ensemble. Don't you instinctively start tapping your foot to the "beat" of the music? Do you find yourself unconsciously clapping your hands, or bobbing your head along with the rhythmical patterns of the music? Don't you sway in synchrony with the "flow" of a lovely ballad, or feel the urge to dance when listening to upbeat Latin rhythms or Strauss waltzes?

These, and more, are further examples of *physiological rhythm entrainment.* When your body can't seem to help moving to the "beat," that's rhythm entrainment! Is it any wonder, then, that *rhythm* should be the most basic element of human-invented music? As we have seen, and what can now be "officially" offered as *Anatomical design principle number 9: the human body is all about rhythm!*

And, in reverse, should it therefore be surprising to learn that musical *rhythms* have the ability to drive the body to change its operating set-points in response to them? Indeed, when people listen to music, various aspects of their *body rhythms* display a dynamic embodiment of, i.e., *entrain*, the temporal structure inherent in the incident musical rhythms (Schneck and Berger 2006). Auditory cues can arouse and raise the excitability of (i.e., *bias*) spinal motor neurons. This excitability is mediated at the reticulo-spinal level by *auditory to motor efferent circuitry*, which has particular relevance and applicability to clinical situations where motor planning is an issue (Schneck and Berger 2006 and Berger 2015).

Furthermore, the heart rate of patients experiencing auditory cues delivered at "preferred" musical tempi—*rhythmical pace*—tends to "lock onto" (*entrain*) and share a common harmonic relationship with that rhythmical pace. Heart rates tend to equilibrate in the 70–100 beats/minute range when individuals are listening to "familiar" tunes. It jumps to an erratic 105–200 beats/minute when they are exposed merely to simple, rapidly repeating, unfamiliar, pure tones (such as a 440 Hz, 60-dB "concert A") delivered machine-gun style to their auditory architecture.

Finally, when "mood adjustment" is an appropriate clinical intervention, auditory cues can capture one's attention in ways that drive the brain into a "pleasing resonance" state of consciousness. This happens as its neural networks are induced to pulsate at the same, mood-altering frequency as the driving, binaural beat frequency of the music. Thus *entrained*, the driving frequencies can elicit an entire range of human emotions, as elaborated on further below.

4. *Redirecting central nervous system information-processing modes:* Many of the entrainment effects discussed thus far are the result of mechanisms that influence how sensory inputs and motor outputs are handled by the reticular activating system and brain. For example, as discussed in Chapters 6 and 10, a person reacts to any stimulus, such as musical rhythms, according to:

- how that stimulus *tracks* through the central nervous system

- his or her unique *information-processing rate,* i.e., inner, *psycho-biological clock*

- how that clock can be affected (*biased*) by a variety of ambiensomatic influences (in particular, *music*)

- how it is *integrated* and *evaluated.*

Thus, any type of entrainment that affects one or more of the above modes for handling sensory data will, in turn, affect the entire functional adaptation process. In this respect, of particular interest are those mechanisms that can cause the handling of such data to "switch tracks" en route through the CNS, i.e., *redirect* how it flows from sensory input to motor output. Thus, although not necessarily ratifying a lateralized, left-brain/right-brain information-processing paradigm, the following observations do confirm that different types of sensory stimulation can trigger different modes of cerebral information processing. Indeed, electroencephalographic (EEG), and oxygen-consumption studies reveal that the brain processes *musical* inputs differently than it does, for example, *verbal* (speech, language) inputs. Therefore, music can elicit an entire spectrum of profound responses, to the extent that, as its elements are *entrained* by the physiologic system, it can cause the brain to:

- *redirect* the path of information transmission (i.e., "switch tracks"):

  ○ *from* having sensory data flowing through the amygdala proceed on to neural networks that drive emotional, "fight-or-flight" responses

  ○ *to* having such data proceed instead to course through neural networks in the hippocampus, from which rational, cognitive responses derive

- *reconfigure existing* neural networks by:

  ○ hyper- or hypopolarizing the resting state of neurons (i.e., *biasing* them)

  ○ stimulating the growth of additional receptor sites on the nerve cells (i.e. *facilitating* which nerves respond to which stimuli)

  ○ disabling and purging such sites on other neurons (essentially taking them out of the network); and so on

- *reprioritize* (optimize) the process of *sensory integration*, driving it toward more desirable outcomes by:

  ○ *activating collateral nerve pathways* that give the process more options

  ○ *recruiting additional nerve networks* to give the process access to greater resources and more alternatives. (*Note:* this might also help to explain *harmonic entrainment*, wherein *consonant* intervals are processed more favorably, and therefore perceived to be more pleasant, than are dissonant ones, with their associated high-frequency "beats," strident tone clusters, and harmonic "disorder." We shall get back to this thought in Chapter 13.)

- experience *temporal distortion* (see Chapter 10), i.e.:

  ○ underestimate the passage of time—it might be "flying" or "dragging" in response to musical *entrainment*

  ○ one might lose track of it completely

- *disable distractions* (treating them as "background noise"), and thus improving its ability to concentrate and stay focused or…*just the opposite*, depending on the music! That is to say:

  ○ lower decibel levels (*dynamic entrainment*) in the range 0–60 dB ("soft" music) tend to be preferred over higher ones, in the range 60–120 dB (hard" rock and techno-music)

  ○ lower frequency registers (*pitch entrainment*), in the range 32–2048 Hz, are generally preferable to higher ones, in the range 2048–8192 Hz

  ○ sound qualities (*timbre entrainment*) that are less "shrill" are preferred over those that "squeal" and "grate on our nerves!"

Various types of music entrained by the brain can also cause it to:

- exhibit cerebral alpha rhythms—characterized by the appearance on an EEG of 8–12 Hz signals at about 50 microvolt-amplitudes—representing the relaxed, tranquil *alpha state of pleasing resonance* described above

- become drowsy, signified by the appearance on the EEG of 4–7 Hz, variable-amplitude "theta-waves"

- drift into a state of deep sleep, with the appearance on the EEG of 1–5 Hz, 20–200 microvolt "delta-waves."

If none of the above entrainment mechanisms succeed in generating desirable adaptive responses to persistent stimulation, the body resorts to:

5. *Neoneurogenesis:* Similar to *neo-vascularization* (the growth of new blood vessels as described earlier in this chapter), *neoneurogenesis* refers to the establishment (*-genesis*) of brand new (*neo-*) neural (*-neuro-*) networks in response to persistent, entrained adequate stimuli that "have nowhere else to go!" Technically, this is referred to as *anatomic plasticity*, the body's ability to be "molded" in order to accommodate changing demands on its operating systems. It is also a concept embedded in *Anatomical design principle number 10: neogenesis*, which asserts that: *Neogenesis endows the human body with the property of anatomical plasticity—the ability to generate new tissue as necessary, in order to meet the organism's need to adapt to persistent, entrained stimulation.*

Note that the above design principle complements *Anatomical design principles number 2: redundancy*, introduced in Chapter 2…and *number 5: synaptic junctions*, introduced in Chapter 4.

In summary, then, the paradigm for *physiological adaptation* proceeds:

- from repetitive, persistent stimuli through…
- various mechanisms of entrainment, including:

- ○ memory of sensation
- ○ facilitation
- ○ stimulated gene expression of first messengers
- ○ activation of second messenger systems
- ○ embodiment of rhythm
- ○ redirecting CNS IT modes
- ○ reconfiguration of existing neural pathways
- ○ recruiting of collateral nerve networks
- ○ reprioritization of sensory integration objectives
- ○ navigating the brain into altered states of consciousness

...to name just a few...to:

- the generation of *conditioned* reflex pathways (programmed learning...as opposed to *instinctive* ones) and/or...
- the generation of *new* neural networks through the attribute of *anatomical plasticity*...to, ultimately...
- the establishment of a new set of operating set-points.

And so, adaptation is the body's way of "coping," which also goes to factors involved in developing one's self-image and attitudes towards life. Considering its clinical relevance, this thought deserves a few additional remarks.

Conditioning: something else to think about

Very early in life, one is programmed with *negativism*. Perhaps second only to hearing words like, "mamma" and "papa," a young infant is bombarded with: "no...do not... don't touch..." and so on. As the child grows, he or she soon learns: "you can't do that... you must not... that's stupid..." etc. Not to mention being continuously exposed to news media that always begin with "good morning," or, "good evening," and then proceed to tell you why it isn't! Indeed, all of these experiences and exposures are persistent *negative* stimuli that may lead to adaptations resulting in self-image, self-belief, and self-esteem operating set-points that program one to *expect* defeat, and therefore, make it a self-fulfilling prophecy, whether one consciously realizes it, or not. In other words, by virtue of the adaptation paradigm, our bodies are susceptible, and vulnerable to being negatively programmed following exposure and constant reinforcement of such pessimistic attitudes and perceptions.

Brainwashing—such as being constantly told that you are a "sinner"—is a perfect example of this negative programming. But in an everyday sense, we are constantly being "brainwashed" to *think* the worst, *expect* the worst, *hope* for the best (almost *against* hope), but *plan* for disaster! Those disasters are almost sure to come because we unwittingly *arrange* for it to happen that way. *Expect* the worst—embedded in programmed, negative emotional operating set-points—and you will inevitably *get* the worst, manifest in behavioral patterns and actions that "make it happen that way!"

But all is not lost. If one subscribes to the idea of programmed learning, then it follows that a corollary to that idea is *deprogramming,* which can change the set-points with *positive* reinforcement as a persistent adequate stimulus. Remember: *physiologic adaptation is a reversible process.* Thus, at any stage in life, one can effectively "erase" the old disk and program in a new one, using the same principles of repetition, entrainment, conditioning, and adaptation. *Biofeedback* offers an effective means for doing just that, as do techniques of *autohypnosis, transcendental meditation,* those that promote *relaxation responses*...and yes, *music therapy!* Indeed, with a fundamental understanding of physiologic function as it relates to the establishment of operating set-points, one can embark on a campaign to ultimately code genetically for a kinder, gentler, more positive generation of compassionate, caring individuals. The only prerequisite is a *desire* and *willingness* to do so, along with a basic comprehension of physiologic information as it is coded and transported via the "body language" of action potentials.

That having been said, it is time to move on. We do so by noting that, while we are on the subject of adaptation and optimization schemes, if we combine *Physiological optimization principle number 3* (the idea of *minimizing the cost of doing business,* i.e., establishing constraints on the *effective* metabolic use of *energy*) with *Anatomical design principle number 3* (the idea of *maximizing the effective use of space,* i.e., establishing constraints on the anatomical architecture of branching networks) there emerges yet another *Anatomical design principle number 11.* Because of its particular relevance to the elements of music—being intimately connected to such things as musical intervals, harmony, and the associated concepts of consonance and dissonance—we must dedicate an entire chapter to this latest design criterion, which brings us to an examination of the body in space and the last of the six basic processes by which the general features of our living engine/instrument become manifest. Read on...

CHAPTER 13

Anatomical Design Criteria, Among Them Self-Similarity

The Body in Space

At the end of Chapter 11, we noted that the fifth of the six basic processes by which the general features of our living engine/instrument become manifest is embedded in a group of *physiological optimization schemes* that were lumped together, summarized, and expanded on in Chapter 12. These deal primarily with the optimization of *function—physiology*. We now note that the sixth of these basic processes is similarly embedded in several *anatomical design principles* that deal essentially with the optimization of *structure—anatomy*. These, too, can be lumped together and considered as a group. In fact, to this point, we have formulated some ten of them, criteria that govern the *architectural design* of human body structure. Let's briefly review them:

1. **Dimensional expansion** (Chapter 2) is a very effective way to "squeeze" a huge geometric shape—like the cerebral cortex—into a very confined space, like the inside of the human skull. This is accomplished by making the shape's boundary very tortuous and irregular, thereby "mapping" it into the next higher dimension...1-D into 2-D; 2-D into 3-D, etc. This design principle actually complements corresponding *Physiological optimization principle number 5: reductionism.*

2. **Redundancy** (Chapter 2) endows a system with multiple, duplicate, complementary and/or supplementary systems that can "take over" if the main system fails. Thus is provided "back-up" that protects and guards against loss of function in the case of a major breakdown (although this criterion is constrained by *Physiological optimization principle number 8: use it, or lose it!*).

3. **Cascading branching pattern** (Chapter 2): Complementing *Physiological optimization principle number 2: cascading reactions*, this anatomical design criterion is a very effective way to maximize the lateral surface area available for trans-boundary transport in a region confined to a very limited space. The idea is to hollow-out the interior of that region, in such a way that a

complex branching network of increasingly larger numbers of smaller and smaller conduits is generated.

4. **Kinematic leverage** (Chapter 3): The mechanical equivalent of *Physiological optimization principle number 11: biasing*, this anatomical design principle endows the body with kinematic variables that promote speed, agility, range of motion, and locomotion, at the expense of *kinetic* variables such as force and power. This is accomplished by having skeletal muscles insert relatively close to the joints around which they act, thereby allowing the body to do best, those activities that need to be accomplished very *fast*—like escaping from predators—but involving the use of only very light objects.

5. **Cascading synaptic junctions** (Chapter 4): Also going along with *cascading reactions* and *cascading branching patterns*, this anatomical design principle:

    -   allows more than one neuron to influence the next one(s), thus generating integrated, net, compound action potentials, while also

    -   establishing an elaborately organized nerve complex whose branching pathways are amenable to *control*, in order to affect an intended result through directed transmission of action potentials.

6. **Transduction** (Chapter 5): Also complementing *reductionism*, this anatomical design principle ensures that the senses will *only* convert (transduce) the adequate stimuli (forms of energy) to which they respond into *digitized*, compound action potentials—raw data—nothing more.

7. **Molecular chirality** (Chapter 7) is a design principle that minimizes the element of chance in establishing consistent geometric structure, thereby ensuring that the same product will be produced time after time, with no exceptions. It thus guarantees the *uniqueness* of any given individual—an attribute exploited by the immune system.

8. **Selective stimulation** (Chapter 12) is an anatomical design principle that also complements *biasing*, by making target tissues more *sensitive* to protein-specific stimulation. This it does by structurally increasing (through *mitogenesis*, i.e., protein-triggered mitosis) the number of available receptor sites that are geometrically congruent—hence compatible—with the respective protein stimulant.

9. **It's all about rhythm!** (Chapter 12) is an anatomical design principle that complements *Physiological optimization principle number 10: phase regulation*, by rhythmically coordinating/synchronizing body *function* with ambient cues; and body *structure* with body function.

10. **Neogenesis** (Chapter 12) endows the body with the anatomical *plasticity* that allows it to generate *new* nerve networks, as necessary, in order to *adapt* to persistent, entrained stimulation.

In this chapter, we will add to our growing set of *anatomical design principles*. First, we will consider one that follows directly from *Physiological optimization principle number 3: minimum energy*, and *Anatomical design principle number 3: cascading branching pattern*. The criterion goes by the name of *Number 11: self-similarity*, which, too, should be of particular interest to the music therapist, as we shall see.

Anatomical, geometrical self-similarity

To understand what is meant by *geometrical self-similarity*, consider the following question: What attribute do the retina of the eye, the utinary collecting tubules of the kidney, lining of the gastrointestinal tract, bile ducts, various neural networks, brain, bile ducts, placenta, lungs, heart, etc., all share in common? Answer:

> *When any one of these organs/systems is examined with progressively stronger and stronger magnifying lenses, the smaller scale structures appear remarkably "similar" to the larger scale ones, in that all relative proportions are uniformly preserved, across all scales of perception!*

That is to say, in each case, basic patterns *within* a given level of perception are maintained and these patterns persist—to within a *scaling factor*—across all magnification levels (Schneck 2011a). This results in a spatial/temporal/functional *ordering* that is called *proportional self-similarity*. Why is there a need for such an anatomical design principle?

Well, a clue is embedded in *Physiological optimization principle number 3: minimum energy* as it applies to musculoskeletal mechanics (Schneck 1992); and the branching configurations of vascular, respiratory, renal, and other systems of the body (Schneck 2000b, 2009a, 2011a; Schneck and Voigt 2006). That is to say, as a design principle, self-similarity is required in order for anatomical structures to satisfy certain underlying physical constraints. Among these are minimum-energy considerations (see *Physiological optimization principle number 3*), and others imposed by various optimization schemes that prevail, *independent of the size of the unit of observation* (Schneck 1992). Indeed, it turns out that a constraint such as "pumping blood through the vascular system at least energetic cost" can be effectively satisfied by establishing branching pattern scaling relationships wherein all generations of the vascular network "look roughly the same," regardless of *which* specific generation is being observed. Thus, in examining this network, one encounters a "nesting" of "similar" anatomical structures, within all scales of perception. All of them have consistent *proportions* when compared to one another, across all scales of perception. In the simplest terms, one can say that:

> *The structures of the human body are constructed in accordance with Anatomical design principle number 11: self-similarity, because they have to be! It's the only effective way to satisfy the constraints that are imposed on them.*

Going one step further, when the structures involved have *irregular geometries*, in accordance with *Anatomical design principle number 1: dimensional expansion*, the relevant geometric dimensions of note are called *fractals* ("fractional" dimensions "in between" integer values 1, 2, and 3). An important defining property of fractals, and the geometries associated with them, is, indeed, self-similarity. All of which is to say that the geometry of anatomical systems such as the CNS, kidneys, lungs, and cardiovascular, are all *self-similar*. In fact, in addition to those already mentioned, systems of the human body in which anatomical/physiological self-similarity prevails include such highly organized ones as the:

- tree of airway passages of the lungs, that progressively branch from trachea (wind pipe) to terminal alveoli (see Chapter 2)

- structure and organization of connective tissue

- many nerve networks

- structure and organization of the genome, itself

- configuration of glandular duct work

- cochlea, which retains its original proportions while *spiraling* in logarithmic, "snail-shell" fashion to form the cavity of the inner ear that houses auditory nerve endings

...to name but a few!

All of that having been said, we do need to qualify this discussion somewhat, although the details are beyond the scope of this book (see Schneck 2011a). For the sake of accuracy, we should mention that general engineering principles of biological scaling recognize that, depending on one's level of observation:

- *additional* criteria might have to be met *specific to that particular level*, in order to satisfy *differing functional objectives* on *different scales of perception*.

Therefore, in self-similar systems—where basic *relative proportions* are preserved across all magnification levels—the *individual* scaling parameters from level to level might have to be *weighted* to allow for a certain degree of *variability*, depending on which of several constraints take(s) precedence at any given scale of observation. In other words, although the *general topography* "looks the same" across all levels of magnification, when viewed more specifically:

- at one level, it might appear to be scaled to *half* the original dimensions of the pattern, whereas

- when examined at another level, the pattern might reveal scaling to only *one-third* of its macroscopic dimensions; and

- even "tighter" focusing might show scaling to only *one-tenth* of the original pattern.

However, all the time, and at all levels of observation, the *same relative proportions* continue to prevail. That is to say, the overall *pattern* still looks the same across all levels of perception, even though, moving from level to level, the scaling factor might have to be *tweaked* to accommodate "local" conditions, i.e., there might not be a *constant* overall scaling factor that is maintained from step to step. The latter is, indeed, the case for "traditional," *classical* similitude. But in "real life" systems, fractal imperfections, together with additional constraining criteria, lead one to encounter a scaling factor that is variably *weighted* relative to the original pattern, even though, again, within each level and across all of them, the same *proportions* prevail (Schneck 2009a and 2011a). Self-similar systems with weighted scaling factors are said to possess the property of *fractal similitude*, also known as *structured randomness* (commonly called, "chaos"), which is quite typical in most biological systems, human ones included! Keeping all of this in mind, we can summarize the entire contents of this section as follows:

> *The anatomical design of the human body is such that: (i) structural ratios of bigger-to-smaller geometric imensions; and, similarly, (ii) longer-to-shorter timescales and, moreover, (iii) in ratios involving growing numbers of anatomical elements (such as successive generations of branching), the organism is a self-similar system, showing generalized scaling proportionalities.*

Which leads us to yet another question: Is there anything *special* about these "scaling proportionalities?" You bet there is!

The golden ratio

The more one studies the detailed geometry of anatomical systems, the more an interesting pattern begins to emerge as it relates to geometric scaling factors. As we shall see, this pattern carries over directly into the time domain, and into the structure of musical intervals. For example, consider the branching pattern of the human vascular system. Suppose we define for this system, an *anatomical geometric scaling factor*, R. R is a measure of the structural proportionality, i.e., *similarity* between successive downstream generations, m (m = 1, 2, 3...), of the vascular network. It is determined from the scaling law: $L_m = L_o R^m$, where L^m is a characteristic length in the m'th generation daughter vascular bed (e.g., the diameter of a "typical" downstream blood vessel in branching generation "m" of the network)...and Lo is the same characteristic length in the parent (m = 0) from which said generation derives (e.g., the diameter of the upstream blood vessel). Then...from a wide variety of measured values for L_m and L_o taken all over the vascular system, we find that, with remarkable consistency, the calculated geometric scaling factor, i.e., the *similarity parameter* R, comes very close to 0.618 in all cases! That is to say, all geometric lengths in the daughter branches of any generation, *on average*, are scaled by a factor of 0.618 compared to the parent branch from which they derive. Furthermore, that scaling ratio holds true across the entire system under investigation, as well as other systems studied (Schneck 2000b, 2008b, 2011a).

That being the case, one can't help notice the glaring similarity between this geometric scaling factor and the value of a scaling factor that routinely appears in studies of self-similar systems—one that was first identified a very long time ago by the famous Greek mathematician, Euclid (ca. 365–265 B.C.). Any two quantities for which this geometric scaling relationship holds are said to be in *golden ratio*, more formally defined by the irrational quotient $[2/(1 + \sqrt{5})] = 0.618033989$.

As shown further by a leading European mathematician of the late Middle Ages (ca. 1202), Leonardo of Pisa (also known as Filius Bonacci, shortened to just *Fibonacci*), the golden ratio happens to be the limiting value of sequential ratios in the numerical series, 0, 1, 1, 2, 3, 5, 8, 13, 21, 34, 55,…as shown in Table 13.1. Note from the table, that—in what has come to be known as the *Fibonacci Series*—each successive term is the sum of the previous two, i.e., $1 = 1 + 0$; $2 = 1 + 1$, etc.

Table 13.1 En route to the golden ratio		
FIBONACCI NUMBER	FIBONACCI RATIO	DECIMAL EQUIVALENT
$0 + 0 = 0$	--------	--------
$0 + 1 = 1$	--------	--------
$1 + 0 = 1$	1: 1	1.0000
$1 + 1 = 2$	1: 2	$1/2 = 0.5000$
$2 + 1 = 3$	2: 3	$2/3 = 0.6667$
$3 + 2 = 5$	3: 5	$3/5 = 0.6000$
$5 + 3 = 8$	5: 8	$5/8 = 0.6250$
$8 + 5 = 13$	8: 13	$8/13 = 0.6154$
$13 + 8 = 21$	13: 21	$13/21 = 0.6190$
$21 + 13 = 34$	21: 34	$21/34 = 0.6176$
$34 + 21 = 55$	34: 55	$34/55 = 0.6182$
$55 + 34 = 89$	55: 89	$55/89 = 0.6180$
$89 + 55 = 144$	89: 144	$89/144 = 0.6180$
Golden ratio	$2/(1 + \sqrt{5})$	0.618033989_

Note: Each element in column 1 of the above table is the sum of the immediately preceding two entries.

Generalizing the above reasoning, if one thinks of the human experience as unfolding in a space/time continuum then it follows that some basic insights derived from *spatial* phenomena can be extrapolated to yield corresponding insights into *temporal* phenomena, and vice versa. This realization allows one to exploit, for example, the general concept and attributes of *spatial, geometric self-similarity*—as embedded in *golden ratio scaling paramters, fractal "space-filling dimensions,"* and *Fibonacci numbers/*

ratios—to explain, as well, the inherent properties of *musical intervals*, and concepts such as *consonance* and *dissonance*.

Extrapolating from physical geometry to temporal relationships

In physical *space*, we talk about geometrical scaling factors, self-similarity, and proportionalities embedded in anatomical design. However, as there is no such thing as physical *perfection*, there arises an additional consideration that has to do with how these spatial geometries *vibrate* when mechanically disturbed from some equilibrated state. In this book so far we have said a great deal about vibration, especially in Part I, and quite specifically with respect to musical pitch and the resonance frequencies of anatomical organs and tissues (see Chapters 1, 4, 5 and Tables 5.2 and 5.3). Now, we ask the following question: Is there some underlying connection among physical vibration phenomena, anatomical *space* considerations, musical pitch frequencies, Fibonacci numbers, musical intervals, concepts such as *consonance* and *dissonance*, and…acoustic scaling, in *time?*" The answer is a resounding, "Yes! There is!" And the connection has to do with those very physical imperfections that do not allow a body to vibrate *uniformly* at any given *fundamental frequency, f.* That is to say, when you pluck, for example, the "A string" on a (tuned) violin, it is made to vibrate at a nominal, *fundamental frequency* of, say 440 Hz ("concert A").

But…not *all* parts of the A string are vibrating at exactly 440 cycles per second, which would be a pure tone. Indeed, whereas the *whole string* is vibrating at a "nominal," *average* frequency of 440 Hz—which is clearly the strongest, loudest, most prominent and *dominant* vibration elicited—some parts of it (due to unavoidable imperfections in the material) are vibrating faster than 440 Hz, while other parts of the string are vibrating slower than 440 Hz. The same can be said of the bridge on the instrument, the sounding post inside the body of the violin, and the wood of which it is made—all, in their own *unique* way, resonating with the vibrations transmitted to them by the vibrating A string. Indeed, no two instruments are *exactly* alike!

Vibrations above 440 Hz are called *harmonic overtones*, which show up as integer multiples of the fundamental frequency, f, i.e., $2f$, $3f$, $4f$, and so on. Those vibrations below 440 Hz are called *harmonic undertones*. Of the two, the harmonic overtone series is of greater interest to the musician because, as we shall see below, it gives birth to the concept of *musical intervals*. Note, however, that the *entire* range of undertones and overtones that are generated when a material is made to vibrate is called the *frequency spectrum* for that material; and the frequency *range* encompassed by this frequency spectrum is called its *bandwidth*. Furthermore, the frequency spectrum and bandwidth of a vibrating body are responsible for giving the sound it generates its *unique* "quality," called *timbre*—another of the basic elements of music. (*Note: timbre* is distinguished from *sonority*, which refers to the fullness and richness of the sound generated, as opposed to its qualitative identify.)

Bottom line: because various materials have different imperfections and a wide range of physical properties they display different *frequency spectra* and *bandwidths* when made to vibrate. Such variance accounts for why the materials *sound* different, even when they are made to vibrate at the same *fundamental* (or "center") *frequency* (i,e., *pitch*). It's why, for example, a trumpet sounds different to a violin, which sounds different to a piano, which sounds different to a flute, etc., even though they all might be playing the "same" 440 Hz concert A. Different frequency spectra/bandwidths is why a soprano voice sounds different to an alto, which sounds different to a tenor, which sounds different to a bass, even though they might all be singing the same melody. And different frequency spectra/bandwidths are *perceived* differently by different *listeners*. Indeed, it's all about the frequency spectrum and the bandwidth—the harmonic overtones—the *timbre*. Thus, music therapists, take note:

> *Be especially cognizant of how your clients might be reacting to the timbre of the music to which they are being exposed. It's quite possible—indeed, probable—that the same song played, for example, on the piano, might be less effective than if it is played on a guitar. Some clients might consider the piccolo to be a "shrill" instrument, compared, say, with a cello. Others might prefer a tympani to a snare drum, so be aware, and be sensitive!*

Musical intervals

Moving on then, other than accounting for sound quality—*timbre*—what additional useful information can be gleaned from the frequency spectrum of a given sound? The answer is embedded, again, in observing that harmonic overtones appear as integer multiples of the center frequency, f. Thus, as promised, we point out that this observation gives birth to the concept and general theory of *musical intervals*. An "interval" is the "distance" in pitch between any two tones, of fundamental frequencies f_1 and f_2, respectively. Most generally, that interval is defined by the *ratio* of f_2 to f_1, where, by convention, f_2 is the greater frequency.

For example, the first harmonic overtone is recorded at a frequency exactly *twice* that of the fundamental, i.e., $2f$. Thus, the *ratio* of this frequency to that of the center-frequency, f, is exactly 2:1, which defines the musical *interval* called an *octave*. The next overtone has a frequency three times that of the fundamental, i.e., $3f$, so that the ratio of *its* frequency to f is 3:1, which defines the musical *interval* called a *major twelfth*. Of greater interest, however, is the ratio of the second overtone, $3f$ to the first overtone, $2f$, which is the ratio 3:2—defining the musical *interval* called a *perfect fifth*. And so we can continue, to construct via the overtone series, a table such as Table 13.2, where the harmonic overtones are listed in column 1, ratios of consecutive overtones are given in column 3 (we'll define "CON," and "DIS" below), and corresponding musical intervals are defined in column 4.

Table 13.2 Overtone series and musical intervals			
HARMONIC OVERTONES	FIBONACCI NUMBER	FREQUENCY RATIO	MUSICAL INTERVAL
Fundamental f (Hz)	0 + 1 = 1		
1f	1 + 0 = 1	1:1	Unison
2f	1 + 1 = 2	2:1 CON	Octave
3f	2 + 1 = 3	3:1 CON	Major twelfth
		3:2 CON	Perfect fifth
4f		4:3 CON	Perfect fourth
5f	3 + 2 = 5	5:4 CON	Major third
		5:3 CON	Major sixth
		5:2 CON	Major tenth
6f		6:5	Minor third
7f		7:6	Augmented second
		7:5	Augmented fourth
		7:4	Augmented sixth
		7:3	Augmented ninth
8f	5 + 3 = 8	8:7	Supermajor second
		8:5	Minor sixth
		8:3	Major eleventh
9f		9:8 DIS	Major second
		9:7	Diminished fourth
		9:5 DIS	Minor seventh
		9:4	Major ninth
10f		10:9 DIS	Sub-major second
		10:7	Diminished fifth
11f		11:9	Neutral third
		11:8	Super fourth
12f		12:11	Neutral second
		12:7	Diminished seventh
		12:5	Minor tenth
13f	8 + 5 = 13	13:12 DIS	Diminished second
		13:8	Neutral sixth

14f		14:13	Sub-minor second
		14:9 DIS	Augmented fifth
		14:5	Augmented eleventh
15f		15:14	Semi-tone
		15:8 DIS	Major seventh
		15:7	Minor ninth
16f		16:15 DIS	Minor second
		16:11	Sub-fifth

Take a close look, now, at column two of Table 13.2 and compare it to columns 1 and 2 of Table 13.1. The sought-after correlation between *spatial* scaling factors and *temporal* proportionalities should start to become evident. That is to say, observe that the *spatial* ratio of the third Fibonacci number—i.e., 2—to the second Fibonacci number—i.e., 1—is exactly equal to the *temporal* frequency ratio 2:1 of the *harmonic overtone series* that defines the musical octave. Likewise, the ratio of the fourth Fibonacci number—i.e., 3—to the third Fibonacci number—i.e., 2—corresponds to the musical frequency ratio, 3:2 for the perfect fifth, and so on, down the line:

- 5:3 defines the musical major sixth

- 8:5 defines the musical minor sixth

- 13:8 defines the musical neutral sixth (i.e., in between major and minor, but not exactly either)

- though not shown in the table, the ratio of the next Fibonacci number—i.e., 21—to 8—i.e., 21:8 defines the musical augmented tenth.

By now, you should get the point—this apparent one-to-one correspondence between *anatomical* geometric proportionalities, as embedded in ratios derived from the Fibonacci number sequence, and *musical* intervals, as embedded in ratios derived from the acoustic overtone series, certainly lends credence to the intimate connection between physiologic function and the basic elements of music, one that may be rooted (at least in part) in the underlying *self-symmetry* that prevails in the human body across various scales of perception (Schneck and Berger 2006, Schneck 2011a).

But that's not all. Thinking further in terms of musical intervals, what happens if we now pluck (or bow) *at the same time* (i.e., *together*), the A string and the D string on the violin, spaced a perfect fifth apart? This creates what is called a *double stop*—two notes sounded *simultaneously*, as elements of a *chord*. Read on…

Consonance and dissonance

In Table 13.2, note that certain frequency ratios are followed by "CON" and others by "DIS." This refers to the fact that the corresponding frequency ratios, when sounded together, are *perceived* by the listener to be "consonant," i.e., "with sound;" *pleasing* to the ear, or "dissonant"—literally, "apart from sound;" connoting a "clashing," harshness in tone quality that is displeasing to the ear, not harmonious. Why not?

Well, consider what happens when two pure sounds of different frequencies, f_1 and f_2 ($f_2 > f_1$) are sounded together. Each one propagates through space, having an effect on the other. The superposition of these effects creates a *composite wave* that has a *resultant frequency* ("pitch") that is the *time-average*, $\frac{1}{2}(f_1 + f_2)$, of the two individual waves, and a time-dependent amplitude ("loudness") that alternately rises and falls, giving it a "wavy" sonority. That waviness is, itself, cyclic, having a net frequency that depends on the *difference* between the two individual frequencies, i.e., $(f_2 - f_1)$. That difference, i.e., the undulating rhythmic, "wah-wah" changes in composite wave "loudness," is called the *beat frequency* of the composite wave, which, in turn, derives from *wave interference patterns* that are generated when two waves of different frequencies are superimposed on one another (Giancoli 1989).

When the difference in frequency between the two sounding waves is very small, the amplitude undulations (alternating rises and falls in loudness) take very long to cycle, and so the effect on the ear of the listener is almost unnoticeable, certainly not objectionable; it's just a very slow *wah-wah* of insignificant changes in loudness. Indeed, *individual* beats between two tones, i.e., single amplitude cycles of the composite wave, can be unobtrusively detected by the human ear up to a beat frequency of six or seven cycles per second. Beyond that it becomes difficult for the hearing apparatus to distinguish among individual beats, and they begin to merge into a continuous, pulsating "hum."

Perception of *individual beating* disappears altogether after the beat frequency surpasses 15 Hz, at which point it is perceived, instead, as being simply a *consonant* or *dissonant* experience, depending on the frequency ratio of the tones involved (Roederer 1975). The unpleasantness of the effect seems to reach its most objectionable state when the beat frequency hovers around 24 cycles per second. It then begins to subside, disappearing completely when the beat frequency surpasses a "critical bandwidth." The latter spans the range from 10 to 20 percent of the fundamental frequency, f, for f greater than 500 Hz, which is to say, tones sounded simultaneously are perceived to be "smooth" and "pleasing" when the beat frequencies generated are greater than 50–100 Hz.

But why the unpleasantness? We used to think that the concordance (degree of consonance) between tones comprising musical intervals depended on the absence of disagreeable beats between them (Roederer 1975), and that is certainly still a prominent assumption in the field of acoustics. But recent research (Lots and Stone 2008) into the existence of specific neural pathways that are devoted exclusively to dissonance computations, suggests that there is more to it than that. It turns out that consonance is *not* just the absence of "roughness" due to the presence of objectionable beats. Rather, it is also determined by neural *processing* in the auditory cortex—in the right superior temporal gyrus (convolution of the cerebral cortex), where, it is believed, much of the analysis of pitch and timbre takes place. Processing and analysis of what? Let's dig a little deeper.

Communication among neurons: coupled oscillations and synchronization (resolution)

We talked earlier about what happens when two pure (for simplicity) *tones*, having fundamental frequencies f_1 and f_2, respectively, are sounded simultaneously, and how they affect one another (through *interference patterns*) as they travel through space. In *music*, such simultaneous tonality defines *intervals* (see Table 13.2). In *physics*, such simultaneous superposition of energy vibrating at different frequencies, and the consequences that result therefrom, is called *coupled oscillations;* "coupled," in the sense that each set of vibrations has an intimate relationship with and significantly affects the other.

Thus, carrying the above reasoning to its next logical step, it seems appropriate to explore what is likely to happen when two *auditory neurons*—having responded to and transduced f_1 and f_2 into corresponding sensory action potentials, respectively— fire simultaneously. Analogous to how two sound waves will interact and affect one another, these two neurons, too, will interact and communicate with one another in a process called *neural coupling*. However, whereas the interaction of pure tones involves the superposition of *mechanical, acoustic energy*, the coupling of neurons involves the superposition of *electromagnetic energy* derived from the transmission of *ionic action potentials* (which act like electric currents) through neural networks.

Nevertheless, just as tones sounded simultaneously produce a net resultant, neurons firing simultaneously *also* generate a coupled firing pattern. This pattern, in turn, depends on how well the firing frequencies of each nerve *mode-lock* with one another (Table 13.2). "Mode-locking" is just a fancy way of saying that the firing frequencies of the two neurons are *synchronized* to produce a net, *coupled firing pattern* that is, itself, purely (or *nearly purely*) periodic (cyclic). If this coupled firing pattern repeats with the same, *fixed* period of oscillation, the two neurons are "locked onto one another" and firing *in synchrony*. Moreover, if the coupled frequency comes close to being in-phase with the *resonance ("natural") frequency* of the coupled network, the acoustic experience is perceived to be "pleasurable." That is to say:

> *Consonance appears to result from the structured stability inherent in synchronized wave patterns that are mode-locked to the intrinsic firing frequencies of the corresponding nerve network through which the waves are travelling.*

As it turns out, synchronization of coupled neuronal firing patterns depends on the acoustic firing rates, f_1 and f_2, specifically, their interval ratio, f_2/f_1. In other words, it is the degree of stable synchronization, identified as the *strength of coupling*, and how that synchronization is handled by the auditory cortex that determines consonance and dissonance. Furthermore:

> *Mutually coupled neuronal firing patterns are more likely to be optimized, stable, and synchronized, and the acoustic experience perceived to be "consonant," if f_1 and f_2 are in low-number, simple firing ratios, i.e., 2:1 (octave), 3:2 (perfect fifth), 4:3 (perfect fourth), 5:4 (major third),6:5 (minor third), 5:3 (major sixth), etc.*

There is thus a correspondence between musical intervals, and synchronized, mode-locked states, such that the fundamental, and all harmonics up to the sixth, when sounded together in various combinations, produce harmonious, pleasing-to-the-ear *consonant* sensations. In fact, the consecutive sequence of frequencies: 4:5:6—composed of a major third (5:4), followed by a minor third (6:5), spanning the interval of a perfect fifth (6:4 = 3:2)—defines the *major consonant triad*, which is one of the basic elements of *harmony*, another of the six basic elements of music. Those chord progressions that end on a major triad are said to *resolve;* and the human brain strives for that sense of *resolution* in all aspects of life, not just music!

Higher-number frequency ratios, by contrast, produce a displeasing, *dissonant* experience (see Table 13.2). Although the exact mechanism responsible for such displeasure is still under investigation, based on everything we do know about how the central nervous system processes information (see Chapter 10) it is quite likely that the *absence* of synchronized, mode-locked states—or the *presence* of *disorganized* states—triggers an amygdala-driven *fear response*. Stress hormones then start running all over the place, setting off *general anxiety symptoms*, and consequent "fight-or-flight" behavior (see Chapters 7 and 8). Remember, according to the Gestalt Laws of human perception (see Chapter 10), the brain *seeks* order, stability, and self-consistency in the afferent signals that it processes, and thus, humans generally *prefer consonance* (i.e., intervals with low-frequency ratios) to dissonance, although, admittedly, one can *learn* (adapt) to "like" the latter.

One final point: neural synchronization no longer appears to be a factor at acoustic frequencies above 5000 cycles/sec (roughly between the notes D and E that are above the C that is four octaves above "middle C," when the latter is 256 Hz). Above these frequencies, our sense of musical pitch and our ability to discriminate among specific intervals is also significantly impaired (Lots and Stone 2008), but fortunately we rarely experience acoustic stimulation at these high frequencies (see Table 5.2). We do, however, frequently experience *more* than two, three, or four simultaneous pitches, which, speaking of discordance and disorder among afferent signals to the CNS, brings us to yet another source of acoustic discomfort…noise!

Noise!

We know it when we hear it: that undesired, *disturbing*, intrinsically unpleasant sound that is often harsh and loud, to the point of interfering with and/or masking other sounds to which one is listening. That is because one's brain has difficulty "picking out" the *desired* acoustic signal from the *background noise*. In fact, the very word, *noise*, which describes such an objectionable, subjective acoustic experience, derives from the Latin, *nausea*, which generally refers to "unpleasant conditions of various kinds." Most notably, the unpleasant conditions referred to involve the stomach's "queasiness"—associated with *sea*sickness (-*sea*), and, the vessel that caused it, from the Greek, *nâus*, meaning "ship," hence, *nau*- and the resulting *nausea*. Generalizing the meaning of *nausea* then, we have in *noise* the "unpleasant condition" experienced by the hearing apparatus forced to listen to a disagreeable acoustic signal. But what makes this signal displeasing to the ear?

Answer: noise is a conglomeration of *random, unpredictable* groups of sound waves that impact the outer ear drum (*tympanic membrane*) with no single, fundamental frequency ("pitch") or "pitch components." Rather, the sound contains *irregular, unsynchronized vibrations*, which include a very wide spectrum (*broad bandwidth*), of many, aperiodic, non-harmonic frequency components of comparable (if not equal) amplitudes. These frequency components are randomly distributed throughout the incident signal. When the random signal impacts the acoustic architecture of the body, the brain has difficulty "making head or tail of it," and, again, it does not like that one bit! Hence, we experience an "unpleasant sensation," a feeling of discomfort.

More generally, "noise" refers to *any* disturbing sound, regular *or* otherwise, but that reference is a highly subjective, individual-specific perception that is virtually impossible to quantify objectively, especially as it relates to pain, fatigue, discomfort, and the compromising of mental and motor efficiency that results therefrom. Be that as it may, and taking a leaf out of the "Book of Light" for vision, *white* noise, in the *acoustic* literature, is defined to be a signal containing (hypothetically) *all sonic frequencies, f,* between 20 and 20,000 cycles per second—just as *white* light contains all *electromagnetic frequencies* between 400 and 800 *Terahertz* in the *visible* spectrum. (*Note:* a "terahertz" is a million million cycles per second; see also Chapters 4 and 5.)

In *pure* white noise, each frequency component has the same "loudness," i.e., all of them contain the same amount of energy. In other words, the total acoustic energy of the signal is distributed *equally* among all frequencies contained therein, producing what is known as a *flat* frequency spectrum. The latter is a graph of wave amplitude ("loudness") versus wave frequency ("pitch") for all of the components contained in the composite, "white" sound wave. "Flat" means, for example, that in the 30-cycle/sec range between 20 Hz and 50 Hz *all* sound "pitches" are as "loud" (i.e., contain the same amount of acoustic energy) as they are in the 30-Hz range between 9220 and 9250, and, for that matter, in *any* 30-Hz range within the entire audible spectrum between 20 and 20,000 Hz. All the pitches in this spectrum are "equally loud," hence the cacophony (harsh, clashing sound) associated with noise!

Of course, *simultaneously* sounding 20,000 *different* tones of equal intensity is a purely "hypothetical" construct, because to generate so many pitches randomly, with energy distributed uniformly across all frequencies, would require an enormous amount of power; indeed, in the extrapolated limit of total, pure "white noise," composed of *all* sonic frequencies, as the frequency goes to huge values, so does the power necessary to generate all of them simultaneously. Thus, in "real life," a "noisy" signal is considered to be "white" if it has a uniform or nearly uniform *energy spectrum*, expressed as "loudness per pitch," calculated over any well-defined frequency range (bandwidth) within the spectrum.

Now, suppose we have a situation where equal power does *not* exist in all frequency bands of constant *increments*—such as the above 30-Hz bands. Instead, what we have is equal power in "laddered" bands separated by a constant *proportionality factor*, rather than a *specific bandwidth*. For example, the power might be the same in all frequency bands separated by a factor of two—expressed as "equal power *per octave*, 8^{ve}," rather than "equal power *per bandwidth*." Is this beginning to sound a lot like our previous discussion of geometric scaling factors in self-similarity? It should, because the *spatial* principles involved in *geometric self-similarity* carry over directly to the *temporal* principles involved in *harmonic self-similarity*. Indeed, the space/time expanse is inundated with self-similarity all over the place! Thus, instead of having constant energy in each band of, say, width 30 Hz, as was the case earlier for pure white noise, we now have the *same amount of energy* in:

- the band from 20 Hz to 40 Hz, i.e., in the bandwidth that *doubled* (increased by a *scaling factor* of two) over a frequency range of 20 Hz, i.e., 40−20 = 20... as we do in

- the comparable band from 9220 Hz to 18,440 Hz, i.e., the bandwidth that *also doubled*, but this time, over the much wider frequency range of 9220 Hz, i.e., 18,440−9220 = 9220.

Both the 20–40 Hz span *and* the 9220–18,440 span contain the *same* amount of energy, as do all frequency intervals that increase by a factor of two, which is partly why the octaves all "sound the same." Moreover, the same holds true for other regions of the spectrum that share a common scaling factor, i.e., the frequency ratios involved all contain the same amount of energy, and so "sound the same" to the auditory cortex.

The above considerations help to explain the auditory phenomenon of *pitch equivalence*. That is to say, as one travels up the frequency ladder, since the *power is equal* among all octave bandwidths, all pitches separated by one or more perfect "octaves" (i.e. all acoustic frequencies that are related by powers of two) are *perceived* to be equivalent, regardless of the actual frequencies involved. That is why the upper note of an octave, for example, "sounds the same" as does its lower note, regardless of the register in which the octave is sounded.

Taking the above reasoning still one step further, in the current "self-similarity scaling" case, as opposed to the previous, "pure white-noise" case, each bandwidth of equal energy involves a constant *proportionality factor* (such as 2, for octaves), not a constant *frequency increment* (such as 30 Hz). Consequently, compared to pure *white* noise—where *each frequency component* (pitch) is assumed to have equal power (loudness), yielding a *flat* energy spectrum—we now have a situation where each *individual* frequency component actually *loses* energy as we move up the frequency spectrum in octaves. For instance, note that, for an octave in the low register of the audible range—say, 20–40 Hz—a given amount of energy is shared by only 20 frequency components, so each one gets $(1/20)^{th}$ of the energy available. But nine octaves above that, at the higher end, say 10,240–20,480 Hz, that *same amount of energy* is shared by 10,240 frequency components so *each* frequency *component* at the high end gets only $(1/10,240)^{th}$ of the energy available—far less than $(1/20)^{th}$!

That's a fancy way of saying, simply, that for a complex acoustic wave of given total intensity, the lower-pitched components (sounds) contained in that wave are much louder than the higher-pitched ones; or, equivalently, that the higher harmonics gradually fade out as one moves up the ladder. In other words, sound intensity fades with increasing frequency, which is often expressed in terms of "decibels, dB loss, per octave" above the center frequency, f. Often, that loss averages *three decibels per octave*, which amounts to a 50 percent loss in "loudness" per pitch, per octave, as we travel in octaves up the frequency spectrum (Schneck 2011a). That partially explains why, as we move up the frequency ladder, the higher harmonics, which yield large frequency ratios that tend toward dissonance, are generally not heard. Other reasons are beyond the scope of this book (see, Giancoli 1989).

We will close this section by merely mentioning that, just as *white light* can be broken down into a *visible* spectrum that includes red, orange, yellow, green, blue, violet, and many colors in between, so, too, can *white noise* be broken down into an *audible* spectrum that includes red (or brown), orange, yellow ("sunlight noise"), green ("background noise" of the world), blue (or azure), violet (or purple), pink, gray, black, and also many sounds in between. Once again, details are beyond the scope of this book, so the reader is referred to the literature (e.g., Schneck 2011a) for more information.

It is definitely worth repeating, however, that noise, in the time domain—and, by inference, music, as well—has many of the same properties of self-similarity as does geometric configuration in the space domain. This means that, as we move up the frequency spectrum from bandwidth to bandwidth, we encounter proportionally scaled time-dependent behavior, related to energy considerations per bandwidth. Moreover, *music therapists take note:* the intimate relationships between these self-similarity considerations in space/time, music included, and the anatomy/physiology of the human body, clearly provide a basis for understanding why and how music can elicit such profound human responses. Further research is expected to establish a foundation for *applying* this understanding to the management of diagnosed populations, using *music* as a clinical tool. Keeping that in mind, let's say a few words about some other significant considerations of the body in space.

Anatomical design principle Number 12: decussation

Decussation was mentioned briefly in Chapter 5, but deserves further comment here. From the Greek *déka*, meaning "ten," and the Roman-numeral symbol for *ten*, i.e., the upper case letter "X," the word *decuss* connotes an intersection configured to look like the Roman numeral ten, hence, an "X-crossing." *Decussation*, then, refers to the crossing of lines, fibers, neural networks, etc., so as to form an X-like intersection. Most sensory and motor pathways, including more than half of somato-sensory, spino-thalamic, cortico-spinal, and cortico-rubral (frontal lobe to red nucleus of the brain) anatomical tracts in vertebrates (including humans) *decussate*—cross the midline of the body to the opposite (*contralateral*) side. The question is, "Why?" The answer is, "Who knows!" But everybody has a "theory," three of which are discussed in Schneck (2009b).

Suffice it to say here that, according to *Anatomical design principle number 1*, the body economizes on the utilization of limited space by exploiting the advantages of *enfolding*—"wrapping up" a relatively large, two-dimensional surface (like the cerebral cortex) into a confined, three-dimensional volume (like the interior of the skull). To illustrate how enfolding relates to decussation, take a sheet of paper (a two-dimensional surface) and draw on it several parallel lines of different colors, for easy identification. These will represent sets of *non*-decussating neural tracts. Now, either randomly "crumple-up" the flat sheet into a tight ball of paper, or keep folding it in half, into smaller and smaller pieces, thus *enfolding* the lower, two-dimensional surface into the next higher dimension, a three-dimensional volume. You have thus essentially formed the *gyri* (bulges), *sulci* (furrows), fissures, and "lobes" of the brain! When done, note that quite a few of the color-coded lines that started out to be parallel will automatically have decussated! In other words, decussation is a natural *topological consequence* of enfolding elaborate neural networks into complex, three-dimensional, constrained configurations.

But that's not all. In this experiment, we were purely *arbitrary* in the way we crumpled-up/folded the paper. By contrast, in the human body, decussation is *not* random; the enfolding is highly structured, *optimized*, and specific. Indeed, decussation is characteristic of information-processing pathways (neural tracts) that deal primarily with *spatially organized data* (Shinbrot and Young 2008). That is to say, if one is to achieve optimized, reliable results, topological constraints *require* three-dimensional, spatially organized data to be processed through decussating networks (Shinbrot and Young 2008)! This is because decussating networks have distinct advantages over non-decussating ones, to wit:

- *Pathfinding errors are minimized,* which is to say, as the number and complexity of wiring schemes increases, decussating arrangements are especially accurate in properly "targeting" axons so that they efficiently and effectively reach their intended destination (known as *neuronal projection*) during development, and/ or following regenerative therapy.

- *Collisions are avoided,* which is to say, crossing patterns minimize the risk that nerve impulses traveling in one direction will collide with others moving in the opposite direction along the same tract. This is further guaranteed by designing an *asymmetry* into the crossing network, which also ensures reliability and stability.

- *Traffic patterns can be effectively regulated,* which is to say, introducing "path flexibility," and several cross-over branch points/nodes in decussating systems optimizes the body's ability to control *information transport*—analogous to a similar point made in our discussion of cascading *biochemical reactions.* This is true *provided* the system is also optimized to have as few crossings as are necessary, because each takes up space and adds length to connections.

- *Processing speeds are faster,* which is to say, when decussated crossings are *absent,* information-processing speeds slow down, resulting in a lack of coordinated motion and control flexibility.

- *Singularities (discontinuities) in the conformal mapping of kinematic data are eliminated,* which is to say, consider the question, "How does the two-dimensional brain communicate with the three-dimensional body?" Answer: by employing sophisticated, decussating topographic principles. Information thus derived from a *three-dimensional domain,* such as the location and movement of certain anatomical structures (e.g., your hands and feet), can be effectively *mapped* onto the enfolded *two-dimensional surface* of the brain *in a one-to-one correspondence.* This is sort of the *reverse* of crumpling up the piece of paper—we are now *unfolding* it to "map" the volume it occupies from three to two dimensions. Indeed, decussated networks are essential for conveying and mapping such information accurately and unambiguously.

- *The architectural blueprint for decussated data-handling systems requires a minimum amount of genetic specification,* which is to say, the number of *genes* required to code for an optimized information-processing system is least when the geometric configuration of that system is decussated (Shinbrot and Young 2008).

- *Information entering or leaving the central nervous system is not contradictory, confusing, or erroneous,* which is to say, decussating networks minimize these potential errors by allowing "triangulation, typing, and cross-matching" of data as it is processed. Such effective "cross-talk" among *ipsilateral* (same-side) tracts is virtually impossible and non-existent, making them vulnerable to miscues and confusion.

Decussating networks are not confined solely to the nervous system; they are also observed in many groups of muscles of the mouth, trunk, and extremities. For example, most of the fibers of the *ipsilateral* abdominal *superficial transverse perineal muscle*, in the region of the anus, proceed medially (toward the midline of the body) in a criss-crossing pattern with the muscle fibers of the corresponding *contralateral* muscle. Similarly, the fibers of the *deep transverse perineal muscle* decussate with their counterparts from the opposite side.

The *arytenoideus obliquus muscle* of the larynx consists of two fasciculi (bands of fibers) that cross each other as they pass from the base of one arytenoid cartilage to the apex of the opposite one. The fibers of the central portion of the *buccinator muscle* (an important accessory muscle of mastication, i.e., chewing) also cross each other. Those fibers from above the lip continue on to merge with the *orbicularis muscle* of the lower lip, while en route traversing across the fibers from below that become continuous with the musculature of the upper lip. And, extra slips from opposite sides of the anterior belly of the *digastricus muscle* that assists in opening the jaw can cross one another as they traverse the mandible (jaw bone). All of these musculoskeletal crossing patterns presumably ensure that when the muscles on both sides of the "X" contract simultaneously, they will act as a single unit, i.e., the result will be a type of biomechanical functional synchrony.

But before we get complacent and start generalizing too much, we must quickly note that decussation is not universal in the body. Indeed, among the neural pathways that do *not* decussate are those belonging to the olfactory (smell), vestibulo-spinal (VES), reticulo-spinal (RES), and rubro-spinal (RUS) systems. VES tracts descend from the lateral vestibular nucleus of the medulla oblongata, down the front side of the spinal cord's white matter. RES tracts descend to the spinal cord from the reticular formation of the brain's pons and medulla oblongata. The RUS tracts are motor pathways that project *ipsilaterally* from the red nucleus to specific spinal motoneuron pools. The significance of these *non*-decussating systems is that they are phylogenetically *older* than those that *do* decussate. If we add to this the fact that some of the molecules responsible for *orchestrating* the decussation of neural pathways are quite "young" (again, from an evolutionary point of view), there emerges the clear suggestion that the *need* for such anatomical configurations only developed quite "recently." Thus, it may very well be that decussation became a necessity with increasing evolutionary complexity… but the jury is still out on that one, so let's move on.

Anatomical design principle number 13: lateralization

As a design concept, *lateralization*, too, has been addressed several times in this book. For example, recall our brief vision experiment of Chapter 5, where we distinguished between your ipsilateral "sighting" eye and the contralateral one that "triangulates." In Chapter 2, we distinguished between the right and left sides of the heart; and in Chapter 4 we talked about the triune brain, and lateralization theories of "right-brain" and "left-brain" function (we'll get back to that below).

We know all about "right-handedness" and "left-handedness." Roughly ten percent of the general population is left-handed, the vast majority being right-handed or, in even fewer cases, *ambidextrous* (which, ironically, literally means, "doubly right-handed"), referring to individuals capable of using both hands equally well to perform most tasks. As is the case for L-amino acids and D-carbohydrates (see discussion of *chirality* in Chapter 7), theories abound to explain *why right* D-, as opposed to *left* L- and why *right*-handedness should prevail so overwhelmingly over *left*-handedness, but nobody knows for sure.

What we do know, is that, when viewed in a macroscopic sense, our body might *appear* to be anatomically symmetric about a vertical plane that divides it into equal right and left halves. However, given that observation, the two sides of the body, when examined in greater detail—"below the surface"—exhibit quite different *functions*, which is what we mean by *lateralization*. Moreover, what *does seem plausible*, is that lateralization—or *laterality*, the attribute of having "preferred" sides of the body, each responsible for distinctly different tasks—most likely represents the body's attempt to *economize on the use of space and resources*, and *optimize performance*. That's why there exist these various *Physiological optimization principles* and *Anatomical Design principles*, from which we can learn a great deal. Indeed, engineers have exploited these principles in a field called *bionics* (remember "The Six Million Dollar Man" television series?). *Bionics* is a term coined at the Aerospace Medical Research Laboratories of the United States Air Force to define a field wherein nature's designs are used as prototypes for human-made products, such as totally implantable artificial organs.

But we digress. Getting back to our earlier promise, consider, for example, the human brain…again. It is very efficiently organized in terms of how much space is reserved for encoding complex activities. That is to say, the more intricate the activity, the more room is required to program it into this organ. Thus, given the enormous number of nerve networks required to perform activities such as writing, using tools, formulating theories, doing complicated things, talking, etc., and despite giving due respect to *Anatomical design principle number 2: redundancy*, once *one side* of the brain has been programmed to perform these complex activities effectively, it makes no sense to take up valuable space in a restricted, confined skull by programming the *other side* of this organ to do exactly the same thing, most especially if you really don't need such duplication of effort!

Furthermore, to preserve space and optimize performance, it makes no sense to organize cerebral neural networks in a way that requires signals to "run back and forth from left side to right side" in order to accomplish a task. Thus, *all* of "handedness" motor function is restricted to one cerebral hemisphere, most often the left, which, according to decussation principles, controls the right side of the body.

Going one step further—and analogous to our earlier "eye-experiment"—we observe here, again, that although both sides of the brain might *look* alike under gross inspection, the right and left halves *seem* to be responsible for specialized, totally different (though carefully synchronized and coordinated) functions, to wit (see Edwards 1989, and Ornstein and Thompson 1984):

- The "left brain" seems more *process-oriented*, being concerned mainly with *sequential, temporal* events. It likes to name and categorize, reason *linearly*, analyze and perform cognitive functions, without necessarily deriving any inherent *understanding* of basic principles. The left brain is comfortable dealing with digitized data, structure, order, *deductive modes of information processing*, and manipulating symbols (letters, words, syntax, numbers), hence its important role in language, reading, writing, mathematics, and symbolic-based cognitive functions.

By contrast:

- The "right brain" seems more concerned with *holistic, spatial* events. It prefers to deal with "worldly," ubiquitous issues and seeks *understanding based on experience*, as opposed to *deductive reasoning based on process.* Thus, here we have the seat of intuitive, perceptive-based logic that is metaphoric, sensuous, existential, and representative of "outside-the-box, *thing*-thinking," hence the importance of right-brain function in the more imaginative, abstract, not-necessarily-verbal, creative activities associated with, for example, the visual and performing arts, and with more *inductive modes* of information processing.

Obviously, the above generalizations are gross over-simplifications, and investigators still argue about their "black-and-white" validity. Certainly, the experimental evidence is not without a certain degree of controversy. But the paradigm does serve to illustrate certain advantages of lateralization in matters related to information processing.

Lateralization also helps effectively to "distribute the load," and "back up the effort." In that sense, it *does*, too, subscribe to the idea of *redundancy.* For example, having *two* kidneys—one on each side of the body—allows some 1100–1250 ml of blood/minute (21–24% of total cardiac output) to be cleansed of toxins and wastes, "the sooner the better!" Attempting the *same thing* with only one organ would require it to be rather large and cumbersome. Thus, it is better to "split" this large organ in two, placing each lima-bean-shaped "half" on either side of the spine (for balance), behind the abdominal (*peritoneal*) cavity. Recall from Chapter 2, that within this cavity, the kidneys occupy a space called the *retroperitoneum*, a region lying somewhat between the twelfth thoracic and third lumbar vertebral levels. Because of the presence of the liver, the left kidney is typically slightly larger, somewhat higher, and more medial than the right. The point is, that this *lateralized kidney pairing* not only makes the total blood-cleansing job easier, but, while economizing on space utilization, provides the added advantage of having each kidney benefit from a lateral "back-up"—*redundancy*—in case it fails. That is, if we had only *one*, large, cumbersome kidney, and it were to fail, the blood-cleansing process would come to a complete halt, leading to fatal consequences! Splitting the organ in two insures that, it is hoped, at least half of the renal system will keep functioning if the other half fails, as evidenced by the fact that one can survive quite well (although not as efficiently), with only one, over-worked kidney.

A similar argument—i.e., increased capacity, "back-up" insurance, space-saving, optimized function, etc.—can be developed for why we have *two*, cone-shaped lungs that fill the left and right sides of the chest (*pleural cavity*)—from the level of the diaphragm to about 1.5 inches above the collar bone (*clavicle*). Again, they are lateralized for "balance," although, because of the presence of the heart, the right lung has three "lobes" (*superior, middle,* and *inferior*), compared to the smaller left lung's two (*superior* and *inferior,* see Chapter 2). And again, although life would be tough, and one would not have the same endurance as one had with two lungs, it is possible to live with only one. In fact, because of the redundancy built in to our anatomical structure, it would be terribly inconvenient, but we can survive with only one of most of the laterally paired organs and tissues in the body—one arm, one leg, one eye, one ear, one kidney, one lung, one ovary, one breast…and so on.

Some closing remarks

The list of anatomical design principles could go on and on—there are many, such as:

- The way the kidney goes about filtering the blood of waste products. Recall (Chapter 2) that it *first* empties the plasma of just about *everything,* and then *puts back* what it wants to save. This ensures that it will not have inadvertently "missed" ridding the body of wastes that might have "snuck in, unnoticed," a very clever way of "covering all bases," rather than *just filtering!*

- The way the trachea rises to seat against the epiglottis, and falls to open the airway passage every time we swallow (Chapter 2). This allows the entrance to both the esophagus and trachea to originate from the same part of the pharynx, an interesting design concept.

- The way the coronary circulation of the heart is configured so that this vital organ receives *its* blood supply during the *diastolic* phase of the cardiac cycle—rather than the systolic phase, when the coronary vasculature is "blocked off" by *extravascular compression* due to contraction of the myocardial musculature (again, see Chapter 2 for details).

- The way the *valves* in the heart and venous system are designed and configured to prevent back flow

…and so on. However, since we only considered a baker's dozen (13) of physiologic optimization principles in Chapter 12, realizing that there are many more, it seemed only fair to concentrate in this chapter on only a baker's dozen of anatomic design principles, keeping in mind that there are many more, as well. Moreover, to ensure that this book does not encumber the reader with a plethora of anatomic and physiologic principles, we shall move on in Chapter 14 to "wrap it up," recapitulate our 7–6–5–4–3–2–1 paradigm (with special emphasis on the four major *constraints* within which the human body is forced/obliged to operate), summarize, and attempt to "tie all of this together" from the point of view of the practicing music therapist.

CHAPTER 14

Recapitulation, Summary, and Music Therapy Perspective

The paradigm *reviewed and developed further*

Our hypothesis in this book has emphasized that to study and understand the anatomy and physiology of the human body, it is convenient to formulate a 7–6–5–4–3–2–1 paradigm, to wit:

Seven: The body is viewed as having seven general *features* that, collectively, account for *all* of its organs and systems, i.e., it is a:

1.   sophisticated living/isothermal/electrochemical engine/instrument (Chapter 2) that has an…

2.   optimized, digitized, mechanical output (Chapters 3 and 4).

The body is:

3.   sentient (Chapters 4 and 5), allowing it to monitor/control and "direct" its optimized performance

4.   responsive (Chapter 6), in order to maintain stationarity

5.   controlled (Chapter 7), leaving nothing to chance.

Moreover, the organism is able to:

6.   adapt (Chapter 12), through entrainment mechanisms

7.   procreate—make other engines/instruments just like it, a feature addressed in context throughout Parts I and II thus far.

Six: All of the above, the body accomplishes through six basic *processes* that include:

1.   metabolism (Chapter 8)—energy transport and conversions

2. transduction, transmission, and central nervous system processing of digitized data (Chapter 10), i.e., "IT," that is then…

3. differentiated, translated and integrated into useful information, eventually reaching *consciousness* (Chapter 10).

The body operates:

4. in *time* (Chapter 11), in accordance with well-defined *biorhythms*

5. in *space* (Chapter 13), in accordance with specific anatomical design principles, and it complies with

6. well-defined physiological optimization principles (Chapter 12).

As pointed out in context, all of these processes have, as well, intimate connections with the six basic *elements* of music:

- Rhythm (pulse, pace, pattern)
- Melody (pitch, prosody, phrasing, profile, perceptive processing)
- Harmony (overtone series, intervals, chords, concordance, consonance, dissonance, noise)
- Dynamics (loudness, softness, decibels)
- Timbre (sound quality, frequency spectra, bandwidths)
- Form (*musical* structure analogous to and symbiotic with *anatomical* structure).

In fact, speaking of *biorhythms*, although it is beyond the scope of this book (and so, we have not said much about it), it should be pointed out that there exists an important corollary to this entire concept/process—one that should be of particular interest to the practicing music therapist. That is to say, the *process* encoded into biorhythms, as applied, goes hand in hand with the *notion* of *rhythm and movement* as exploited by the growing field of *Dalcroze eurhythmics.* The interested reader is referred to Schneck and Schneck (1997), the fine text by Findlay (1971), and the forthcoming volume by Berger (2015) for more details. Suffice it to say here, that the pulse, pace, and patterns of *musical* rhythms, when anatomically/physiologically *entrained* (Schneck and Berger 2006), surface as corresponding rhythms of *body movement.* This was observed by the late Emile Jaques-Dalcroze to have significant application in the development of motor consciousness and listening skills, particularly in children. Dalcroze's system of rhythmic education/entrainment teaches the body to be the "interpreter" of musical rhythm—to have the latter become manifest in physical movement. This has come to be known worldwide as *eurhythmics*—literally, "good rhythm!" (Findlay 1971). That having been said, we continue with our paradigm.

Five: All of the above are governed by five basic *laws* of:

Physics (Chapter 8):

1. Conservation of Energy (First Law of Thermodynamics)

2. Conservation of Mass (continuity principles)

3. Conservation of Linear Momentum (translational inertia)

4. Conservation of Angular Momentum (rotational inertia)

5. The Second Law of Thermodynamics (irreversibility).

And Gestalt *laws* of perception (Chapter 10):

1. Proximity (spatial/temporal *resolution*)

2. Directionality (spatial/temporal *tracking*/continuity)

3. Similarity (spatial/temporal identification/*discrimination*/scaling)

4. Closure (spatial/temporal *completeness*/"wholeness")

5. Pragnanz (spatial/temporal differentiation/integration/synthesis/*interpretation* of information).

All of the above are *constrained* by:

- *Four* levels of *control*
- *Three* levels of *organization*
- *Two sexes*, all seeking to fulfill
- *One au fond purpose.*

Some specific elements of the four levels of control were actually discussed individually, in context, throughout the book thus far, for example, in Chapters 2 (*isothermal* constraints), 5 (*adequate stimuli* limitations), 8 (*enzyme-kinetic* restrictions), 9 (constraints to *knowing*), and so on. However, a closer look at all of these constraints, and more, reveals that they may be conveniently grouped into *four levels of control*, these being: things over which one has:

1. literally *no* control; absolutely *nothing* you can do about them

2. *some* control, but very limited; *perhaps* you can "tweak" them, but that's all; your influence, if any, is quite restricted

3. *minimal to significant* control, *enough* to make a difference

4. *total* control, *entirely* at your discretion; it's *all* up to you!

The above reminds one of the famous, so-called *Serenity Prayer:*

God, grant me the:

Serenity to accept the things I cannot change;

Courage to change the things I can; and

Wisdom to know the difference!

We'll get back to these considerations in a moment. But first, it is also significant to note, speaking of "four," that *we* live in a *four-dimensional, space/time* universe that includes three spatial dimensions (width, height, and depth), and one time dimension. Within this four-dimensional universe, our body is organized spatially into three basic dimensional *scales* (see Chapter 1):

1. Atomic (almost entirely the elements carbon, oxygen, hydrogen, and nitrogen).

2. Molecular (basically, carbohydrates and fats for fuel and insulation, proteins for structure and function, and nucleic acids for control, reproduction, and heritage).

3. Continuum (larger scale cells, tissues, organs, and systems).

These three levels of organization, in compliance with *Feature 7* (Procreation), and the concept of *sexual* reproduction, have resulted in a division of human gender into two distinct *sexes*. Thus, the human species is comprised of the:

- *male* gender (boys, and men anatomically designed to fertilize an egg)
- *female* gender (girls, and women anatomically designed to bear offspring).

Unfortunately, extrapolations derived from (among others): the dichotomy of *gender*, the right/left *lateralization* of the body (Chapter 13), *diurnal* day/night cycles, and so on, have caused some to divide the *entire human experience*, into two distinct parts, often diametrically opposed. Recall that this either/or theory was promulgated by Descartes and has come to be known as *dualism* (see Chapter 9). The bad news is that points of view that are narrowminded enough to be constrained by a dichotomy formulation, lead to unnecessarily heated debates between, for example, science and religion; "rational" thinking and "emotional" reacting (the old mind/body nemesis); the *arts* and the *sciences*, and so on, but we will not go there in this book (the interested reader is referred to Schneck 2011, 2012).

Rather, as advertised, we complete the paradigm with the body's ultimate drive to *survive*—its single, *au fond* purpose! And again, "survive" is actually an umbrella term for the organism's efforts to satisfy its basic needs. Recall that these are reflected in systemic *operating set-points (*see "Paw-to-jaw" reflexes in Chapters 5 and 8; stationarity in Chapter 6; survival of the self, species, and soul in Chapter 8 (including "fight-or-flight" instincts); and all of Chapters 9–13). That having been said, and realizing that we have already spent a great deal of time on the 7–6–5 and 3–2–1 steps of our paradigm, it is now appropriate to go back and take a closer look at the four levels of control itemized above, because they should be of particular interest to the music therapists. Before we do so, however, a disclaimer.

We have emphasized all along that specific numbers and quantified data reported for the human body are "typical" averages—"norms" that can vary widely in real life. They are offered only as statistical means, and not as "hard and fast" values that are without exception. So, here again, we note that the following itemized categories of control are for purposes of discussion only, and are not "black and white." Several of the items listed can easily fit into more than one category, and others are clearly in "gray areas." Indeed, the traditional answer to any question related to anatomy and physiology is, "It depends!" With that in mind, consider the following "levels of control."

Control level 1: things you are "stuck with," like it or not

There are certain aspects of the human experience over which we have absolutely no control. Indeed, there are surprisingly many of them, more than you might realize, hence, "God grant me the serenity to *accept* the things I *cannot* change, no matter what!" A few of these are:

- The basic laws of physics (nature, see Chapter 8). When you step off the edge of a cliff, it doesn't much matter whether you believe in or subscribe to the laws of gravity, or not, does it? They are what they are, and we must live with them, period! We have no choice, no control.

- Who your biological parents were. In fact, here's a sobering thought, if your biological parents had never met, and if proper conception, followed by a successful pregnancy, had never been consummated, you would not be reading this right now because you would never have existed! (see Schneck 2001a, 2011, 2012). Thus, you have absolutely nothing to say about the "hand you were dealt," your heredity, your *LEGO set*, your genome.

- Similarly, regardless of whether you were actually raised by your biological parents, your adoptive ones, a foster home or whatever, you have no choice about who your relatives are, even if you choose to have little or nothing to do with them. They are who they are, period! You inherited *them*, as well as your genome.

- History! This is often a hard one to accept, but try as you might, what's happened, *happened*, what's done, is *done*—it's fact—it's undeniable, irrefutable. The historical landscape that is our heritage is etched in stone. Today is the first day of the rest of your life, and whatever happened prior to today is something you will simply have to live with. There is nothing you can do to change it; its only value might be pleasant (or *unpleasant*) memories, and perhaps, the valuable lessons you learned from your experiences to date. You cannot turn back the hands of time to undo (or relive) the past. Time starts *now* and moves only *forward*, which brings up yet another constraint over which we have no control.

- The merciless, relentless *forward motion of time.* Time marches on, whether we like it or not! *Tempus progrĕdĭor!* Sometimes it is *perceived* to move faster, sometimes slower (see Chapter 10: *The physiology of relativity*), but always forward, never backward! Science fiction might speculate about "time travel"…forget it!

- You had no control over *how* you were raised—nurtured—early in life, say, from birth through pre-school to age 5. Thus, during some of your most formative and impressionable periods in life, the "strings were being pulled" by somebody else.

- Similarly, you had nothing to say about *where* your early childhood was spent, especially if you were a child raised in a military (or any) family that moved a great deal. You might not have liked it, but there was absolutely nothing you could do about it (except run away from home, if you were so inclined, but that's not likely at such a young age). Nobody ever asked your opinion about where *you* wanted to live, and you had no input relative to the decisions that were made.

- The weather! Everybody talks about it, news programs spend a great deal of time reporting and "predicting" it, but nobody can do anything about it (or can they? See the second category below).

- Congenital/hereditary conditions, to wit, for example:

  ○ Albinism—absence of skin, hair, and eye pigments

  ○ Congenital hypothyroidism

  ○ Cystic fibrosis—pancreatic insufficiency; chronic pulmonary disease

  ○ Down syndrome, see Chapter 1

  ○ Haemophilia—greatly prolonged blood coagulation time

  ○ Rett syndrome—neurological disorder that affects girls almost exclusively

  ○ Spina bifida—lack of intervertebral union of laminae

  ○ Color blindness—inability to distinguish among primary colors (generally expressed in sets of three, i.e., cyanmagenta yellow; red yellow blue; red green blue, etc.)

  ○ Porphyria—inborn error of metabolism

  ○ Muscular dystrophy—wasting away of muscle tissue

…to name but a few!

- Aging—and the inevitability of death (or not).

Death and taxes... or just taxes?

The native son of Nova Scotia, Canada, lawyer, writer, politician, and judge Thomas Chandler Haliburton (1796–1865), once said, "Death and taxes are inevitable." More than likely, he was wrong…or at least not aware of future possibilities. That's because some 300 years later, say, by about circa 2150, his quote would have to be modified. By then, it will be simply, "Taxes are inevitable." Indeed, at the rate we are going, by 2150, we will have conquered the inevitability of our ultimate physiologic demise. Far be it for me to even attempt to discuss here the wisdom of seeking immortality; such discussion would result in a list of pros and cons that would fill volumes! But there is some merit in exploring why this goal is rapidly becoming realizable. Consider, for example, how the criteria for defining "death" have evolved and changed over the centuries.

In the earliest of times, simple *bodily movements* sufficed to establish a person's state of animation. If you moved, if you responded reflexively to sensory stimulation, then you were officially alive, otherwise, you were dead; that's it! Thus, those whose responsibility it was to determine the presence or absence of reflexive activity carried around with them such primitive diagnostic devices as knives, pins and other sharp objects with which they would poke the victims in an attempt to elicit some response.

Of course, this simple criterion was eventually recognized to be seriously flawed—one could be quite motionless and unresponsive, yet be still very much alive—and so a new "life gauge" had to be established, which was: if you were actively *breathing*, then you were "officially" alive, otherwise, you were dead. Moreover, just in case your breathing was too shallow to be observed visually by the heaving motions of your bosom, sharp, knife-like diagnostic instruments were replaced by mirrors. That is to say, those examining you would place a cool reflecting surface under your nose to see if it fogged up from the water vapor in your warm breath. If it did, there was hope; if it did not, your eventual fate was sealed, even if it meant being buried alive! Too bad!

As technology moved forward, there soon came into existence artificial respirators, heart-lung machines, and other breathing-assist devices that soon proved the then-current criterion for properly and accurately defining "death," to be equally inadequate. Along with that came an improved understanding of physiologic function, and more sophisticated diagnostic equipment—such as electrocardiograph (ECG) machines—to replace sharp instruments and reflective surfaces. Thus, the revised, new definition of death was now based on the presence or absence of a *pulse*, together with some degree of measureable electrical (ECG) activity to suggest that the heart was still functional, even if unaided breathing had, in fact, stopped. So now, police and private detectives in the movies and on television shows could be seen entering a room in which was lying a motionless body, feeling for a pulse in the carotid arteries or jugular veins of the neck, and declaring, "He's dead!"

But still further progress brought us cardio-tachometers, artificial heart-assist devices, cardioverters, defibrillators, pacemakers, and other resuscitation equipment that proved beyond a reasonable doubt that the absence of an ECG signal or pulse did not *necessarily* indicate that an individual was in a non-recoverable state of demise. On the contrary, we now know that the heart can be revived and kept functioning in situations where previously you would have been declared legally dead. In fact, we can even replace this vital organ with an anatomical transplant or totally implantable artificial heart, and you're practically as good as new!

So, now attention turned to the absence of brain activity as the new criterion for "death." Surely, if we detect no brain function, as measured by *electroencephalic (EEG)* recordings of cortical brain activity, you must certainly be dead! Or must you? Note that the brain activity that is routinely recorded in a clinical EEG is from the *cerebral cortex*, not the deeper regions of this organ, within which are located centers responsible for many life-sustaining activities. Thus, we now know that there can be an absence of *cortical* activity in situations where the patient continues to show signs of still being able to carry out unaided vital life functions—in some cases, even to the point of recovering fully from a long-term comatose condition.

A classic historical example of such longevity (although she did *not* eventually recover) is the highly publicized 1976 case of Karen Ann Quinlan, a 22-year-old who, by the above definition, was pronounced "legally dead" after lying in a moribound, comatose state for over a year at St. Clare's Hospital in Denville, New Jersey. Since she was in a vegetative state, devoid of any cognitive function, and since she had an abnormal, essentially flat EEG showing minimal cerebral activity, the New Jersey Supreme Court authorized her health-care providers to "pull the plug" on the resuscitation devices that were keeping her artificially alive—without the legal fear of being accused of medical malpractice subject to judicial reprisal. The hospital so-complied with the wishes of her parents. The plugs were pulled. Karen Ann Quinlan did eventually die—in June 1985—*after surviving nine years off resuscitation machines and life-support equipment!* So much for cortical brain function as a criterion for death!

In fact, in the wake of technological advancements and physiological research, so elusive has the concept of death become, that the health-care industry has essentially abandoned the use of this word in favor of an earlier criterion that went by the name of "irreversible coma" (Harvard Medical School 1968). The latter basically adds together all of the previous criteria. That is to say, it defines irreversible coma to be a state wherein:

- the patient shows complete *unreceptivity* and *unresponsitivity* to externally applied stimuli or internal needs (remember our sharp diagnostic instruments?)

- for at least one continuous hour, the patient exhibits no perceptible *movement*, including spontaneous, unaided breathing (remember our diagnostic mirrors?)

- the patient shows no *electromyographic* (EMG, muscle) activity, including any evidence of reflexive action

- an essentially flat ECG (*electrocardiogram*) exists in the absence of extracorporeal circulatory-assist devices (sound familiar?)

- an essentially flat *electroencephalogram* (EEG) exists, indicating minimal cortical brain activity (Harvard Medical School 1968)

- the above-defined state is confirmed by at least two other physicians completely unrelated to the case in question (i.e., not standing by, for example, waiting for an organ to become available to be transplanted into another one of their patients!).

Finally, if these six criteria are satisfied, the final decision to "pull the plug" does *not* become the responsibility of the patient's family, but of the physician in charge of the case, in consultation with one or more physicians who have been directly involved to that point.

But wait! What happens if we can "fix" what's wrong? You say the patient has a flat EEG, well how about we by-pass the damaged portions of the brain with synthetically engineered microchips that can be surgically implanted to completely restore structure and function? You say the patient has a flat ECG, how about we just put in a brand new, implantable, biocompatible, totally synthetic heart, complete with a permanent power pack, carefully controlled and paced so as to respond perfectly to the metabolic needs of the organism at any given time, and, of course, guaranteed for life? You need new sensory transducers—eyes, ears—we've got 'em! You need new joints—ankles, hips, knees—we've got 'em! Need new limbs—arms, legs—we've got those, too! Need a new liver, a new pancreas, a new kidney? No problem!

The fact is that thanks to incredible achievements in biomedical engineering and allied health sciences, we can replace just about every single organ or tissue in the human body—teeth, skin, larynx, heart valves, blood vessels, muscles, tendons, blood…you name it, we can replace it. Furthermore, not only do we have available synthetic, human-made, totally implantable artificial parts, but in many cases these are even better than the ones they are replacing! Indeed, the "bionic man or woman" is no longer science fiction. Going still one step further, we can supply these organs and tissues in various colors, models, designer styles, configurations, shapes, and sizes (children, adults, etc.).

Physicians (if there are any) in the mid-21st century will routinely write prescriptions for any and all such artificial body parts. Patients will have these orders filled in the human anatomical technology section of their nearest Radio Shack or Walmart store (maybe even mailorder houses), where they can buy their new organs or tissues right off the shelf. Then, they will take these in to their local health-care facility to have them implanted on an out-patient basis "while you wait." Or, if you are perhaps one of those "do-it-yourself" types who would rather install the devices in the privacy of your own home, that, too, could be arranged through a quick "crash course" and user-friendly instruction paraphernalia. Whatever your preference, the technology is either already state of the art, or soon will be. What we are talking about is not purely hypothetical, it may even happen within our lifetime.

Back in Greek and Roman times, the average lifespan was about 20 years. Today, it is nearing 80 years; and it is expected to climb to over 85 years by 2030. By the year 2050, folks will routinely live well past 100! More than likely, by 2150, biomedical engineering technology, advances in stem-cell research, the marvels of genetic engineering, breakthroughs in innovative arenas that don't even exist yet, and "who knows what else" will basically make "death" an obsolete concept. One will have the choice of living just about as long as one wants to, provided, of course, that one will be able to afford the taxes! So, perhaps the "inevitability" of death belongs more appropriately in one or more of the following categories, as does taxation.

Control level 2: things over which you have very minimal, limited control, regardless of how hard you try

Included in this category are things such as:

- Your body's operating set-points that comply with its need to survive itself! (see Table 8.3, and vital signs).

- *Nature*, as expressed through anatomical/physiological constraints such as those discussed in:
    - Chapter 2: *An isothermal living engine*
    - Chapter 3: *Our optimized living engine*
    - Chapter 3: *Levers and principles of leverage*
    - Chapter 5: Anatomical limitations due to *adequate stimuli transduction constraints*—microscopic and telescopic technology can help here, hence the "minimal" control
    - Chapter 6: *Stationarity/homeostasis* constraints
    - Chapter 7: *Chirality*
    - Chapter 9: *Constraints to knowing*
    - Chapter 10: *Gestalt Laws of perception*
    - Chapter 10: *The physiology of relativity*
    - All of Chapter 12: *Physiological optimization principles*
    - All of Chapter 13: *Anatomical design principles*

…you get the point! This category is all about *being human* and accepting/dealing with all of the frailties that go along with it!

- *Nurture*—how you were raised, say, from the age of 6 through to 12 (primary education years), including your school teachers.

- *Natural disasters*, such as earthquakes, hurricanes, tornadoes, tsunamis, and so on. In fact, technically, these should be listed in category 1 above, because we really have *no* control over them. Putting them in this category is just a way of saying that, with sufficient advance warning, we can at least *prepare* for them and take remedial action to anticipate and minimize the consequences. Indeed, one can make the same argument for our having a *minimal* control over the weather, even thought the latter *is, arbitrarily,* listed in category 1.

- Unforeseen, unanticipated, unexpected events—*serendipity* being among them (Schneck 2008b).

- How *others* behave. Try as you might, in the end, you actually have very limited (almost *no*) control over how other people live *their* lives. The only life you can live is your *own*.

- Our global/universal *ecosystem(s)*, including how we deal with natural resources, the environment, the effects of global warming, factors related to climate control, etc. (This item, too, could just as easily be included in the next category, as well.)

- Death and taxes, but see earlier discussion of irreversible coma.

- Certain congenital/hereditary/medical conditions, perhaps effectively controlled by surgical, pharmaceutical, or other means of intervention (including music therapy?), for example:
  - cleft lip/palate—fissure/crevice formation
  - club foot—non-traumatic foot deviation
  - congenital diaphragmatic hernia (tear in tissue)
  - congenital heart defects
  - neonatal jaundice—yellowness due to bile pigment deposits
  - nystagmus—constant involuntary movement of the eye balls
  - umbilical hernia (tear)
  - orthopaedic issues
  - food allergies/intolerance (see Chapter 2)
  - learning/behavioral/hyperactive/autistic issues

...to name just a few!

- The sex of your offspring. One has rather limited control over whether a child born naturally of biological parents will be a boy or a girl. For the most part, it's a roll of the dice! Except, of course, in cases of artificial insemination, *in vitro* fertilization, etc.

Control level 3: things over which you have *substantial* control

We come now to constraining factors over which we have substantial, if not total, control, *provided* we choose to exercise it! It is hoped, these, and those that follow in control level 4 below, are situations for which *the courage to change the things that I can* apply. Included, for example, are:

- Electing political and other leaders—voting.

- Choosing a mate (it is hoped, by mutual consent!), and consummating the drive for sexual fulfillment. This goes to establishing the operating set-points for satisfying the second strongest of all human drives—that for *survival of the species*. It also presumes that you are not bound by cultural norms and/or religious traditions. The choice is entirely yours.

- Your friends/role models/acquaintances/colleagues—the "circles" with which you choose to associate yourself and those with whom you decide to "hang around" and allow to influence you. (This item could also easily be included in control level 4 below.)

- How you raise your children, including the role model *you* choose to be, for them, and for others to emulate. How you choose to live *your* life, as opposed to trying to live somebody else's. What you *do* with the "LEGO set" (genome) with which you have been entrusted; what part(s) of it get expressed, what part(s) are *suppressed*.

- Your destiny (the control of which is the fourth strongest of all human drives). This includes things such as: your higher education, career path, employment, lifestyle, etc.

- All of the operating set-points that are established to satisfy anthropocentric needs, such as those described in Chapter 9.

- Your health; your energy levels; your stress levels (see Chapter 8), including how you *handle* controversy, the unexpected, and set-backs. In control levels 1 and 2, we addressed health issues over which you have little, or no control. Here, we have in mind more mundane health concerns, such as:
  - the common cold
  - everyday aches and pains
  - minor headaches
  - fatigue
  - eye, ear, nose, and throat (EENT) issues
  - routine dental maintenance
  - foot problems such as bunions, plantar fasciitis, etc.

- ○ "tennis elbow" and other forms of tendinitis

- ○ seasonal pollen allergies

- ○ "acid stomach" and other gastrointestinal issues

…again to name just a few.

- Your faith—what you choose to believe, and the means you pursue to satisfy the third strongest of all human drives, the need for *spiritual fulfillment.* The reason this item is included here, and not in control level 4, is that depending on how you were raised, your mentors, role models, etc., you might not have *total* control over your faith, but certainly, *substantial* control.

- Where you decide to ultimately settle down, live, retire, etc.

- Proper exercise.

Which brings us to control level 4.

Control level 4: things over which you have *total* control

Again, there are many in this category, but to name just a few:

- How you treat *yourself!* Don't become your own worst enemy. Indeed, *nosce te ipsum—know thyself first!* Recognize that, "Each of us is a minority of one!" (Schneck 2001a); and for heaven's sake, don't "should" yourself. Get acquainted with the "you" that resides within your own body (see Chapter 9) and strive to genuinely *like* that person! Answer in a very personal way the questions posed in this book, i.e., "What is this thing called 'me,' and How does 'me' work?" (It would help to review Chapters 8 and 9, and see also Schneck 2012).

- How you treat *others*, especially as it relates to your *expectations* of them and your consideration of *their* various limitations and frailties. Would *you* do what you ask of *them?* Are you fair?

- The *extent* to which you *allow* yourself to be influenced by others, such as the news media, books, your peers, social media, radio, movies, television, magazines, family, friends, relatives, clergy, etc.

- *Bad habits*, such as smoking, drinking, drug abuse, laziness, a, shall we say, less-than-admirable lifestyle?

- *Good habits*, such as living by the *Golden Rule*, punctuality, reliability, *honesty*, forthrightness, generosity, and so on.

- Your body mass index (BMI, see Table 8.3 of Chapter 8 for details). Your weight (or losing it!).

- Your diet and eating habits, especially as they relate to food sensitivities and allergies; maintaining a "healthy" weight; staying away from "junk foods," etc. (see Chapter 2).

- Proper rest and relaxation, especially getting enough sleep daily.

- Your hobbies and leisure activities.

- Your "worldly" possessions—cars, houses, furniture, etc.

Notice something interesting about these last two levels of control? They all involve *you!* You have *no*—or, at best—very *limited* control over the laws of physics, the weather, the universe, history, natural disasters, cycles of the Earth, your genome, etc. But you have *substantial*, and in many cases, *total*, control over *yourself* and how you choose to live your life.

So, having thus completed our paradigm, let's close with a final question for the music therapist to consider: "Knowing what I now know about the structure and function of the living human body/instrument, how can I intervene clinically to effectively exploit the role of music in affecting physiologic function, in order to treat and manage diagnosed populations?" In other words…

From theory to practice

As was pointed out in the Introduction, the role of the music therapist is to *resolve* physiologic dissonance (an "out-of-tune" anatomical *instrument* which is the human body) into physiologic consonance (a "tuned-up" engine that is "hitting on all cylinders"). In the limit, the therapist endeavors to come as close as possible to establishing a physiological state of *coenesthesia*. What, exactly, is that?

Coenesthesia or, for short, cenesthesia

Cenesthesia is a theoretical physiological state that can only be approached asymptotically. As we shall see, it is not an actual realization. Derived from the prefix *coen-*, which means "common, general" and the word-root, *-esthesia*, which means "sensibility, feeling," *coenesthesia* refers to a "common feeling," connoting well-being. It is used clinically to describe the physiologic state of euphoria, wherein all organ systems are functioning in perfect, synchronized harmony, in "common" with one another. Their activities are perfectly coordinated; they are all in perfect health; and the individual experiencing this state is totally happy, stress-free, and "without a care in the world!"

Obviously, this is a hypothetical, idealized state, because it is easily upset by any form of disease, malfunction, and/or *stress*. In particular, the latter is an unavoidable fact of life! (See Chapter 8 and our earlier discussion of the four levels of control within which one is constrained to function.) That having been said, one cannot deny that certain forms of music can bring an individual closer to this euphoric condition. Furthermore, history has shown that music can certainly do so better than any other form of human experience. Why? The short answer is to advise you to reread Part II of this book, "How Does 'Me' Work?" to explore some possibilities for how music (and the music therapist) can help to resolve the issues raised in diagnosed populations.

The longer answer is to recognize, as also pointed out in the Introduction, that the key to effective clinical intervention using music therapy is to:

First figure out what's wrong

1. Through proper *assessment, diagnose* and *define* the *operating set-points* (Chapters 8 and 9) that are driving this person.

2. By clinical history, diagnostic tests, and observation, establish the *means*—behavioral or otherwise—by which this individual is attempting to function, in an effort to *satisfy* the needs reflected in those operating set-points.

3. Utilizing the knowledge gleaned from Parts I and II of this book, develop an anatomical/physiological *paradigm* that "connects the dots" between steps 1 and 2 above.

4. *Integrate* the results of your assessment thus far to determine which of this individual's operating set-points are at issue (i.e., problematic), and thus need to be changed, preferably by exploiting mechanisms of *musical entrainment* and *functional adaptation* (such as are discussed in Chapter 12). Ask yourself:

   a) Are we dealing here with *anatomical* problems—structural, congenital, those having to do with *nature?*

   b) Are we dealing here with *physiological* problems—functional, behavioral, those having to do with *nurture?*

   c) Are we dealing with some combination of *both?*

   d) What are all of the variables, including confounding ones, that are contributing to the problems at issue here? Then:

      ° Do we have a complete list of them?

      ° Which ones can be controlled?

      ° Which ones can't, and how do we deal with them?

   With respect to the sensory and central nervous systems (Chapters 4, 5, 10, and 11:

   e) Are the problems on the *input* end, i.e., related to sensory stimulation and/or *transduction* issues?

    f) Do the problems involve faulty *processing* of information, i.e., issues related to:

- sensory *transmission;* neurotransmitters, neural networks

- cerebral *information-processing rate;* dropouts; tagging; primary, secondary and/or tertiary memory; etc.

- sensory *integration; translation;* Gestalt Laws, reconstruction.

    g) Are the problems on the *output* end, dealing with issues of physiologic entrainment and accommodation?

Are there known contributing/confounding variables, such as:

    h) Inherited genetic disorders (see Chapter 1 Down syndrome, Chapter 2 food allergies, Chapter 3 congenital hypothyroidism and Grave's disease, and conditions listed earlier in this chapter, etc.).

    i) Family/peer/social problems.

    j) Endocrine issues, especially involving stress hormones (see Chapters 7 and 8).

    k) Musculoskeletal issues involving motor planning, balance and equilibrium, leverage, etc. (see Chapter 3).

    l) Issues associated with the autism spectrum.

    m) Issues related to the *fear cycle* (Schneck and Berger 2006).

The list is, indeed, long, but needs to be addressed in detail if the ensuing intervention is to be meaningful and effective.

5. Continuing with the assessment/diagnosis, inquire as to whether or not there are *measureable* clinical parameters that can be (or have been) *operationally* defined (i.e., *quantifiable*), and have direct relevance to all of the above. Parameters that define relevant anthropometric/anatomic variables, as well as physiological/morphological ones. If so, obtain as many of these clinical records and diagnostic procedures as can be made available to you. If not, recommend them!

6. Ask yourself, "What additional information would help me make a clear, unambiguous diagnosis as to what, exactly, is wrong with my client, so that I can develop an effective treatment plan/intervention protocol based on objective, "hard" evidence, rather than guessing?"

7. Finally, using a type of *differential diagnosis*, by process of elimination, determine what *type* of musical intervention will prove to be most effective in changing the "problem set-points" defined. Ask yourself, "Based on my assessment of this client:

- what elements of music

- in what combinations

- delivered in what forms

- in accordance with what established dose-response criteria

- under what types of conditions

- for how long

- how often

- for how many total sessions

will be most effective in accomplishing my objectives with this client, i.e., will reasonably ensure that the right 'medicine' is being prescribed for the right condition, and that the problems identified are being satisfactorily resolved?" Having answered this question, you can now move on.

Second, do something about it!

On dose-response relationships

Based on:

- the anatomical/physiological considerations, and corresponding formulations developed in this book

- thorough, effective clinical diagnosis, as described above

- available, published criteria in the technical literature, reporting on proven methods of effective clinical intervention using music...

the practicing music therapist should be able to develop successful clinical intervention protocols—including *dose-response relationships*—that take into consideration and account for the following (corresponding elements of music, where appropriate, are shown in parentheses):

1. The *type* of music that should be used to treat *this specific client*, i.e.:

    - Its historical *period*—Middle Ages (450–1450); Renaissance (1450–1600); Baroque (1600–1750); Classical (1750–1820); Romantic (1820–1900); Contemporary (1900–1950); Modern (1950 to date).

    - Its musical *form*—repetition, contrast, variations, tertiary (three-part, ABA form); binary (two-part, AB form); continuous, undivided forms; fugue; sonata, symphony, concerto, broadway musicals, mono-/polyphonic, ballet, opera, operetta, oratorio, suites, rondo.

- Its musical *style*, e.g., improvisation, vocal chants, madrigals, a capella, orchestral, secular, sacred, gospel, jazz, pop, hip-hop, big band, country and western, rock and roll, reggae, blue-grass, ballad, Appalachian, dance/disco, folk, song, ragtime, "classical," Latin American, non-Western (koto, raga, African, Indian, Middle East).

- The *modality* of presentation—audio, visual, tactile, some combination of these; distracting influences (noise, smell, other things going on in the room; client's mood at the time, etc.).

- The *medium* of presentation—indoor, outdoor, large concert hall, small chamber auditorium, smaller music room; instrumental, vocal, specific performers (singers, instrumentalists, groups, etc.); record albums, CDs, DVDs, audio tapes, videotapes, radio, TV.

2. The *dose*, i.e., the:

- *quantity* of music to which the client is exposed (how much?)

- *frequency* of such exposure (how often?)

- *duration* of each session (how long?)

- *time of day* at which the exposure occurs (when?)

- *time of year* during which the exposure takes place (when?)

- number of *breaks*—during each session and between sessions—and *how long* each one is. There may be an optimum to both.

3. The *elements* of music exploited to achieve the desired results:

- Loudness/softness (*dynamics*)

- Vocal ranges and/or instruments employed, including optimum registers (*timbre; clefs*)

- Specific key signatures (*harmony*), keeping in mind that (see Schneck and Berger 2006):

    ○ *tonic modes* (e.g., the key of *C Major* and the chords, chord progressions and harmonies that define this key)—because of their inherent *stability* and "grounding" (they are, indeed, the *strongest* tonal factor in music)—can be quite effective in controlling highly aggressive, *passionate* behavior (associated with the color, *red*) or, its opposite extreme: timidity and shyness. Prophet and Spadaro (2000) suggest that the body organs and systems most responsive to *tonic modes* are the heart and blood vessels (i.e., the cardiovascular system) and the thymus gland. The authors also suggest that the most effective instrument for expressing these modes is the *harp*.

o *super-tonic modes* (e.g., the key of *D Major*), which tend to become absorbed into sub-dominant modes (see below), might have some (as yet ill-defined) relationship to the human drive for sexual fulfillment and so, quite logically, are most associated with the organs and systems of reproduction (and their cousins, those of elimination, including the kidneys). These modes are most associated with the color *orange*; and, according to Prophet and Spadaro (2000), the *woodwind* family of instruments are very effective in expressing super-tonic moods.

o *mediant modes* (e.g., *E Major*)—because of their *moody* and "sobering" nature—can be a beneficial intervention when dealing with the need to balance one's egotistical sense of superiority, or its opposite: inferiority (traditionally associated with the color, *yellow*). These modes tend, also, to be very cerebral, and hence, the body's nervous system, cerebral cortex, and pineal gland *entrain* mediant modes the best, as expressed most effectively by the entire *string* family.

o *sub-dominant modes* (e.g., *F Major*)—by virtue of their inherent sense of balance and equilibrium—can induce feelings of joy and expansiveness (not unlike those derived from sexual fulfillment). These modes, associated with the blend of colors, *yellow-green*, tend to evoke a positive image of one's self and, as such, are also associated with certain portions of the brain and the *master* (pituitary) gland. The musculoskeletal system, too, is recruited for issues related to *proprioception*, balance, and equilibrium. The *piano* seems to be the instrument of choice for expressing these modes (Prophet and Spadaro 2000).

o *dominant modes* (e.g., *G Major*), as a balancing complement to mediant modes, and in support of tonic modes, have a *centering effect* on physiologic function, driving the body toward a better sense of balance, equilibrium, stability, and calmness. The *brass family* of instruments that seem to express this mode best are reflective of its association with the lungs and respiratory system, the throat, and the thyroid and parathyroid glands located in this same anatomical region. And here, again, *entrainment* through the musculoskeletal system can also address issues of balance and equilibrium. The blend of colors most associated with dominant modes are *green-blue*.

o *sub-mediant modes* (e.g., *A Major*), as a complement to super-tonic modes (but with much less influence on tonality), can, because of their ability to invoke feelings of tranquility and peace, be an effective intervention in managing sleep/wake activity. Interestingly, the system of the body with which these modes are most associated is the digestive system, along with its complementary organs, the liver and pancreas. The blend of colors associated with sub-mediant modes are *blue-violet;* and the instrument of choice for expressing them is the *organ.*

○ finally, *leading-tone modes* (e.g., *B Major*), as a complement to tonic modes and because of their drive towards the tonic, can contribute to the sense of satisfaction derived from *resolution.* Recall that this is also associated with the same physiological/physical principles that relate to one's seeking *closure* of dissonant harmonies into consonant ones. As such, therefore, the brain, autonomic nervous, and endocrine systems play a major role here, especially the adrenal glands; and *percussion instruments,* perhaps because of their endogenous rhythmic *drive,* seem best suited to express these modes. Similarly, the blend of colors, *violet-red,* coming full circle in the visible spectrum ("resolving"), tend to be most associated with leading-tone musical modes.

Indeed, we have come full-circle in the major instrumental sections of a symphony orchestra, the diatonic scale of major key signatures, and the visible spectrum, except to mention the in-between steps of the 12-tone scale. Thus, we have the blend of colors:

- *red-orange,* associated with $C^{\#}$ (or D^{b} in a tempered system)
- *orange-yellow,* associated with $D^{\#}$ (or a tempered E^{b})

and the pure colors:

- *green,* associated with $F^{\#}$ (tempered G^{b})
- *blue,* associated with $G^{\#}$ (tempered A^{b})
- *violet,* associated with $A^{\#}$ (tempered B^{b}).

Thus, continuing with the elements of music:

- Specific time signatures and meter settings (*rhythm:* pulse, pace, pattern; tempo: lento, largo, allegro, allegretto, presto, vivace, etc.).
- Specific moods (*melody, harmony, rhythm, timbre, dynamics, form*).
- Specific articulation (*prosody*—tenuto, marcato, staccato, legato, accents, ties, repeats, crescendo, diminuendo, fermata, retard, etc.).

Clinical intervention, "driving the system," "playing the instrument," anticipating results

Okay, so you now have a plan:

- You've diagnosed and assessed your client.
- Based on that assessment, you've developed a protocol for musical intervention.

- You exercise that protocol, "driving the system;" "playing the instrument;" subjecting the body to a "forcing function" that is persistent sensory stimulation through music.

The major mechanisms of action of musical stimulation is via its effects on: (i) sensory *transduction;* (ii) sensory *transmission;* (iii) sensory *translation;* (iv) anatomic *entrainment;* (v) physiologic *adaptation;* and, as a result, (vi) a resetting of *operating set-points* to more optimum values.

Sensory *transduction* is affected by persistent musical stimulation, to the extent that exposure to such repetitive stimulation can eventually re-set *existing* (see Chapters 1, 4, and 5) neural:

- resting potentials
- receptor potentials
- threshold potentials
- depolarization potentials
- action potentials
- sensory adaptation mechanisms, and hence
- response characteristics and sensitivity of the nerves involved, optimizing their performance.

The *transmission* of sensory data *to* (afferent) the central nervous system is affected by musical stimulation, to the extent that exposure to such repetitive stimulation can eventually influence (see Chapters 1, 3, 6, and 10) the:

- generation of *new* neural networks (*plasticity; neogenesis*)
- re-direction of information-processing networks via existing *collateral* neural pathways and trajectories
- reconfiguration and *biasing* of existing neural pathways
- *synchronization* and *coordination* of neural and neuro-musculoskeletal activity through *rhythm entrainment*
- excitation/inhibition/expression of genetic material, such as proteins, hormones, neurotransmitters, antibodies, second messengers, and enzymes, via *resonance* phenomena
- transport and utilization of energy
- metabolism of the body, as a result of all of the above.

Sensory *translation* is affected by persistent musical stimulation, to the extent that exposure to such repetitive stimulation can influence (see Chapters 4 and 6–13):

- information-processing rates
- conversion of afferent data into meaningful information
- sensory differentiation/integration
- cognitive processing of information; *consciousness*
- the body's response to stress and the *fear cycle* (Schneck and Berger 2006)
- the generation of efferent motor signals
- primary, secondary, and tertiary *memory*
- the establishment of optimized operating set-points.

As discussed in the text (especially, Chapter 12), all of the above affect systemic outputs through mechanisms of anatomical/physiological *entrainment* and *functional adaptation*, which lead to:

- memory of sensation, and *facilitation*, which eventually becomes a
- *conditioned* (as opposed to instinctive) reflex pathway, which ultimately triggers the
- *adaptive* process, wherein "rewired" neural networks now establish
- revised, optimized homeostatic/stationary/behavioral operating set-points (Chapters 12 and 13).

But we are not done yet…

Finally, track and evaluate how well you and the client are doing

Ask yourself the following. Have I:

- established an effective means for *tracking* both *my* progress, and that of my *client*, in achieving the objectives of the clinical intervention program?
- successfully "hit" client-specific target goals and plateaus?
- been able to relate our progress *specifically* to the musical intervention protocol? That is to say, is there a well-defined, clearly manifest cause/effect relationship in evidence here? Good science and credibility criteria demand it, if music therapy is to be recognized as a viable, effective means for clinical intervention; and if music therapist expect to be accepted as clinical professionals among their health-care colleagues?
- based on progress, or lack thereof, identified what criteria to use to make "mid-course corrections" as necessary?
- developed a "Plan B" protocol for administering those mid-course corrections?

- made sure to integrate and coordinate my form of musical intervention with other treatments/therapies that the client is receiving, e.g., vocational, physical, art, etc. therapies?

- made sure to do the same with respect to whatever else is going on in my client's life at the time, e.g., problems at home, in school, with his/her peers, and so on?

In summary

We began this book with a quote from Shakespeare: *"What a piece of work is a man!"…* *"The paragon of animals!"* Realizing, of course, that although he used the word "man" Shakespeare meant "*human*" (i.e., it was not uncommon in Shakespeare's day to describe *all* humans using the biblically motivated male gender, as in *mankind*) and he used the word "*paragon*" to express, "a model of excellence or perfection." Indeed, the word derives from the Greek prefix *para-*, meaning "on the side," and *akónē*, meaning "whetstone," as in "a stone for sharpening knives or tools." Hence, *paragon* connotes having been sharpened—refined, perfected, optimized. Having read this book, I hope you developed the same respect, admiration, and appreciation for the beauty and perfection of this human "instrument" that I have in over 50 years of studying it. The human body is, indeed, an *incredible machine.*

But…so is *music*—the *incredible sensory stimulus* invented by this *incredible machine!* True, birds sing and other manifestations of acoustic energy can be described as being *melodic* and "lyrical." But *music*—defined as consisting of basic elements that include rhythm, melody, harmony, timbre, dynamics, and form—is strictly a human-made commodity. It was invented by humans as a useful, convenient, effective means for satisfying basic human needs and drives.

The transformative power of music derives from several things:

- First, it is a *passive* form of perception, in the sense that it requires only to be *experienced*, not interpreted, as is the case, for example, with verbal language. There is no specific education, training, or preparation required to "just" experience music!

- Second, music exploits the fact that we are creatures of *emotion*, not reason. Music "plays" on our emotions, "yanks" at our heart strings, "soothes" the savage beast, communicates with the body via stimuli to which it is most responsive, and anatomical pathways/networks that are unique to this specific type of syntax.

- Third, music shares a *symbiotic* relationship with the human body; it wouldn't exist without us (i.e., we *create* it), and we cannot exist without it (i.e., it *satisfies* basic human needs), which is to say, we *both* benefit from each other. Indeed, historically, there has never existed a civilization devoid of some form of music!

- Fourth, as pointed out throughout the book (especially in Part II), music and the human body share in common many structural and functional attributes, not the least of which are "natural" tempos (the *rhythm of life*), and architectural scales (*similarity*).

- Fifth, it's readily, and relatively easily accessible. It's everywhere: radio, television, movies, CDs, DVDs, concert halls, etc.

- Sixth, music and the human body *speak* a common *universal language*. It doesn't matter whether you are young or old, male or female, African-American or Albino, suffering from Down syndrome or autism, tall or short, fat or skinny, Western-European or from the Middle-East, the 7–6–5–4–3–2–1 paradigm works the same way for *all* of us. Music understands and works within that paradigm to elicit profound responses!

So, the answer to the question, "Why music?" is, simply, "Why not?"

Furthermore, having read this book, I also hope that you will have developed an appreciation for how important it is for the practicing music therapist to have an understanding of "What is this thing called 'Me?'," and "How does 'Me' work?" Without a fundamental knowledge of basic anatomy and physiology, one cannot effectively determine "what's wrong?" much less "do something about it!" and even less, meaningfully "track and evaluate how well you and the client are doing!" Indeed, it is my hope that this book will help to establish the criteria by which one can achieve effective management of diagnosed populations, using music as the mode of clinical intervention.

References

Ackerman, D. (1990) *A Natural History of the Senses*. New York: Random House.

Alexjander, S. and Deamer, D. (1999) "The infrared frequencies of DNA bases." *IEEE Engineering in Medicine and Biology*, 18, 2, 74–79.

Berger, D.S. (2002) *Music Therapy, Sensory Integration and the Autistic Child*. London: Jessica Kingsley Publishers.

Baker, C. and Miller, J.B. (eds) (2006) *The Evolution Dialogues: Science, Christianity, and the Quest for Understanding*. Washington, D.C.: American Association for the Advancement of Science.

Berger, D.S. (2015) *Eurhythmics for Autism and Other Neurophysiologic Diagnoses: A Sensorimotor Music-Based Treatment Approach*. London: Jessica Kingsley Publishers.

Berger, D.S. and Schneck, D.J. (2003) "The role of music therapy as a clinical intervention for physiologic functional adaptation." *Journal of Scientific Exploration, Winter Edition*, 17, 4, 687–703.

Buser, P. and Imbert, M. (1992) *Audition* (translated by R.H. Kay). Cambridge, Massachusetts: MIT Press; A Bradley Book.

Coren, S. and Ward, L.M. (1989) *Sensation and Perception, Third Edition*. San Diego, California: Harcourt Brace Jovanovich Publishers.

Cutler, A.G. and Hensyl, E.R. (co-managing eds) (1976) *Stedman's Medical Dictionary, 23rd Edition*. Baltimore, Maryland: Williams and Wilkins.

Dennett, D.C. (1991) *Consciousness Explained*. Boston, Massachussetts: Little, Brown and Company.

Deutsch, S. and Micheli-Tzanakou, E. (1987) *Neuroelectric Systems*. New York: New York University Press.

Duck, F. (1990) *Physical Properties of Tissue: A Comprehensive Reference Book*. San Diego, California: Academic Press, Inc.

Edwards, B. (1989) *Drawing on the Right Side of the Brain*. New York: G.P. Putnam's Sons.

Findlay, E. (1971) *Rhythm and Movement: Applications of Dalcroze Eurhymics*. Van Nuys, California: Summy-Birchard, Inc.

Frazier, A.A. (1974) *Coping With Food Allergy*. New York: Quadrangle Books.

Giancoli, D.C. (1989) *Physics for Scientists and Engineers: With Modern Physics*. Englewood Cliffs, New Jersey: Prentice Hall.

Goss, C.M. (ed.) (1966) *Gray's Anatomy of the Human Body, 28th Edition*. Philadelphia, Pennsylvania: Lea and Febiger.

Graedon, J. and Graedon, T. (2007) *Best Choices from the People's Pharmacy.* New York: Rodale Press.

Harvard Medical School (1968) "A definition of irreversible coma: report of an ad hoc committee." *JAMA,* 205, 6, 337–340.

Jacob, S.W., Francone, C.A., and Lossow, W.J. (1982) *Structure and Function in Man: Fifth Edition.* Philadelphia, Pennsylvania: W.B. Saunders Company.

Junge, D. (1981) *Nerve and Muscle Excitation, Second Edition.* Sunderland, California: Sinauer Associates, Inc.

Kinne, R.K.H. (1989) *Structure and Function of the Kidney.* New York: Karger.

Lentner, C. (ed.) *Geigy Scientific Tables:* (1981) *Volume 1: Units of Measurement; Body Fluids; Composition of the Body; Nutrition.* (1982) *Volume 2: Introduction to Statistics; Statistical Tables Mathematical Formulae;* (1984): *Volume 3: Physical Chemistry; Composition of Blood; Hematology; Somatometric Data;* (1986): *Volume 4: Biochemistry; Metabolism of Xenobiotics; Inborn Errors of Metabolism; Pharmacogenetics and Ecogenetics* (1990): *Volume 5: Heart and Circulation.* West Caldwell, New Jersey: CIBA-GEIGY Corporation.

Liebert, R.M. and Spiegler, M.D. (1994) *Personality: Strategies and Issues; Seventh Edition.* Pacific Grove, California: Brooks/Cole.

Lots, I.S. and Stone, L. (2008) "Perception of musical consonance and dissonance." *Journal of the Royal Society: Interface;* Published online: doi: 10.1098/rsif.2008.0143; Available at: http://journals.royalsociety.org. Accessed 10 October 1998.

MacLean, P.D. (1990) *The Triune Brain in Evolution: Role in Paleocerebral Functions.* New York: Plenum Press.

McGovern, T. and Waldbaum, R.S. (1985) *The Kidneys: Balancing the Fluids.* New York: Torstar Books, Inc.

Nin, Anaïs (1961) *Seduction of the Minotaur* (self-published).

Orlock, C. (1993) *Inner Time: The Science of Body Clocks and What Makes Us Tick.* New York: Birch Lane Press.

Ornstein, R. and Thompson, R.E. (1984) *The Amazing Brain.* Boston, Massachussetts: Houghton Mifflin Company.

Plato (1992) *The Republic.* Trans. Grube, G.M.A. (1948) revised Reeve, C.D.C. (1992) Indianapolis, Indiana: Hackett Publishing Company. Original work written ca. 380 B.C.E. Indianapolis, Indiana; Hackett Publishing Company.

Prophet, E.C. and Spadaro, P.R. (2000) *Your Seven Energy Centers.* Corwin Springs, Montana: Summit University Press.

Roederer, J.G. (1975) *Introduction to the Physics and Psychophysics of Music.* New York: Springer.

Rose, K.J. (1989) *The Body In Time.* New York: John Wiley & Sons.

Schneck, D.J. (1990) *Engineering Principles of Physiologic Function.* New York: New York University Press.

Schneck, D.J. (1992) *Mechanics of Muscle, Second Edition.* New York: New York University Press.

Schneck, D.J. (2000a) "Mind/Body…both, or neither?" *American Laboratory,* 22, 14, 6–7.

Schneck, D.J. (2000b) "Cardiovascular Mechanics." Chapter 19 in J.D. Enderle, S.M. Blanchard, and J.D. Bronzino (eds) *Introduction to Biomedical Engineering.* San Diego: Academic Press.

Schneck, D.J. (2001a) "Each of us is a minority of one." *American Laboratory,* 33, 1, 6–8.

Schneck, D.J. (2001b) "On the seven elements of knowledge." *American Laboratory,* 33, 15, 4.

Schneck, D.J. (2004) "Food allergies." *American Laboratory News Edition,* 36, 9, 4–6.

Schneck, D.J. (2005a) "What is this thing called, 'me'? Part 2: Attributes that classify the human body as being 'alive'." *American Laboratory News Edition,* 37, 11, 4–6.

Schneck, D.J. (2005b) "What is this thing called, 'me'? Part 3: The living *isothermal* engine." *American Laboratory,* 37, 14, 4–8.

Schneck, D.J. (2005c) *SEARCHING.* Shelton, Connecticut: International Scientific Publications.

Schneck, D.J. (2006a) "What is this thing called, 'me'? Part 4: The *buffered,* isothermal living engine." *American Laboratory News Edition,* 38, 2, 4–8.

Schneck, D.J. (2006b) "What is this thing called, 'me'? Part 5: The *stationary,* buffered, isothermal, living engine." *American Laboratory,* 38, 10, 4–10.

Schneck, D.J. (2007a) "What is this thing called, 'me?' Part 7: The *organic* living engine." *American Laboratory, 39, 2, 6–10.*

Schneck, D.J. (2007b) "Dualism." *American Laboratory News Edition,* 39, 17, 6–8.

Schneck, D.J. (2007c) "On the seven paths to knowledge." *American Laboratory News Edition,* 39, 15, 4–6.

Schneck, D.J. (2008a) "Serendipity." *American Laboratory,* 40, 10, 4.

Schneck, D.J. (2008b) "What is this thing called, 'Me?' Part 13: *The Optimized, Temporally-Synchronized, Binary, Organic Living Engine,"* American Laboratory 40, 12, 4–6.

Schneck, D.J. (2009a) "What is this thing called, 'me?' Part 14: The *self-similar,* optimized, living engine." *American Laboratory,* 41, 4, 4–6.

Schneck, D.J. (2009b) "What is this thing called, 'me?' Part 16: The *decussating,* spatially-ordered, self-similar, optimized, living engine." *American Laboratory,* 41, 11, 4–6.

Schneck, D.J. (2011a) "Music, the body in time, and self-similarity concepts." *J. Biomusical Engineering,* 1, 1, 2–10. Article ID# M110102; doi:10.4172/2090-2719.1000102; Available at: www.omicsonline.com/open-access/ArchiveJBE/mostly-viewed-articles-biomusical-engineering-open-access.php. Accessed 15 September 2011.

Schneck, D.J. (2011b) *OMNIOLOGY: A Unified Approach to the Study of Everything.* Charleston, South Carolina: CreateSpace, a DBA of On-Demand Publishing, LLC.

Schneck, D.J. (2012) *Simple Wisdom: Alphabetical Reflections on the Nature of the Human Experience.* Floyd, Virginia: Wilder Publications, Inc.

Schneck, D.J. and Berger, D.S. (1999) "The role of music in physiologic accommodation: its ability to elicit reflexive, adaptive, and inscriptive responses." *IEEE Engineering in Medicine and Biology,* 18, 2, 44–53.

Schneck, D.J. and Berger, D.S. (2006) *The Music Effect: Music Physiology and Clinical Applications.* London: Jessica Kingsley Publishers.

Schneck, D.J. and Schneck, J.K. (1997) *Music In Human Adaptation*. Blacksburg, Virginia: Virginia Polytechnic Institute and State University Press/MMB Music, Inc.

Schneck, D.J. and Tempkin, A. (1992) *Biomedical Desk Reference*. New York: New York University Press.

Schneck, D.J. and Voigt, H.F. (2006) "An Outline of Cardiovascular Structure and Function." Chapter 1 in J.D. Bronzino *The Biomedical Engineering Handbook: Third Edition, Volume I: Biomedical Engineering Fundamentals; Section I: Physiologic Systems*. Boca Raton, Florida: CRC Press, LLC.

Seldin, D.W. and Giebisch, G. (eds) (1985) *The Kidney: Physiology and Pathophysiology*. New York: Raven Press.

Shenk, D. (1999) "Why You Feel The Way You Do." *The Magazine For Growing Companies 21*, 1, 56–67.

Sherrin, T., Blank, T. and Todorovic, C. (2011) "c-Jun N-terminal kineses in memory and synaptic plasticity" *Rev. Neurosci. 2011*, 22,4,403–410; Epub. doi: 10.1515/RNS.2011.032.

Shiffrin, N. and Bailey, S.L. (1976) *Acupressure*. Canoga Park, California: Major Books.

Shinbrot, T. and Young, W. (2008) "Why decussate? Topological constraints on 3D wiring." *Anat. Rec. (Hoboken)*, 291, 10, 1278–1292; doi: 10.1002/ar.20731.

Siegel, G.J., Albers, R.W., Agranoff, B.W., and Katzman, R., (eds) (1981) *Basic Neurochemistry, Third Edition*. Boston, Massachusetts: Little, Brown and Company.

Singhal, S., Henderson, R., and Horsfield, K. (1973) "Morphometry of the human pulmonary arterial tree." *Circulation Research*, 33, 190–197.

Springer, S.P. and Deutsch, G. (1981) *Left Brain Right Brain*. San Francisco, California: W.H. Freeman and Company.

Sweatt, J.D. (2004) "Mitogen-activated protein kineses in synaptic plasticity and memory." *Current Opinion in Neurobiology*, 14, 2, 311–317.

Taylor, C.C.W. (1995), "Politics," in Barnes, Jonathan (ed.) *The Cambridge Companion to Aristotle*. Cambridge: Cambridge University Press.

Thomas, C.L. (ed.) (1981) *Taber's Cyclopedic Medical Dictionary*. Philadelphia, Pennsylvania: F.A. Davis Company.

Thommen, G.S. (1987) *Biorhythms*. New York: Crown Publishers.

Tortora, G.J. and Grabowski, S.R. (1993) *Principles of Anatomy and Physiology, Seventh Edition*. New York: HarperCollins.

Trivers, H. (1985) *The Rhythm of Being: A Study of Temporality*. New York: Philosophical Library.

Tsuei, J.J. (guest ed.) (1996) Special Topic Issue: "The science of accupuncture – theory and practice." *IEEE Engineering in Medicine and Biology*, 15, 3, 52–76.

Twain, M. (1996) in Baetzhold, H.G. and McCullough, J.B., *The Bible According to Mark Twain*. New York, NY: Simon and Schuster.

Woody, C.D. (1982) *Memory, Learning, and Higher Function*. New York: Springer-Verlag.

Some other books written by Daniel J. Schneck

Simple Wisdom: Alphabetical Reflections on the Nature of the Human Experience. Floyd, Virginia: Wilder Publications, Inc. (2012).

Omniology: A Unified Approach to the Study of Everything. Charleston, South Carolina: CreateSpace, LLC (2011).

SEARCHING. Shelton, Connecticut: International Scientific Publications (2005).

Mechanics of Muscle: Second Edition. New York: New York University Press (1992).

Biomedical Desk Reference (co-authored with Alan Tempkin). New York: New York University Press (1992).

Engineering Principles of Physiologic Function. New York: New York University Press (1990).

Subject Index

Sub-headings in *italics* indicate tables and figures.

Author Index

Ackerman, D. 129, 147, 163, 164, 214, 241
Alexjander, S. 283

Bailey, S.L. 88
Baker, C. 215
Berger, D.S. 13, 20–1, 28, 44, 50, 91, 106,
    109–10, 126–7, 133, 137, 144–5, 155,
    166–7, 200, 203, 218, 227, 233, 241,
    245–6, 254, 258, 280, 282–3, 285,
    299, 314, 328, 330, 334
Blank, T. 280
Buser, P. 137

Coren, S. 147, 164, 167, 214, 241
Cutler, A.G. 16

Deamer, D. 283
Dennett, D.C. 242
Deutsch, G. 116, 161
Deutsch, S. 109, 110
Duck, F. 33

Edwards, B. 116, 161, 215, 310

Findlay, E. 314
Francone, C.A. 14
Frazier, A.A. 62

Giancoli, D.C. 205, 216, 300, 305
Giebisch, G. 84
Goss, C.M. 14, 16, 84, 179
Grabowski, S.R. 14, 16, 41, 81, 84, 120,
    164, 179, 203, 205, 233
Graedon, J. 62
Graedon, T. 62

Harvard Medical School 320, 321
Henderson, R. 81
Hensyl, E.R. 16
Horsfield, K. 81

Imbert, M. 137

Jacob, S.W. 14, 16, 33, 41, 81, 84, 120, 179,
    233
Junge, D. 44, 110

Kinne, R.K.H. 84

Lentner, C. 33
Liebert, R.M. 226
Lossow, W.J. 14
Lots, I.S. 300, 302

MacLean, P.D. 112
McGovern, T. 84
Micheli-Tzanakou, E. 109, 110
Miller, J.B. 215

Nin, A. 163

Orlock, C. 262
Ornstein, R. 116, 241, 310

Plato 19, 20
Prophet, E.C. 88, 208, 330, 331
Roederer, J.G. 300
Rose, K.J. 260